OXFORD MEDICAL PUBLICATIONS

Paediatric Anaesthesia

T0177578

Published and forthcoming Oxford Specialist Handbooks

General Oxford Specialist Handbooks
A Resuscitation Room Guide
Addiction Medicine
Day Case Surgery
Parkinson's Disease and Other Movement Disorders 2e
Perioperative Medicine, 2e
Pharmaceutical Medicine
Postoperative Complications, 2e
Renal Transplantation
Retrieval Medicine

Oxford Specialist Handbooks in Anaesthesia
Anaesthesia for Medical and Surgical Emergencies
Cardiac Anaesthesia
Neuroanaesthesia
Obstetric Anaesthesia
Ophthalmic Anaesthesia
Paediatric Anaesthesia
Regional Anaesthesia, Stimulation and Ultrasound Techniques
Thoracic Anaesthesia

Oxford Specialist Handbooks in Cardiology
Adult Congenital Heart Disease
Cardiac Catheterization and Coronary Intervention
Cardiac Electrophysiology and Catheter Ablation
Cardiovascular Computed Tomography
Cardiovascular Magnetic Resonance
Echocardiography, 2e
Fetal Cardiology
Heart Failure, 2e
Hypertension
Inherited Cardiac Disease
Nuclear Cardiology
Pacemakers and ICDs
Pulmonary Hypertension
Valvular Heart Disease

Oxford Specialist Handbooks in Critical Care
Advanced Respiratory Critical Care
Cardiothoracic Critical Care

Oxford Specialist Handbooks in End of Life Care
End of Life Care in Cardiology
End of Life Care in Dementia
End of Life Care in Nephrology
End of Life Care in Respiratory Disease
End of Life in the Intensive Care Unit

Oxford Specialist Handbooks in Infectious Disease
Infectious Disease Epidemiology
Manual of Childhood Infections 4e

Oxford Specialist Handbooks in Neurology
Epilepsy
Parkinson's Disease and Other Movement Disorders, 2e
Stroke Medicine, 2e

Oxford Specialist Handbooks in Oncology
Practical Management of Complex Cancer Pain

Oxford Specialist Handbooks in Paediatrics
Paediatric Dermatology
Paediatric Endocrinology and Diabetes
Paediatric Gastroenterology, Hepatology, and Nutrition
Paediatric Haematology and Oncology
Paediatric Intensive Care
Paediatric Nephrology, 2e
Paediatric Neurology, 2e
Paediatric Palliative Medicine, 2e
Paediatric Radiology
Paediatric Respiratory Medicine
Paediatric Rheumatology

Oxford Specialist Handbooks in Pain Medicine
Spinal Interventions in Pain Management

Oxford Specialist Handbooks in Psychiatry
Addiction Medicine, 2e
Child and Adolescent Psychiatry
Forensic Psychiatry
Medical Psychotherapy
Old Age Psychiatry

Oxford Specialist Handbooks in Radiology
Interventional Radiology
Musculoskeletal Imaging
Pulmonary Imaging
Thoracic Imaging

Oxford Specialist Handbooks in Surgery
Cardiothoracic Surgery, 2e
Colorectal Surgery
Gastric and Oesophageal Surgery
Hand Surgery
Hepatopancreatobiliary Surgery
Neurosurgery
Operative Surgery, 2e
Oral and Maxillofacial Surgery, 2e
Otolaryngology and Head and Neck Surgery
Paediatric Surgery
Plastic and Reconstructive Surgery
Surgical Oncology
Urological Surgery
Vascular Surgery, 2e

Paediatric Anaesthesia

Second edition

Edited by

Steve Roberts

Consultant Anaesthetist
Jackson Rees Department of Anaesthesia
Alder Hey Children's NHS Foundation Trust
Liverpool, UK

OXFORD
UNIVERSITY PRESS

OXFORD
UNIVERSITY PRESS

Great Clarendon Street, Oxford, OX2 6DP,
United Kingdom

Oxford University Press is a department of the University of Oxford.
It furthers the University's objective of excellence in research, scholarship,
and education by publishing worldwide. Oxford is a registered trade mark of
Oxford University Press in the UK and in certain other countries

Published in the United States of America by Oxford University Press
198 Madison Avenue, New York, NY 10016, United States of America

British Library Cataloguing in Publication Data
Data available

Library of Congress Control Number: 2018966028

ISBN 978–0–19–875579–1

Printed and bound in China by
C&C Offset Printing Co., Ltd.

Contents

Detailed contents

First edition contributors

Graham Bell
Consultant Paediatric
Anaesthetist, Royal Hospital for
Sick Children, Glasgow, UK

Alison Carlyle
Anaesthetic Department, Royal
Hospital for Sick Children,
Edinburgh, UK

Emma Dickson
Consultant Paediatric
Anaesthetist,
Royal Hospital for Sick Children,
Edinburgh, UK

Pamela Eccles
Royal Hospital for Sick Children,
Edinburgh, UK

Anne Goldie
Consultant Paediatric
Anaesthetist, Royal Hospital for
Sick Children, Glasgow, UK

Fiona Kelly
Department of Anaesthesia,
Royal Hospital for Sick Children,
Edinburgh, UK

Volker Lesch
Consultant Anaesthetist,
Kantonsspital,
St. Gallen, Switzerland

Anthony Moores
Consultant Paediatric
Anaesthetist, Royal Hospital for
Sick Children, Glasgow, UK

Andrew Morrison
Fellow in Paediatric
Anaesthesia, Vancouver, British
Columbia, Canada

Manchula Navaratnam
Royal Hospital for Sick Children,
Glasgow, UK

Steve Roberts
Consultant Paediatric
Anaesthetist, Royal Liverpool
Children's NHS Trust,
Liverpool, UK

Mandy Sim
Clinical Nurse Specialist, Royal
Hospital for Sick Children,
Edinburgh, UK

Carolyn Smith
Consultant Paediatric
Anaesthetist, Royal Hospital for
Sick Children,
Edinburgh, UK

Francois Taljard
Royal Hospital for Sick Children,
Edinburgh, UK

Second edition contributors

Acute Pain Service

(Jennie Craske, Frances Dooley, Catherine Walker, Jennie McHugh, Helen Neary, Rishi Diwan, Stephanie Sinha) Alder Hey Children's NHS Foundation Trust, Liverpool, UK

Phil Arnold

The Jackson Rees Department of Anaesthesia, Alder Hey Children's NHS Foundation Trust, Liverpool, UK

Laura Bowes

Consultant Anaesthetist, Birmingham Children's Hospital, Birmingham, UK

Ed Carver

Consultant Anaesthetist, Birmingham Children's Hospital, Birmingham, UK

Richard Craig

Consultant Anaesthetist, The Jackson Rees Department of Anaesthesia, Alder Hey Children's NHS Foundation Trust, Liverpool, UK

Thomas Engelhardt

Department of Anaesthesia, Royal Aberdeen Children's Hospital, Aberdeen, UK

Anne Hunt

The Jackson Rees Department of Anaesthesia, Alder Hey Children's NHS Foundation Trust, Liverpool, UK

Doug Johnson

Consultant Anaesthetist, Birmingham Children's Hospital, Birmingham, UK

Barry Lambert

Anaesthetic Department, Birmingham Children's Hospital, Birmingham, UK

Nuria Masip

The Jackson Rees Department of Anaesthesia, Alder Hey Children's NHS Foundation Trust, Liverpool, UK

Anthony Moores

Consultant Anaesthetist, Royal Hospital for Sick Children Glasgow, Glasgow, UK

Naveen Murali

Consultant Anaesthetist, Birmingham Children's Hospital, Birmingham, UK

Pete Murphy

North West and North Wales Paediatric Transport Service (NWTS), Newton House, Birchwood Park, Warrington, UK

Naveen Raj

The Jackson Rees Department of Anaesthesia, Alder Hey Children's NHS Foundation Trust, Liverpool, UK

Steve Roberts
The Jackson Rees Department
of Anaesthesia, Alder Hey
Children's NHS Foundation
Trust, Liverpool, UK

Sarah Stibbards
Consultant in Emergency
Medicine, Salford Royal Hospital,
Salford, UK

Kate Thomas
Consultant Anaesthetist,
Birmingham Children's Hospital,
Birmingham, UK

Elizabeth Wright
The Jackson Rees Department
of Anaesthesia, Alder Hey
Children's NHS Foundation
Trust, Liverpool, UK

Symbols and abbreviations

➔	cross-reference, 'see'
↑	increase
↓	decrease
→	leading to
2,3-DPG	2,3-diphosphoglycerate
2D	two-dimensional
3D	three-dimensional
5-HT$_3$	5-hydroxytryptamine (serotonin)
A+E	Accident and Emergency
AAG	alpha-1-acid glycoprotein
AAGBI	Association of Anaesthetists of Great Britain and Ireland
ABC	airway, breathing, and circulation
ABCD	airway, breathing, circulation, and disability
ABCDE	airway, breathing, circulation, disability, and exposure
ABG	arterial blood gas
ABR	auditory brainstem response
ACE	angiotensin-converting enzyme
ACh	acetylcholine
AChR	acetylcholine receptor
ACT	activated clotting time
ADH	antidiuretic hormone
ADHD	attention deficit hyperactivity disorder
AED	antiepileptic drug
AHA	American Heart Association
AIDS	acquired immune deficiency syndrome
AIR	anaesthetic-induced rhabdomyolysis
AKI	acute kidney injury
ALL	acute lymphoblastic leukaemia
ALTE	apparent life-threatening events
AML	acute myeloid leukaemia
AMM	anterior mediastinal mass
ANA	antinuclear antibody
AP	antero-posterior
APA	Association of Paediatric Anaesthetists GBI
APLS	advanced paediatric life support
APTT	activated partial thromboplastin time
ARC	arthrogryposis, renal dysfunction, and cholestasis
ARDS	acute respiratory distress syndrome
ARF	acute renal failure
ASA	American Society of Anesthesiologists
ASD	atrial septal defect
ASD	autistic spectrum disorder
ASGE	American Society for Gastrointestinal Endoscopy
ASIS	anterior superior iliac spine
ATLS	advanced trauma life support
ATP	adenosine triphosphate
AV	atrioventricular
AVM	arteriovenous malformation
AVPU	alert to Voice, responds to Voice, responds to Pain, Unresponsive
AVSD	atrioventricular septal defect
BAL	bronchoalveolar lavage
BiPAP	bilevel (or biphasic) positive airway pressure
BIS	bispectral index
BLS	basic life support
BMT	bone marrow transplantation
BP	blood pressure
BSA	body surface area
BT	Blalock–Taussig
Ca^{2+}	calcium

CBD	common bile duct
CBF	cerebral blood flow
CBV	cerebral blood volume
CCAM	congenital cystic adenomatoid malformation
CDH	congenital diaphragmatic hernia
CE	capsule endoscopy
CF	cystic fibrosis
CHAOS	congenital high airway obstruction syndrome
CHARGE	coloboma, heart defects, choanal atresia, retardation of growth/development, genital/urinary abnormalities, ear abnormalities/deafness
CHD	congenital heart disease
CI	cochlear implant
CICO	can't intubate can't oxygenate
Cl$^-$	chloride
C_{max}	maximum serum drug concentration in a compartment
CMRO$_2$	cerebral metabolic rate of oxygen
CMV	cytomegalovirus
CNS	central nervous system
CO	cardiac output
CO$_2$	carbon dioxide
CP	cerebral palsy
CPAP	continuous positive airway pressure
CPB	cardiopulmonary bypass
CPK	creatinine phosphokinase
CPP	cerebral perfusion pressure
CPR	cardiopulmonary resuscitation
CRF	chronic renal failure
CRP	C-reactive protein
CRPS	complex regional pain syndrome
CRT	capillary refill time
CSE	convulsive status epilepticus
CSF	cerebrospinal fluid
CT	computed tomography

CTEV	congenital talipes equinovarus
CV	closing volume
CVA	cerebrovascular accident
CVL	central venous line
CVP	central venous pressure
CVS	cardiovascular system
CVVH	continuous veno-venous haemofiltration
CXR	chest radiograph
D$_2$	dopamine receptor
DC	direct current
DDH	developmental dysplasia of the hip
DHCA	deep hypothermic circulatory arrest
DI	diabetes insipidus
DIC	disseminated intravascular coagulopathy
DKA	diabetic ketoacidosis
DM	myotonic dystrophy (dystrophia myotonica)
DMD	Duchenne muscular dystrophy
DS	Down syndrome
DSU	day surgery unit
DVT	deep vein thrombosis
ΔarSO$_2$	regional arteriovenous oxygen difference
EB	epidermolysis bullosa
EBUS	endobronchial ultrasound
EBV	Epstein–Barr virus
ECF	extracellular fluid
ECG	electrocardiogram
ECHO	echocardiogram
ECLS	extracorporeal life support
ECMO	extracorporeal membrane oxygenation
ED	Emergency Department
ED	external diameter
EEG	electroencephalogram
EMG	electromyogram
EMLA	eutectic mixture of local anaesthetics
ENT	ear, nose, and throat

EOM	external oblique muscle
ERCP	endoscopic retrograde cholangio-pancreatography
ETCO$_2$	end-tidal carbon dioxide
ETT	endotracheal tube
EUA	examination under anaesthesia
EXIT	ex utero intrapartum treatment
FB	foreign body
FBC	full blood count
FEIBA	factor eight inhibitor bypassing activity
FETO	fetoscopic endoluminal tracheal occlusion
FFP	fresh frozen plasma
FGF	fresh gas flow
FiO$_2$	fraction of inspired oxygen
FIX	factor IX
FLACC	face, legs, activity, cry, consolability (scale)
FOAR	fronto-orbital advancement and remodelling
FOB	fibreoptic bronchoscopy
fOE	fractional oxygen extraction
FONA	front-of-neck access
Fr	French gauge
FRC	functional residual capacity
FVC	forced vital capacity
FVIII	factor VIII
FVIIIC	factor VIII coagulation activity
G	gauge
G+S	group and save
GA	general anaesthesia
GABA	γ-aminobutyric acid
GAG	glycosaminoglycan
GCS	Glasgow Coma Scale
GFR	glomerular filtration rate
GIT	gastrointestinal tract
GOR	gastro-oesophageal reflux
GORD	gastro-oesophageal reflux disease
GSD	glycogen storage disease
GU	genitourinary

GVHD	graft-versus-host disease
h	hour
H$_1$	histamine receptor
H$_2$O	water
Hb	haemoglobin
HbA	haemoglobin A
HbAS	sickle cell trait
HbC	haemoglobin C
HbF	fetal haemoglobin
HbS	haemoglobin S
HbSS	sickle cell disease
HBV	hepatitis B virus
HCO$_3$	bicarbonate
Hct	haematocrit
HDU	high-dependency unit
HEV	hepatitis E virus
HFNO	high-flow nasal oxygen
HFOV	high-frequency oscillation ventilation
HHFNC	humidified high-flow nasal cannula
HIV	human immunodeficiency virus
HLHS	hypoplastic left-heart syndrome
HME	heat and moisture exchange
HMEF	heat and moisture exchanger filter
HR	heart rate
HSV	herpes simplex virus
hyperCl$^-$	hyperchloraemia/ hyperchloraemic
hyperCO$_2$	hypercapnia
hyperK$^+$	hyperkalaemia/hyperkalaemic
hyperNa$^+$	hypernatraemia/ hypernatraemic
hypoCa^{2+}	hypocalcaemia/hypocalcaemic
hypoCl$^-$	hypochloraemia/ hypochloraemic
hypoK$^+$	hypokalaemia/hypokalaemic
hypoMg^{2+}	hypomagnesaemia/ hypomagnesaemic
hypoNa$^+$	hyponatraemia/ hyponatraemic
I&C	incision and curettage

IAP	intra-abdominal pressure
IBD	inflammatory bowel disease
ICP	intracranial pressure
ID	internal diameter
IDDM	insulin-dependent diabetes mellitus
I:E ratio	ratio of inspiratory time to expiratory time
IgG	immunoglobulin G
IM	intramuscular
INR	International Normalized Ratio
IO	intraosseous
IOL	intraocular lens
IOM	internal oblique muscle
IOP	intraocular pressure
IP	in-plane
IPPV	intermittent positive pressure ventilation
i-time	inspiratory time
ITU	intensive therapy unit
IU	international units
IUGR	intrauterine growth retardation
IV	intravenous
IVC	inferior vena cava
IVCT	in vitro contracture test
IVH	intraventricular haemorrhage
JCA	juvenile chronic arthritis
J-PEG	percutaneous endoscopic jejunostomy tube
JIA	juvenile idiopathic arthritis
KCl	potassium chloride
kPa	kilopascal
L	litre
LA	left atrium
LA	local anaesthetic
LAARP	laparoscopically assisted anorectal pull-through
LED	light-emitting diode
LET	lidocaine, epinephrine and tetracaine mix
LFTs	liver function tests

LLD	leg length discrepancy
LMA	laryngeal mask airway
LMP	last menstrual period
LOC	level of consciousness
LOS	lower oesophageal sphincter
LP	lumbar puncture
LV	left ventricle/left-ventricular
LVH	left ventricular hypertrophy
MABL	maximal allowable blood loss
MAC	minimum alveolar concentration
MAG3	mercaptoacetyltriglycine
MAP	mean arterial pressure
MAPCA	major aortopulmonary collateral arteries
mcg	microgram
MDT	multidisciplinary team
MELAS	mitochondrial myopathy, encephalopathy with lactic acidosis and stroke
MEN	multiple endocrine neoplasia
MEP	motor evoked potential
MERRF	myoclonus epilepsy associated with ragged-red fibres
Mg^{2+}	magnesium
MH	malignant hyperthermia
min	minute
MIBG	meta-iodobenzylguanidine
mL	millilitre
mmHg	millimetres of mercury
mmol	millimole
MMR	mumps, measles, and rubella vaccine
MODY	maturity-onset diabetes in the young
mOsmol	milliosmole
MPA	main pulmonary artery
MPS	mucopolysaccharidosis
MR	magnetic resonance
MRCP	magnetic resonance cholangiopancreatography
MRI	magnetic resonance imaging
MRV	magnetic resonance venography

MUA	manipulation under anaesthesia
MV	minute ventilation
N_2O	nitrous oxide
Na^+	sodium
NaCl	saline
$NaHCO_3$	sodium bicarbonate
NAI	non-accidental injury
NBM	nil by mouth
NCA	nurse-controlled analgesia
NCEPOD	National Confidential Enquiry into Peri-operative Deaths
nCPAP	nasal continuous positive airway pressure
NEC	necrotizing enterocolitis
ng	nanogram
NG	nasogastric
NGT	nasogastric tube
NHL	non-Hodgkin's lymphoma
NIBP	non-invasive blood pressure
NICE	National Institute of Health and Care Excellence
NICU	neonatal intensive care unit
NIPS	Neonatal/Infant Pain Scale
NIRS	Near-infrared spectroscopy
NIV	non-invasive ventilation
NJ	nasojejunal
NLS	newborn life support
NMDA	N-methyl-D-aspartate
NMJ	neuromuscular junction
NNRTI	non-nucleoside reverse transcriptase inhibitor
NO	nitric oxide
NPA	nasopharyngeal airway
NRTI	nucleoside-analogue reverse transcriptase inhibitor
NSAID	non-steroidal anti-inflammatory drug
NWTS	North West and North Wales Paediatric Transport Service
O_2	oxygen
OA	oesophageal atresia
OCR	oculocardiac reflex
OD	outer diameter
ODP	operating department assistant
OGD	oesophagogastroduodenoscopy
OGT	orogastric tube
OI	osteogenesis imperfecta
OLV	one-lung ventilation
OOP	out-of-plane
OPA	oropharyngeal airway
ORIF	open reduction and internal fixation
OSA	obstructive sleep apnoea
P_{50}	oxygen tension at which haemoglobin is 50% saturated
PA	pulmonary artery
PACU	post-anaesthetic care unit
PAP	pulmonary arterial pressure
PBF	pulmonary blood flow
PCA	patient-controlled analgesia
PCA	postconceptual age
PC-CMV	pressure control–controlled mandatory ventilation
pCO_2	partial pressure of carbon dioxide
PCR	polymerase chain reaction
PCV	pressure-controlled ventilation
PCV-VG	pressure-control ventilation volume guaranteed
PD	pharmacodynamics
PDA	patent ductus arteriosus
PDPH	post-dural-puncture headache
PEA	pulseless electrical activity
PEEP	positive end-expiratory pressure
PEFR	peak expiratory flow rate
PEG	percutaneous endoscopic gastrostomy
PET	positron emission tomography
PEW	Paediatric Early Warning
PFC	persistent fetal circulation
PFO	proximal femoral osteotomy
PICC	peripheral intravenous central catheter

PICU	paediatric intensive care unit
Pinsp	inspiratory pressure
PIP	peak inspiratory pressure
PIS	pinning in situ
PK	pharmokinetics
PLS	paediatric life support
Pmax	maximum pressure
PNB	peripheral nerve block
PNS	peripheral nerve stimulator
pO	per orum
pO_2	partial pressure of oxygen
PO_4	phosphate
PONV	postoperative nausea and vomiting
POP	plaster of Paris
PPHN	persistent pulmonary hypertension of the newborn
PR	per rectum
PRN	pro re nata
PRS	Pierre Robin sequence/syndrome
PS	pressure-supported
PSARP	posterior sagittal anorectoplasty
PT	prothrombin time
PVB	paravertebral block
PVR	pulmonary vascular resistance
pVT	pulseless ventricular tachycardia
QDS	*quater die sumendum*— four times daily
Qp	pulmonary blood flow
Qs	systemic blood flow
RA	right atrium
RAE	Ring, Adair, and Elwyn endotracheal tube
RED	rigid external distraction
rFVIIa	recombinant activated factor VII
RhF	rheumatoid factor
R–L	right–left
ROSC	return of spontaneous circulation

ROTEM	rotational thromboelastometry
RR	respiratory rate
RSI	rapid sequence induction
rSO_2	regional oxygen saturation
rSO_2C	cerebral regional oxygen saturation
rSO_2S	somatic–renal regional oxygen saturation
RTI	respiratory tract infection
RV	right ventricle/right-ventricular
RVH	right-ventricular hypertrophy
RVOTO	right-ventricular outflow tract obstruction
s	second
SAFE	Shout for help. Approach with caution. Free from danger. Evaluate patient's ABCs
SaO_2	arterial oxygen saturation
SBYB	Stop Before You Block
SC	subcutaneous
SCBU	special care baby unit
SCM	sacrococcygeal membrane
SDB	sleep disordered breathing
SDR	selective dorsal rhizotomy
SIADH	syndrome of inappropriate secretion of antidiuretic hormone
SIMV-PC	synchronized intermittent mandatory ventilation, pressure control
SIRS	systemic inflammatory response syndrome
SNOD	Specialist Nurse in Organ Donation
SPECT	single photon emission computed tomography
$SpaO_2$	pulmonary arterial oxygen saturation
SpO_2	oxygen saturation
$SpvO_2$	pulmonary venous oxygen saturation
SSEP	somatosensory evoked potential
$SsvcO_2$	superior caval oxygen saturation

SUFE	slipped upper femoral epiphysis
SV	spontaneous ventilation
SV	stroke volume
SVC	superior vena cava
SvO$_2$	venous oxygen saturation
SVR	systemic vascular resistance
SVT	supraventricular tachycardia
t$_{1/2}$	half-life
TACE	trans-arterial chemotherapy embolization
TA-GVHD	transfusion-associated graft-versus-host disease
TAP	transversus abdominis plane block
TAT	trans-anastomotic tube
TBI	total body irradiation
TBV	total blood volume
TCI	target-controlled infusion
TDD	total daily dose
TDS	ter die sumendum— three times daily
TEG	thromboelastography
TEM	thromboelastometry
TENS	transcutaneous electrical nerve stimulation
TGA	transposition of the great arteries
THRIVE	transnasal humidified rapid-insufflation ventilatory exchange
Ti	inspiratory time
TIVA	total intravenous anaesthesia
tmax	time to maximum plasma concentration
TMJ	temporomandibular joint
TOE	transoesophageal echocardiography
TOF	tracheo-oesophageal fistula
TOI	tissue oxygen index

TPN	total parenteral nutrition
TT	thrombin time
TTO	to-take-out
U+E	urea and electrolytes
UO	urine output
UPJO	ureteropelvic junction obstruction
URTI	upper respiratory tract infection
US	ultrasound
UTI	urinary tract infection
VACTERL	vertebral defects, anorectal anomalies, cardiac defects, tracheo-oesophageal fistula/oesophageal atresia, renal abnormalities, limb abnormalities
VAD	ventricular assist device
VAS	visual analogue score
VATS	video-assisted thoracoscopic surgery
VCFS	velocardiofacial syndrome
VCV	volume-controlled ventilation
V$_d$	volume of distribution
VF	ventricular fibrillation
VMA	vanillylmandelic acid
VP	ventriculo-peritoneal
VQ	ventilation–perfusion
VSD	ventricular septal defect
VT	ventricular tachycardia
V$_T$	tidal volume
vWD	von Willebrand's disease
vWF	von Willebrand factor
WAGR	Wilms' tumour, aniridia, GU malformation, mental retardation
WCC	white cell count
WHO	World Health Organization

Section 1

Basic sciences

System-based anatomy and physiology

Thomas Engelhardt

Overview

- Children have an increased perioperative morbidity and mortality compared with adults.
- Provision of safe perioperative care therefore requires an understanding of neonatal and paediatric anatomy and physiology in addition to other aspects covered elsewhere.
- This chapter outlines major differences in the respiratory, cardiovascular, central nervous, and hepatorenal systems and in thermoregulation.

Airway and respiratory system

Upper airway

- Perioperative airway problems frequently result in significant morbidity and mortality.
- The airway undergoes significant changes from birth to adulthood. These changes affect the development of the skull, the oral cavity, the larynx, and the trachea. Facial structures are small and paranasal sinuses absent.
- The small oral cavity is easily compressed during mask ventilation, resulting in upper airway obstruction.
- The tongue has a flat surface with limited lateral mobility in neonates, complicating direct laryngoscopy unless a retromolar approach is used.
- Neonates are obligate nose breathers owing to the relatively large tongue; 50% of airway resistance is secondary to nasal passages.
- The large head and prominent occiput produce a cephalad (anterior) view of the larynx during direct laryngoscopy. There is a loosely embedded 'anterior' larynx at C2/3, moving to C5/6 in later life
- The epiglottis (long, narrow, U- or Ω-shaped) obscures the laryngeal inlet if not 'picked up' by the laryngoscopy blade.
- Vocal cords are shorter in neonates.
- The ETT is commonly directed against the anterior wall of the trachea, creating an impression that the ETT is too wide to pass through the cricoid ring (ellipsoid, does not expand).
- The ETT must be narrow enough not to exert pressure on the mucosa of the cricoid cartilage, but large enough to provide an adequate seal for ventilation.
- Cuffed ETTs are now considered safe provided cuff pressures are continuously monitored and maintained <20 cmH$_2$O.

Lower airway

- The tracheal length is measured from the cricoid to the carina and is related to age and height but not weight.
- Unintentional bronchial intubation and extubation are a constant threat during positioning. (For ETT sizing, ➋ Chapter 6.)
- A small internal tracheal diameter leads to a significant ↑ in airway resistance, particularly following mucosal injury.
- The alveoli are thick-walled in neonates and amount to only 10% of the adult total. The single terminal bronchiole opens into a single alveolus instead of a fully developed cluster.
- The chest wall of small infants and neonates is primarily cartilaginous and highly compliant. Horizontal alignment of the soft and pliable ribs prevents the 'bucket-handle' action of the adult thoracic cage.
- Weak intercostal and diaphragmatic muscles (due to a lack of type I fibres) with a more horizontal attachment and a protuberant abdomen predispose to fatigue. Sedation, GA and illness ↓ tonic muscular contraction, resulting in a diminished FRC. The latter can be reversed by CPAP or IPPV.

- Chest wall specific compliance is higher in neonates and infants (0.06 mL/cmH_2O) than in adults (0.04 mL/cmH_2O). Therefore, intercostal recession and sternal recession occur readily in neonates and young infants with increased respiratory effort and during episodes of airway obstruction.
- Upper and lower airways are susceptible to a large ↑ in airway resistance (and the work of breathing) in the event of an obstruction.

Respiratory physiology

- Respiratory complications related to GA are highest in infants owing to differences in respiratory physiology (Table 1.1).
- There is a similar V_T per kg in all age groups. The higher RR produces higher alveolar minute ventilation (MV).
- The ratio of alveolar ventilation to FRC is 5:1 in neonates and infants (2:1 in adults), resulting in rapid uptake of volatile agents.
- Changes in the concentration of inspired gases are more rapidly reflected in alveolar and arterial values.
- Risk of atelectasis and tendency for V/Q mismatch is due to closing volume encroaching FRC, resulting in a fall in arterial O_2 tension. The small available intrapulmonary O_2 reservoir (relative to O_2 consumption) can lead to rapid desaturation in the event of airway obstruction or apnoea and is measured in seconds.
- FRC is reduced further during and for a period after GA. Physiological mechanisms to maintain FRC in neonates include partial adduction of the vocal cords during expiration (laryngeal braking), early termination of expiration (tachypnoea), and inspiratory muscle activity during expiration.
- These mechanisms are abolished by GA, sedation, or illness, when FRC falls markedly when compared with awake. This further reduces the O_2 reserves and contributes to the rapid onset of hypoxia in infants and neonates in the event of an airway obstruction.
- The anteroposterior and lateral thoracic diameters are not significantly increased in neonates and infants during deep inspiration.

Table 1.1 Differences in respiratory parameters with age

Parameter	Neonate	Child	Adult
RR (breaths/min)	40–60	20–30	16–24
V_T (mL/kg)	7–8	7–8	7–8
Alveolar ventilation (mL/kg/min)	100–150		60
FRC (mL/kg)	30	30	30
Dead space (mL/kg)	2	2	2
O_2 consumption (mL/kg/min)	6–9		2–3
Airway resistance (cmH_2O/L/s)	40	20	2
Airway compliance (mL/cmH_2O)	5		100

- As the child grows (spending time in an upright position), the chest wall compliance ↓ and FRC is maintained above closing volume (6–12 months onwards).
- The work of breathing is reduced by CPAP and improves oxygenation.
- The anatomical dead space is fixed in humans (2 mL/kg). However, the dead space in anaesthetic equipment is more significant in relation to the small V_T of neonates and infants.
- Neonates and infants rely primarily on diaphragmatic movements. This tonic muscular contraction is lost during GA and hence positive pressure ventilation and PEEP during GA are the norm.
- An ETT reduces the airway diameter more in smaller airways and hence significantly increases the airway resistance, leading to an increased work of breathing. Spontaneous ventilation through a small ETT may therefore be impossible.
- Immature respiratory control: the peripheral chemoreceptor response to hypoxia is weak and the central chemoreceptor response to CO_2 is blunted in premature infants. Neonates are prone to periodic breathing with apnoeic phases (2–10 s). The apnoeic periods in the premature neonate are prolonged, especially after GA.
- Cold and dry gases lead to heat and insensible fluid losses from the lungs (15–20 mL/kg/day).

Cardiovascular system

Fetal circulation

- Fetal gas exchange occurs in the placenta.
- There is preferential streaming of oxygenated blood to the brain and myocardium due to the presence of intracardiac and extracardiac shunts (Fig. 1.1).
- The fetal circulation is said to be 'shunt-dependent'.

Fetal blood flow

- Deoxygenated blood reaches the placenta in the umbilical arteries and returns to the fetus in the umbilical vein.
- pO_2 in the umbilical vein is approximately 4.5–5.0 kPa and fetal blood is 80–90% saturated.
- In the inferior vena cava (IVC), oxygenated blood from the placenta mixes with desaturated blood from the lower body.
- In the right atrium (RA), oxygenated blood from the IVC is directed across the foramen ovale into the left atrium (LA). In the LA, the SpO_2 is around 65%.

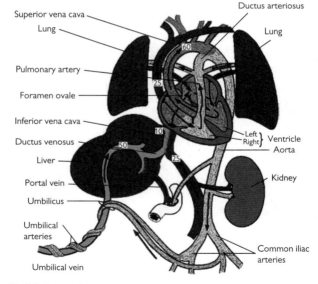

Fig. 1.1 Fetal circulation.

Reproduced with permission from Murphy, PJ. The fetal circulation. *Continuing Education in Anaesthesia, Critical Care & Pain.* 5 (4), 107–12. Copyright © 2005 The Board of Management and Trustees of the British Journal of Anaesthesia, published by Oxford University Press.

- This well-oxygenated blood enters the left ventricle (LV) and is ejected into the ascending aorta. The majority of the LV blood is delivered to the brain and coronary circulation.
- Desaturated blood from the IVC, SVC, and coronary sinus is directed across the tricuspid valve and into the right ventricle (RV). This blood is then pumped into the pulmonary artery (PA).
- Because of the high pulmonary vascular resistance (PVR) in utero, only about 12% of the RV output enters the pulmonary circulation. The remaining 88% passes through the ductus arteriosus into the descending aorta and the lower half of the body; it is relatively desaturated blood (pO_2 2.5–3.0 kPa).
- O_2 delivery in the relatively hypoxic fetus is maximized by:
  - A high haemoglobin concentration, around 16 g/dL at term
  - A high cardiac output (CO), 250–400 mL/kg/min at term.

The presence of fetal haemoglobin (HbF) leads to a lower concentration of 2,3-diphosphoglycerate (2,3-DPG) than HbA and shifts the haemoglobin–oxygen dissociation curve to the left (P_{50} 3.6 kPa).

Changes at birth
- Gas exchange is transferred from the placenta to the lungs, the fetal circulatory shunts close, and the LV output increases.
- With the onset of respiration:
  - pH and arterial O_2 tension ↑.
  - PVR falls by 80% from prenatal levels within a few minutes of commencing ventilation.
  - Blood flow through the lungs and the LA ↑.
  - LA pressure rises above RA pressure closing the foramen ovale.
- With removal of the placenta and closure of the umbilical artery:
  - A large low-resistance vascular bed is excluded from the systemic circulation.
  - SVR ↑ while pressure in the IVC and flow through the RA both ↓.
  - The fall in flow through the IVC and RA reduces RA pressure below that in the LA and contributes to functional closure of the foramen ovale.
- The ↑ SVR and simultaneous ↓ PVR with increasing flow in the pulmonary vascular bed lead to an aortic pressure above that in the PA. The blood flow through the ductus arteriosus reverses direction and now goes from left to right, filling it with oxygenated blood. The ↑ local arterial O_2 tension and lack of prostaglandin E_2 from the placenta cause the muscular tissue of the ductus arteriosus to constrict, leading to functional closure.
- Prostaglandin is used to open the ductus arteriosus in neonates with CHD where the systemic perfusion or the pulmonary blood flow depend on an open ductus arteriosus, e.g. coarctation of the aorta or pulmonary atresia. Conversely, the closure of the duct can be achieved by administration of prostaglandin inhibitors, e.g. indometacin.

Transitional circulation
- The PVR remains high for the first weeks, and the ductus arteriosus may be open for first few days of life. Under some circumstances, a normal

neonatal circulation may revert to a fetal circulatory pattern (persistent fetal circulation).
- This is associated with congenital diaphragmatic hernia, meconium aspiration, and significant respiratory distress of any cause.
- Main stimuli: hypoxia, hypercarbia, acidosis, and hypothermia.
- The pulmonary arterioles constrict in response to these stimuli. PVR rises and right-to-left flow through the functionally closed but anatomically patent foramen ovale and ductus arteriosus may resume. This worsens hypoxia and acidosis (for treatment, ➲ Chapter 13).

Neonatal and infant circulation
- The myocardium contains fewer contractile elements (30% vs 60% in adults) and more supporting tissue. The ventricles are less compliant when relaxed and can generate less tension during contraction. This limits the stroke volume (SV). Therefore, in neonates, LV end-diastolic volume is relatively fixed and CO is largely dependent on heart rate (HR).
- Reduced compliance and contractility of the ventricles lead to heart failure with increasing volume load. Distension of either ventricle results in compression and dysfunction of the contralateral ventricle.
- The neonatal myocardium has a reduced Frank–Starling response. Afterload compensation is finite.
- Bradycardia is not well tolerated and a neonatal HR < 60 beats/min does not provide adequate CO; CPR should be initiated.
- Asystole is the commonest terminal rhythm. VF is rare.
- Tachycardia is well tolerated and the neonate can cope with rates of up to 200 beats/min.
- Sinus arrhythmia is common, but other irregular rhythms are abnormal.
- Term neonates have functional autonomic and baroreceptor control mechanisms. However, the parasympathetic tone mediated by the vagus nerve predisposes them to bradycardia during vagal stimulation, e.g. hypoxia.
- A rough rule of thumb: neonatal MAP in mmHg = gestational age in weeks (Table 1.2).

Table 1.2 Normal cardiovascular parameters for different age groups

Age	Systolic BP (mmHg)	Diastolic BP (mmHg)	Mean BP (mmHg)	HR (beats/min)	CO (mL/kg/min)
Neonate (<1 kg)	40–60	15–35	25–45	80–200	400
Neonate (3 kg)	50–70	25–45	35–55	80–200	200–250
Infant (6 months)	85–105	55–65	65–80	80–140	
Child (2 years)	95–105	55–65	65–80	80–120	
Child (7 years)	100–110	55–70	70–85	80–120	
Adolescent	110–130	65–80	80–95	50–90	80

Central nervous system

Anatomy

- The neonatal CNS is immature and differs from the adult and older child. These differences are relevant to GA and regional techniques.
- At birth the brain weighs approximately 330–350g (10–15% of body weight). Adult proportions (1200–1400 g or 2% of body weight) are obtained at around 12 years of age.
- The cerebral cortex is underdeveloped and synaptic connections are immature. Myelination and dendritic proliferation progress in the last 3 months of pregnancy and during the first years of life.
- The cranial sutures are open, with a large anterior fontanelle that closes by 20 months of age. Palpation of the anterior fontanelle can be used to evaluate ICP in neonates and infants. The posterior fontanelle closes by 3 months of age.
- Increasing ICP is partly relieved by expansion of the fontanelles and separation of the suture lines, so head size ↑ before ICP rises.
- The blood–brain barrier is anatomically and functionally incomplete. Bilirubin, opioids, and barbiturates cross freely.
- In the preterm neonate, cerebral vessels are at risk of rupture, especially in the region of the germinal matrix close to the nucleus caudatus. The germinal matrix has a rich blood supply, scarce vascular supporting tissue, and thin vessel walls, leading to a high chance of intracerebral and intraventricular haemorrhage. With increasing gestational age, the germinal matrix involutes and the risk of bleeding ↓.
- The spinal cord of the fetus initially occupies the entire length of the spinal canal. Differential growth of the canal and spinal cord causes the termination of the cord to move cephalad relative to the vertebral canal: S1 at 28 weeks' gestation, L3 at term, L2/3 at 1 year, and the adult level of L1/L2 around the age of 8 years.
- The intercristal line in neonates is at L5–S1, compared with L4 in adults, and LP is performed below this line. Ossification of the sacral vertebrae is not complete, making a sacral epidural possible.
- The epidural space in the infant contains fat that is loculated, with distinct spaces between individual lobules. A catheter introduced into the epidural space via the sacral hiatus can be threaded to thoracic level to provide epidural analgesia for thoracic dermatomes.
- The sacral hiatus is relatively large compared with later life and is not ossified, allowing easy access to the lower epidural space.
- The volume of CSF is proportionately greater in neonates/infants/adults (10 vs 4 vs 2 mL/kg) and there is a higher relative volume of CSF in the spinal canal (50% in children vs 33% in adults). The pia mater is highly vascular. Therefore, spinal anaesthesia requires a higher dose of LA; and is of shorter duration.
- The cervical and lumbar curves in neonates are undeveloped. The ligamentum flavum is thin compared with that in adults.

Physiology

- Cerebral metabolic rate, blood flow, O_2 requirements, and glucose consumption are all higher in small children than older children and adults (Table 1.3). This makes them vulnerable to any interruption in cerebral perfusion during GA or at other times.

- The global cerebral blood flow (CBF) between 6 months to 4 years of age is twice that of an adult, secondary to the accelerated cerebral development during this period. The low cerebral mass and metabolism in the preterm neonate is reflected in the low CBF.
- Cerebral perfusion pressure (CPP) equals mean arterial pressure (MAP) less central venous pressure (CVP) or intracranial pressure (ICP) (whichever is greater):

$$CPP = MAP - ICP (or CVP)$$

- Autoregulation maintains constant CBF despite changes in CPP within an adult range of 60–150 mmHg. The thresholds of CPP autoregulation in the infant and young child are unknown. Animal models suggest that the limits of autoregulation are lower than those in adults.
- Cerebral autoregulation might be compromised in severely ill children when CBF becomes pressure-dependent. Hypotension may induce cerebral ischemia.
- ICP in neonates and infants (2–5 mmHg) is lower than in older children and adults (8–18 mmHg). Chronic ICP ↑ are compensated to some extent by expansion of sutures and fontanelles (hydrocephalus). Acute ↑ cannot be compensated for in this way.
- Incomplete myelination of nerve tissue in neonates and infants allows effective blockade with low concentrations of LA solution.
- The sympathetic nervous system is not fully developed until the age of 6 years. Central neuraxial blocks (spinal or epidural anaesthesia), therefore, causes little change in HR or BP.
- The baroreceptor reflex is poorly developed in premature neonates and hypovolaemia does not result in tachycardia.

Table 1.3 Cerebral metabolism in children and adults

Age	CBF	O$_2$ consumption	Glucose requirement
Premature	40 mL/min/100 g		
Neonate	40–50 mL/min/100 g	2.3 mL/min/100 g	
Child	**100** mL/min/100 g	5.8 mL/min/100 g	6.8 mg/min/100 g
Adult	50 mL/min/100 g	3.5 mL/min/100 g	5.5 mg/min/100 g

Liver

- Hepatic phase I and II reactions are not fully functional in neonates and premature infants. However, function matures rapidly, reaching adult values at 2–3 months of age (often exceeding that of adults).
- Phase I reactions (cytochrome-dependent) include oxidation, reduction, and hydrolysis. These reactions primarily produce less-active or inactive compounds. These compounds undergo phase II reactions (conjugations), e.g. glucuronidation (opioids) or sulfation (paracetamol) to produce polar compounds; which are eliminated in urine or via the GIT.
- Phase I reactions are catalysed by the cytochrome P450 mixed function oxidase system, which in neonates has about 28% of adult activity.
- Deficient phase I activity is also present for other systems e.g. alcohol dehydrogenase (chloral hydrate metabolism), plasma esterase (amino-ester LA metabolism), and *N*-acetyltransferase (isoniazid and hydralazine metabolism).
- The phase II reactions acetylation, glycination, and glucuronidation are very deficient at birth, but sulfation is highly active. This pathway can metabolize opioids before glucuronidation matures and is also responsible for paracetamol metabolism in neonates.
- Bilirubin is produced from the breakdown of erythrocytes (80%) and from ineffective erythropoiesis (20%). The enzyme that catalyses the transfer of glucuronic acid to bilirubin (uridine diphospho-glucuronosyltransferase) to form glucuronides and allow excretion in bile has only 1% of adult values at term (adult values are reached at 3–4 months of age).
- Physiological jaundice occurs from the second or third day of life, lasting for about 10 days, when most term and virtually all premature infants experience a period of unconjugated hyperbilirubinaemia. This is a consequence of high production (100–140 mcg/kg/day compared with 50–70 mcg/kg/day in adults) from erythrocyte breakdown (neonates are relatively polycythaemic), limited metabolism and excretion, and ↑ enterohepatic recirculation of bilirubin (due to a limited capacity to form urobilinogen and urobilin).
- Kernicterus occurs if plasma bilirubin concentration > 200 micromol/L, resulting in damage to basal ganglia, cerebellum, and hippocampus. Reduced albumin concentration, neonatal infection/sepsis, and haemolysis are risk factors. Phototherapy converts unconjugated bilirubin to photoisomer products, which are excreted in bile or urine without the need for glucuronidation.
- Vitamin K-dependent clotting factors (II, VII, IX, and X) are low in the term neonate. Vitamin K is given to most neonates to prevent haemorrhagic disease of the newborn, and administration is vital preoperatively.
- The ductus venosus (a connection between the IVC, portal vein, and umbilical veins) remains patent for 7–10 days after birth. This shunt bypasses the hepatic vessel bed and decreases hepatic clearance. The effects of drugs with hepatic metabolism are prolonged.

- Hepatic glucose storage is low and activity of the rate-limiting enzyme in gluconeogenesis (phosphoenolpyruvate carboxykinase) is around 10% of adult values. The neonate who is not feeding is prone to develop hypoglycaemia. A glucose infusion is necessary until there is enteral feeding.
- The limited hepatic metabolism in the infant has a limited intraoperative impact. However, the reduced hepatic metabolism is relevant postoperatively with drugs requiring dose modification.

Kidney

- In utero, the kidney is a quiescent organ and the placenta performs all excretory functions. Nephrogenesis is complete at 36 weeks, but nephron formation continues after birth in the premature infant. Production of urine starts between 9 and 12 weeks of gestation. At term the kidneys produce approximately 20–30 mL/h of filtrate.
- High renal vascular resistance largely determines perfusion. The renal blood flow at birth is low (6% of CO increasing, to 18–20% by one month), as is the GFR (10 mL/min/1.73 m^2).
- The renal blood flow and GFR approximately double during the 2nd to 4th weeks of life owing to a fall in renal vascular resistance and an ↑ in BP. Adult values (120 mL/min/1.73 m^2) relative to body surface area (BSA) are attained at 12 months.
- Tubular function is immature: the concentrating ability is limited and urine is only marginally more concentrated than plasma (short loops of Henle, low urea concentration in the medullary interstitium, and limited sensitivity to antidiuretic hormone). Adult concentrating ability is attained within the first months of life.
- The tubular immaturity leads to impairment in modifying the glomerular filtrate for conservation or excretion of solutes. The tubular capacity to absorb Na$^+$ is limited, resulting in a high renal loss. Adequate neonatal Na$^+$ replacement (2-4 mmol/kg/day and 5–10 mmol/kg/day in the preterm neonate) is required.
- Renal tubular acid excretion mechanisms are fully developed in the term neonate but not in the premature. This excretory capacity increases with gestational age. The renal threshold for bicarbonate is lower than in adults, which leads to plasma bicarbonate concentrations of 16–20 mmol/L in preterm infants and 19-21 mmol/L in term neonates (24-28 mmol/L in older children).
- Glucose reabsorption is limited in the preterm neonate and glycosuria may occur. Osmotic diuresis in a patient with marked hyperglycaemia may result in significant dehydration.
- Neonates and young infants have limited renal functions to maintain fluid, electrolyte, and acid–base homeostasis. These effects are more pronounced in the premature infant. In the neonatal period, electrolyte and fluid administration therefore requires careful monitoring and assessments of fluid balance.

Thermal control

- Body temperature results from the balance between heat production and environmental heat loss. The neutral thermal environment is the environmental temperature range within which minimal metabolic heat production can maintain normothermia.
- Thermostasis is important during GA and surgery, directly affecting infant mortality.
- Children are more susceptible to hypothermia.
- The smaller and younger the infant, the higher the required environmental temperature to achieve a neutral thermal environment.
- Thermoregulatory mechanisms are inhibited during GA, with a reduction in metabolic heat production. Peripheral arteriovenous shunts open, causing heat loss from the core to the periphery.
- Radiation accounts for 40–50% of heat loss and is proportional to the difference between body surface temperature and ambient temperature.
- Conduction is direct transfer of heat through direct contact.
- Convection is heat loss through the movement of air, and is usually reduced by covering exposed skin.
- Evaporation is loss of energy through water dissipation from exposed surfaces, e.g. skin, lungs, and visceral organs during surgery.
- Comparison of the neutral thermal environment and critical temperature (lowest sustained temperature compatible with survival) at different ages illustrates the difficulties for the neonate in maintaining an adequate body temperature (Table 1.4).
- Core temperature should be monitored during all procedures in neonates. Axillary temperature measurement is acceptable in low-risk children.
- Measures to ↓ heat loss and actively warm neonates and infants are required to maintain core temperature above 36°C.

Consequences of hypothermia

- Body enzymes slow their speed of action.
- O_2 consumption ↓ by 8% for each degree of temperature drop below 37°C.
- ↑ sympathetic stimulation and shivering, and thus discomfort.
- ↓ drug metabolism, delaying recovery from GA.
- Impaired coagulation.

Table 1.4 Neutral and critical temperatures in neonates and adults

	Neutral temperature (°C)	Critical temperature (°C)
Preterm neonate	34	28
Neonate	32	23
Adult	28	1

Neonates

- Neonates are particularly sensitive to hypothermia, especially when premature. The range of ambient temperatures that they tolerate without hypothermia is narrow.
- Cold-stressed infants develop cardiovascular depression and hypoperfusion acidosis.
- There are relatively high losses of body heat owing to:
  - ↑ thermal conduction due to thin skin and little or no insulating subcutaneous fat;
  - ↑ BSA:body weight (children with < 0.5 m² BSA are especially at risk of hypothermia)
  - High MV and insensible fluid loss (evaporation).
- Ineffective compensatory mechanisms:
  - Shivering is ineffective owing to limited muscle mass.
  - There is a limited vasoconstrictor response.
  - Non-shivering thermogenesis: brown fat is metabolized under adrenergic stimulation (via β_3-adrenergic receptors), leading to significantly increased O_2 consumption. This compensates poorly for the lack of shivering and limited vasoconstriction.
  - Brown fat is deficient in premature neonates.

Fluid compartments

- Total body water content is greater in neonates and infants, becoming comparable to adult values after 1 year of age (Table 1.5).
- As the amount of muscle mass rises, intracellular water content rises.
- Water turnover in the infant is more than double that in an adult. In infants, approximately 40% of extracellular water is lost daily as urine, stool, sweat, and insensible losses via skin and airways and lungs. Dehydration can easily follow a reduction of intake or increased loss of fluids.

Water requirements

- There is a direct association between metabolic rate and water requirements.
- Water requirements (mL/kg body weight) ↑ with decreasing size of the child owing to the higher metabolic rate and higher evaporative losses.
- Evaporate water losses are inversely proportional to gestational age in the premature infants owing to thin and vascularized skin.

Table 1.5 Body water and blood volume with age

	Water (% body weight)	Extracellular volume (% body weight)	Blood volume (mL/kg)
Premature	90	60	100
Term neonate	80	40–45	90
1 year	60	25–30	80
Adult	55	18	70

Further reading

Bissonnette B, Anderson B, Bosenberg A, et al (eds). *Pediatric Anesthesia: Basic Principles—State-of-the-Art—Future*. PMPH-USA, 2012.

Pharmacology and fluids

Thomas Engelhardt

Overview

There are important differences between adults and children in their pharmacokinetics (PK) and pharmacodynamics (PD). These are only clinically important, however, in neonates and infants.

Pharmacokinetics

- Includes absorption, distribution, metabolism, and elimination, all of which are poorly studied in children.
- In neonates and infants, most drugs are metabolized and eliminated slowly owing to immature renal and hepatic function (➔ Chapter 1). They tend to accumulate with repeated doses or during infusions. This is a consequence of reduced protein binding, large volumes of distribution (V_d), prolonged half-lives ($t_{1/2}$), and reduced clearances.
- Neonates have little fat or muscle tissues. Drugs that are normally rapidly redistributed into these tissues may have a high initial peak plasma concentration.

Essential pharmacokinetic parameters

- Volume of distribution:
  - This is an 'apparent' volume derived from the total amount of drug in the body divided by its concentration in plasma.
  - Age-dependent body composition influences drug distribution. A higher proportion of body weight is water in neonates (80%) and premature babies (90%), who therefore have a larger V_d for water-soluble drugs.
  - The relative sizes of body fluid compartments in infants and young children are different from those in adults. The extracellular fluid (ECF) comprises 45% of body weight at birth and 25% at 1 year of age. Drugs that are distributed into this space may need to be given in a larger dose (mg/kg) to achieve a given plasma concentration, e.g. digoxin, theophylline.
  - A drug that is lipid-soluble and widely distributed will have a low plasma concentration and a large V_d. Reduced protein binding results in an increased V_d.
  - A large V_d implies high tissue drug uptake. Only a small fraction of the drug is in the plasma and subject to clearance.
  - The larger the V_d, the longer the elimination $t_{1/2}$.
- Half-life:
  - The time taken for the plasma concentration of a drug to ↓ to 50% of its original concentration is the elimination $t_{1/2}$.
  - To remove a drug from the circulation completely requires five $t_{1/2}$.
  - For a drug to reach steady state requires five $t_{1/2}$.
  - For most drugs, this time is prolonged in neonates and infants compared with adults.
- Clearance:
  - Plasma clearance is the volume of plasma cleared of a drug in unit time. It is proportional to V_d.
  - Reduced in neonates and infants.

Absorption

- Pulmonary absorption is more rapid in infants and children.

- Oral absorption is slower in infants <6–8 months old.
- In infants, there is increased cutaneous absoprtion of topical drugs, e.g. LA.

Distribution

- Movement of a drug from the blood into body compartments.
- High CO means rapid distribution.
- ECF and total body water ↓ in first year of life.
- In early life, V_d is affected by changes in the body fat and protein proportions.
- Neonates have greater total body water and ECF, thus increasing the V_d of highly ionized drugs, e.g. neuromuscular blockers (the effect is offset by the presence of fewer receptors).
- Protein binding determines the amount of free drug able to diffuse from the blood to the ECF and act on receptors or tissues. Albumin and alpha-1-acid glycoprotein (AAG) are reduced in the first 6 months of life, and increased concentrations of unconjugated bilirubin compete for binding sites with acidic drugs.
- A lower level of protein binding means that the free fraction of many drugs in the plasma is high, and therefore lower doses of some drugs, e.g. barbiturates, are needed.
- The blood–brain barrier is less well developed and there is a greater uptake from blood of partially ionized drugs.

Metabolism

- Non-polar, lipid-soluble drugs are converted to water-soluble compounds, which then undergo renal excretion.
- The concentrations and activities of the enzymes involved are reduced. In small infants, most conjugation processes are only fully developed after about 3 months (➲ Chapter 1).
- Hepatocellular enzyme activity and hepatic blood flow are the main determinants of the rate of drug metabolism. Hepatic blood flow can be reduced in the infant by increased abdominal pressure, cardiac failure, and, in the first postnatal days, a patent ductus venosus.
- $t_{1/2}$ of hepatic-dependent drugs in the neonate and small infant are generally prolonged.
- Older infants and children demonstrate rapid elimination of some drugs owing to mature enzyme activity and high hepatic blood flow.
- Extrahepatic elimination occurs through non-specific esterases.
- Non-specific esterase activity in plasma and other tissues is reduced in neonates without a clinically significant effect, e.g. remifentanil.
- Some drugs have active metabolites, e.g. ketamine, morphine, and tramadol.

Elimination

- Drugs and metabolites are excreted by the kidneys through glomerular filtration and tubular secretion.
- GFR relative to BSA is reduced in neonates, increasing to adult values during the first year.
- Proximal tubular secretion reaches adult values by 6 months of age.
- Excretory capacity is similar to that in older children by 6 months of age.

Intravenous anaesthetic agents

Propofol

- A 2,6-diisopropylphenol isotonic emulsion with egg lecithin, soybean oil, and glycerol can be used in 'egg allergy' patients.
- Indications: sedation, induction, and maintenance of GA.
- Usually preferred to thiopental for induction in short cases for improved quality of early recovery.
- Causes more pronounced and prolonged hypotension (especially in neonates), respiratory depression, and suppression of pharyngeal and laryngeal reflexes than an equipotent dose of thiopental.
- Recovery is due to redistribution, but metabolism and elimination are quicker than those of thiopental.
- Advantages:
  - Reduced airway reflexes
  - Rapid emergence
  - Favourable recovery profile
  - Antiemetic properties.
- Disadvantages:
  - Pain on injection (use lidocaine).
  - There is currently no pragmatic real-time measurement of plasma or effective site concentration, and unrecognized infusion pump failure, disconnection, or extravasation might lead to awareness.
  - Propofol infusion syndrome (metabolic acidosis, rhabdomyolysis, cardiac failure, cardiac arrest) has been described after propofol sedation on the PICU. Propofol is now contraindicated for this use.
- Induction dose: 2.5–4 mg/kg in children aged 1 month–16 years.

Total intravenous anaesthesia

- Indications:
  - Absolute: MH and muscular dystrophy.
  - Relative: high risk of PONV, scoliosis surgery, airway procedures and URTI.
- Benefits: less emergence delirium, less laryngospasm.

Models

Manual controlled infusions

- McFarlan model (> 3 years of age) to achieve approximately 3 mcg/mL plasma concentration:

Time (min)	0–15	15–30	30–60	60–120	120–240
Propofol (mg/kg/h)	15	13	11	10	9

Paediatric TCI models

- More than 20 TCI models are available; common models include Paedfusor (1–16 years of age and 5–61 kg body weight) and Kataria (3–16 years of age and 15–61 kg body weight).
- Age is a significant covariate in the Paedfusor model (less propofol for given weight with increasing age), with bias and precision probably being better than those of the Kataria model.

- Effect-site targeting is not possible in children for any model.
- Induction: initial target 5–6 mcg/mL.
- Maintenance: target 3–4 mcg/mL and adjust to effect; combine with opioid (remifentanil) and/or LA as propofol is not analgesic.
- If child is >61 kg, use adult TCI models. In obesity, use of total body weight may result in relative propofol overdose.
- EEG/BIS monitoring is potentially useful if the patient is > 1 year old.

Thiopental

- Ultra-short-acting barbiturate for induction of GA, and potent anticonvulsant.
- Presented as 2.5% solution with pH 10.5; limited pain on injection.
- Plasma protein binding is reduced in neonates and the unbound fraction is twice that in older children (reduced dose required).
- Recovery is due to redistribution. Reduced clearance and prolonged elimination $t_{1/2}$ of 19 hours in neonates, compared with 6–12 hours in older children.
- Accumulation with repeated doses or infusion.
- Hypotension (negative inotrope with limited effect on SVR) and respiratory depression are dose-related and more pronounced in hypovolaemic patients.
- Bronchoconstrictor: caution with recent URTI.
- Decreases IOP, CBF, $CMRO_2$, and ICP.
- Contraindications: porphyria, status asthmaticus.
- Induction dose: neonate 2–4 mg/kg, child 5–6 mg/kg.
- Sleep obtained in 10-30 s, duration 5–10 min.

Ketamine

- Phencyclidine derivative; NMDA receptor antagonist. Produced as a racemic mixture and as the $S(+)$-enantiomer, which is twice as potent.
- Produces dissociative anaesthesia characterized by catalepsy, catatonia, and amnesia. The eyes may remain open and display nystagmus.
- Potent analgesic.
- Administer IV, IM, or orally (low oral bioavailability).
- Rapid redistribution, metabolized in liver to norketamine (active metabolite with 1/3 potency). Clearance depends on hepatic blood flow. Elimination $t_{1/2}$ is approximately 3 h. Neonates have a larger apparent V_d and a lower clearance than older children.
- Advantages:
  - IM administration can be useful in extreme situations.
  - Sympathomimetic effects result in ↑ BP and HR (not dose-dependent). Hypotension occurs if endogenous catecholamines exhausted.
  - Airway maintained with some preservation of protective reflexes, but inadequate to protect against aspiration.
  - Minimal respiratory depression compared with thiopental and propofol.
  - Bronchodilator (use in status asthmaticus).

- Disadvantages:
  - Increased salivation and airway secretions. An antisialogogue (atropine 20 mcg/kg or glycopyrronium bromide 5–10 mcg/kg) may be given concurrently.
  - Distressing nightmares or hallucinations on emergence with GA doses (may be prevented by benzodiazepines).
  - High incidence of PONV with GA dose.
  - Tolerance after repeated exposure.
- Also used in postoperative pain management in combination with opioids by infusion or PCA to influence opioid tolerance.
- Preservative-free ketamine is used as an additive to LA solutions for caudal epidural block (⮑ Chapter 11).
- Induction: 1–2 mg/kg IV, 5–10 mg/kg IM (onset 3–5 min).
- GA duration following a single IV dose 5–10 min (15–30 min after IM), longer analgesic effect.
- Prolong GA: additional boluses (50% original dose), start infusion at 20–40 mcg/kg/min, or use a volatile agent.
- Analgesia: 0.25–0.5 mg/kg IV.
- Oral premedication: 5–10 mg/kg—stay with child, have LMA, trolley, and assistance to hand.

Etomidate

- Carboxylated imidazole derivative with rapid onset and short duration.
- Adrenal suppression (decreases 11β-hydroxylase activity).
- Pain on injection, myoclonus, and PONV.
- Contraindicated in patients with septic shock.
- Dose 0.2–0.3 mg/kg in children 2–12 years of age, with limited effect on haemodynamic parameters; may be useful in non-septic shocked patients.

Inhalational anaesthetic agents

Nitrous oxide

- Commonly used as sole agent or carrier gas for volatile anaesthetic agents.
- Predominantly NMDA receptor antagonist; not metabolized.
- Indications:
  - Second-gas effect for inhalational induction.
  - 'Volatile sparing': reduces the percentage of volatile required to achieve an effect in younger children who are particularly susceptible to myocardial depression and bradycardia.
  - Procedural analgesia as a 50% mixture with O_2.
- Mild cardiovascular depression in neonates.
- Absolute contraindications: pneumothorax, bowel obstruction, and air embolism.
- Relative contraindications: laparoscopic and bowel surgery, middle-ear surgery, some ophthalmic procedures, and emphysema.
- Current use declining owing to:
  - Adverse effects due to absorption into air-filled spaces causing increased pressure in non-compliant spaces, e.g. middle ear, and expansion of compliant spaces, e.g. ETT cuff.
  - PONV in adolescents/adults.
  - Potential toxicity due to effects on methionine synthetase and vitamin B_{12} during prolonged administration.

Volatile anaesthetic agents

- Polyhalogenated ether/alkane derivatives.
- Induction and maintenance of GA.
- Easily titrated to effect.
- Physiological differences of patient (MV, FRC, CO) determine 'wash-in' and 'wash-out' of volatile agent.
- Sevoflurane is recommended for inhalational induction; isoflurane and desflurane are unsuitable.
- MAC values of volatiles vary with age (Table 2.1):
  - Infants and small children need higher concentrations of volatiles.
  - Premature babies and neonates need lower concentrations.
- Contraindications: previous MH, suspected MH, family history or risk factors for MH.

Table 2.1 Age-dependent MAC values

	Sevoflurane	Isoflurane	Desflurane
Preterm		1.3	
Neonate	3.3	1.6	9.1
Infant	3.2	1.9	9.4
Child	2.5	1.6	8.6
Adult	2.0	1.16	6.0

- All volatile agents cause moderate ↓ BP and agent-dependent alteration of HR and QT interval.
- All volatile agents depress spontaneous respiration in a dose-dependent manner.
- Airway resistance is decreased by direct relaxation of bronchial smooth muscle, with the exception of desflurane.

Sevoflurane
- Preferred agent for inhalational induction.
- Very suitable for incremental inhalational induction.
- Commonest maintenance agent in children.
- Benefits:
  - Cardiovascular safety profile: less arrhythmias, less ↓ in myocardial contractility, less bradycardia
  - Respiratory system: absence of pungency, ↓ airway resistance
  - Cerebrovascular dynamics: preservation of CO_2 reactivity, no change in CBF, and preservation of cerebral autoregulation.
- High incidence of emergence delirium, epileptiform activity in high concentrations.

Isoflurane
- Unsuitable for inhalational induction.
- Declining importance but still commonly used.

Desflurane
- Very limited metabolism, with rapid emergence from GA.
- Unsuitable for inhalational induction.
- Used for maintenance in prolonged GA.
- Usually with ETT and IPPV; with experience can be used with spontaneous ventilation and a LMA.
- Use with caution if increased ICP suspected.
- Avoid in irritable airways, e.g. recent URTI, since airway resistance increases.

Neuromuscular blockers

- Act on postjunctional nicotinic acetylcholine receptors.
- The neuromuscular junction (NMJ) in the neonate is immature and maximal acetylcholine release is limited (1/3 of adult levels).
- V_d of neuromuscular blockers is relatively large, but decreases in the first year of life. Therefore, a similar dose in mg/kg results in lower plasma concentrations than in adults. Clinically, the responses are similar owing to lower acetylcholine concentrations and fewer receptors.
- Muscle relaxants are given in similar doses in all ages. The highest doses are required in infants.
- The main difference between neonates/young infants and older children/adults is that organ-dependent elimination takes longer and duration is prolonged (not with atracurium and mivacurium).
- Even minimal residual paralysis can severely compromise neonatal respiratory physiology.
- Always reverse muscle relaxants if $<5t_{1/2}$ since last dose.

Suxamethonium

- Declining use, except as part of a RSI.
- Smaller children have a ↑ V_d and therefore require higher doses to reach sufficient plasma concentrations.
- Duration of action is similar in all age groups.
- Metabolized by plasma cholinesterase. Duration of action is prolonged by enzyme deficiency.
- Side effects and contraindications are the same in all age groups; fasciculations are frequently not seen, especially in young children
- HyperK$^+$ arrest due to depolarization of extrajunctional nicotinic receptors (2–10 times longer openings).
- 3 mg/kg in neonates, 2 mg/kg in infants, 1–1.5 mg/kg in older children.
- Onset 60 s; duration 4–6 min.
- Can also be used IM/IO.

Non-depolarizing muscle relaxants

- Competitive binding at acetylcholine receptor.
- Indications, contraindications, and side effects are similar across all age groups.
- Onset of action is faster in young children owing to higher CO.
- Choice is often a matter of personal preference.

Benzylquinolinium compounds

Atracurium
- Histamine release if injected quickly.
- Hofmann degradation makes it attractive to use in neonates.
- 0.5 mg/kg IV; onset 1.5–2 min; duration 30 min.

Mivacurium
- Short duration, but speed of onset is similar to that of medium-duration drugs.
- Metabolized by plasma cholinesterase. Duration of action is prolonged by enzyme deficiency.

- Significant histamine release.
- 0.2–0.3 mg/kg IV; onset 1.5–2 min; duration 10–15 min.

Aminosteroid compounds

Vecuronium

- No cardiovascular side effects; bradycardia in response to vagotonic stimuli.
- Unstable in solution (requires reconstitution).
- Mostly excreted unchanged in bile.
- 0.1 mg/kg IV; onset 90 s–3 min; duration 30–50 min.

Rocuronium

- Mildly vagolytic; painful on injection.
- Onset very fast and used as alternative for RSI.
- 0.2–0.5 mg/kg IV (infants); onset 2–3 min; duration 30–45 min.
- RSI 0.9–1 mg/kg; onset 60–90 s; duration 60 min.

Sugammadex

- Chelating agent used to reverse rocuronium and vecuronium.
- Synthetic host molecule (γ-cyclodextrin) forms 1:1 complex.
- Complex is excreted in urine.
- Limited data < 2 years of age.
- IV: shallow block: 2 mg/kg; deep block 4 mg/kg; rescue 16 mg/kg.

Anticholinesterases

- Temporary ↑ acetylcholine at NMJ.
- Ultimate reversal requires drug elimination.
- Process is accelerated rather than reversed.
- Combine with anticholinergic (glycopyrronium bromide or atropine).
- IV: neostigmine 50 mcg/kg, edrophonium 500 mcg/kg.

Alpha-2 receptor agonists

- Inhibit release of noradrenaline (norepinephrine) and reduce sympathetic activity.
- Effects are mediated via $G_{\alpha i}$ proteins; bind to receptors in locus coeruleus.
- Clinical effects: ↓ HR and BP, sedation, anxiolysis, and analgesia.
- Sedated children remain rousable (unlike benzodiazepines) → 'steal induction'.

Clonidine

- Selective to α_2 receptor 220:1.
- Poorly known PK data but apparently good bioavailability.
- Tasteless and odourless oral preparation.
- Indications: anxiolysis, acute and chronic pain, reduces emergence delirium, attenuate shivering, and opioid weaning protocols.
- Oral: 4 mcg/kg onset 60–90 min; duration 3 h. Associated ↓ HR uncommon.
- IV: 1–3 mcg/kg (lower dose for infants).
- Sedation ITU: 0.1–3.6 mcg/kg/hour IV or 3–5 mcg/kg 8-hourly orally.
- Frequently used as analgesia adjunct to central blocks, e.g. caudal (1–2 mcg/kg).

Dexmedetomidine

- Selective to α_2 receptor 1620:1.
- Bioavailability: oral 0.16; buccal 0.82.
- Useful for procedural sedation, e.g. MRI or echocardiography.
- Oral: 2–4 mcg/kg; buccal: 1 mcg/kg; intranasal: 1-2mcg/kg; onset 30–60 min.
- IV bolus: 0.4–0.5 mcg/kg (over 5 s).
- Sedation: 1 mcg/kg (over 10 min) followed by 1–2 mcg/kg/h.
- Adult ITU sedation: 0.2–1.4 mcg/kg/h.

Benzodiazepines

- GABA receptor complex agonists; produce dose-dependent anxiolysis, sedation, and amnesia.

Midazolam

- Most common sedative premedication.
- Plasma concentration is correlated with clinical effect: higher doses lead to delayed emergence and recovery; paradoxical excitation is possible.
- Oral preparation has a bitter taste; nasal administration is very irritant.
- Active metabolite: 1-OH-midazolam; clearance is reduced in preterm infants; elimination is age-dependent (0.5–3 h).
- Bioavailability and time to peak plasma concentration:
  - PO: 0.27–0.36 and 30–60 min
  - Nasal: 0.55 and 10–15 min.
- May contribute to emergence delirium.
- PO 0.5 mg/kg, maximum of 20 mg.
- IV sedation 50 mcg/kg (titrate to effect).
- ITU sedation 30–120 mcg/kg/h.

Opioids

- Lower clearance and longer $t_{1/2}$ in neonates.
- Immature liver metabolism and immature blood–brain barrier.
- Similar morphine plasma concentrations result in higher CNS concentrations in neonates and young infants.

Morphine sulfate

- Oral bioavailability 38% (15–65%).
- Age-dependent metabolism to morphine-6-glucuronide (potent analgesic) and morphine-3-glucuronide (inactive).
- Morphine-6-glucuronide accumulates in renal failure.
- Intraoperative: 50–150 mcg/kg IV; 25–50 mcg/kg IV (<3 months).
- Intensive care sedation: > 20 mcg/kg/hour (titrate to effect).
- For PCA/NCA, ➲ Chapter 12.

Diamorphine

- 3,6-Diacetylmorphine. Prodrug and metabolized to morphine.
- Very potent, with rapid onset due to high lipid solubility.
- More commonly used in the palliative care setting.
- Used >1 month of age.
- Intraoperative: 50–100 mcg/kg IV (> 6 months), titrate to response.
- In emergency department, if venous access is difficult, the intranasal route (100 mcg/kg in 0.2 mL 0.9% saline) is useful in children >2 years of age.

Codeine phosphate

- Commonly used in the past for mild to moderate pain. Acts as a prodrug and approximately 10% is converted to morphine.
- Unpredictable and unreliable metabolism (CYP2D6 ultrarapid metabolizers).
- Administered IM, PO, or PR. Never given IV.
- Contraindicated:
  - Breastfeeding mothers
  - Any child undergoing tonsillectomy for OSA
  - Any child <12 years old.
- Postoperative pain: 12–18 years of age only: 30–60 mg every 6 h (maximum 240 mg/d).

Fentanyl citrate

- Synthetic opioid and anilidopiperidine derivative.
- Alternative to morphine sulfate intraoperatively.
- Less frequently used postoperatively.
- Obese patients: calculate on basis of ideal body weight.
- Transdermal patches are unsuitable for acute pain.
- Intraoperative: 1–3 mcg/kg IV; titrate as required.
- Used as additive to LA epidural solutions (➲ Chapter 12).

Alfentanil

- Potent short-acting synthetic opioid (anilidopiperidine derivate).
- Faster onset and offset compared with fentanyl.
- Metabolism through liver oxidation (mono-oxygenase) and accumulates in liver failure; PK profile unchanged in renal failure.
- Intraoperative: 5–20 mcg/kg IV; titrate to effect.
- Infusion: 30–120 mcg/kg/h (usually 60 mcg/kg/h).

Remifentanil

- Highly potent anilidopiperidine derivate with exceptionally short $t_{1/2}$.
- Elimination by plasma and tissue esterases with rapid and predictable offset even in neonates.
- Bolus to facilitate tracheal intubation or very short procedures: 0.1–1 mcg/kg (bradycardia and muscular rigidity may occur). Inadvisable to bolus neonates.
- Intraoperative infusion: 0.01–0.5 mcg/kg/min.
- Paediatric TCI model: Minto (>12 years and >30 kg body weight):
  - Height is a significant covariate.
  - Linear relationship between plasma concentration target and infusion rate.

Tramadol

- Synthetic derivate of codeine opioid.
- Two enantiomers:
  - (+) has weak μ-opioid receptor affinity, inhibits reuptake, and promotes release of serotonin.
  - (−) inhibits norepinephrine reuptake and promotes release.
- Metabolite O-desmethyltramadol is responsible for majority of opioid-related analgesia.
- Children 12–17 years:
  - IV 100 mg (1–2 mg/kg), titrate to effect.
  - PO 50–100 mg (1–2 mg/kg) 4–6-hourly.

Naloxone

- No agonist activity at opioid receptors; no PO availability.
- Useful for treatment of opioid side effects, e.g. pruritus.
- IV/IM/SC: 10 mcg/kg (1 month–11 years), 400 mcg (12–17 years), repeat/double and titrate to effect. Infusion: 0.25 mcg/kg/h (pruritus).

Non-steroidal anti-inflammatory drugs (NSAIDs)

- Heterogeneous group with analgesic, antipyretic and anti-inflammatory properties; frequently combined with paracetamol.
- Commonest for perioperative use in children are ibuprofen, diclofenac sodium, and ketorolac trometamol.
- Elimination $t_{1/2}$ and V_d ↓ with age.
- Not licensed <5 kg or <3 months (ibuprofen) and <6 months (diclofenac), but are frequently used off label.
- Rarely used for analgesia in neonates because of the effects on renal prostaglandins and perfusion of the immature kidney.
- Side-effect profile similar to adults.
- Absolute contraindications: gastrointestinal bleeding, peptic ulcers, allergy, coagulation disorders, renal impairment, hypovolaemia, and NSAID/aspirin-sensitive asthma.
- Asthma is not a contraindication.
- Relative contraindications: surgery with high risk for diffuse bleeding, e.g. neurosurgery. Check local protocol.
- Short-term perioperative use in healthy children causes very few side effects.
- Aspirin is contraindicated in children <12 years of age (Reye syndrome).
- No PK data for COX-2-selective inhibitors in children.

Ibuprofen

- Commonly given preoperatively as an analgesic premedication.
- Orphan license for PDA closure in neonates.
- PO 5–10 mg/kg 6-hourly. Maximum 400 mg single dose or 40 mg/kg/d.

Diclofenac sodium

- Relative equal COX-1/COX-2 selectivity.
- Plasma C_{max} achieved in around 60 min.
- PO 1 mg/kg 8-hourly, PR 1–2 mg/kg 8-hourly, IV 1 mg/kg IV.
- Maximum by all routes 3 mg/kg/d or 150 mg/d >6 months old.

Ketorolac trometamol

- Licensed for short-term management of moderate to severe acute postoperative pain.
- Off-label use in neonates.
- IV 0.5–1 mg/kg (maximum 15 mg per dose, 60 mg per day for 2 days only) in children 6 months–15 years.

Paracetamol (acetaminophen)

- First-line non-opioid analgesic for mild-to-moderate pain.
- Since the introduction of the IV preparation there is an increased risk of overdosing, in particular infants—BE HYPERVIGILANT WHEN CALCULATING THE DOSE.
- Commonly used for pyrexia.
- Enteral and parenteral preparations available
- Bioavailability oral >> rectal; C_{max} 30–45 min.
- Elimination $t_{1/2}$ 1.5–2.5 h (neonates 5–11 h).
- IV preferred if oral route is unavailable.
- In neonates, sulfation rather than glucuronidation is the most important metabolic pathway.
- Hepatotoxicity is a small but serious risk; neonates are relatively protected through immature CYP2E1 and inability to produce toxic N-acetyl-p-benzoquinoneimine (NAPQI).
- Consult formulary for latest dose updates.
- PO loading dose 20–30 mg/kg, followed by 15–20 mg/kg 4–6-hourly; maximum 75 mg/kg/d (maximum 4 g/d for all)
- IV neonates >32 weeks: 7.5 mg/kg 8-hourly; neonates and children < 10 kg: 10 mg/kg 4–6-hourly maximum 30 mg/kg/d; children 10–50 kg: 15 mg/kg 4–6-hourly, maximum 60 mg/kg/d.
- PR loading dose 30–40 mg/kg (30 mg/kg in neonates), followed by 15–20 mg/kg 6-hourly (maximum 75 mg/kg/d).

Local anaesthetics (LA)

- Block propagation of impulses by inactivating voltage-gated Na^+ channels.
- In children, fibrous sheaths around nerves are not well developed and myelination is incomplete until about 2 years of age. This makes immature nerves more sensitive to LA, and less concentrated solutions than are used in adults are equally effective.
- The elimination $t_{1/2}$ of amide LA in neonates is at least twice the adult value; this reflects an ↑ V_d and possibly a reduced clearance.
- LA are bound to plasma proteins, although AAG has a high affinity for LA and a greater mass of drug will be bound (albeit weakly) to albumin.
- Acidosis reduces protein binding and therefore ↑ the proportion of free drug (responsible for toxicity).
- At <6 months of age, immature hepatic metabolism of amide drugs and reduced AAG lead to higher free plasma levels of drug. The recommended dose in neonates is half the adult maximum, both for bolus doses and for infusions. Halving the dose seems arbitrary but does retain the same safety margin (on available pharmacokinetic evidence) for this higher-risk group.
- Children >6 months of age receive the same dose as adults (Table 2.2).

Bupivacaine
- Potent amide LA.
- Hepatic metabolism produces slightly active metabolites that are significantly less toxic than the parent drug.
- Longer $t_{1/2}$ than in adults and may accumulate with infusions.
- An infusion of 0.1% or 0.125% generally provides good postoperative analgesia.

Levobupivacaine
- Single stereoisomer S($-$)-bupivacaine.
- Equipotent to but less toxic than racemic bupivacaine.

Ropivacaine
- Amide LA, single isomer.
- Equipotent but less toxic than bupivacaine.

Table 2.2 Maximum doses of LA in children

Drug	Bolus (mg/kg)	Bolus <6 months (mg/kg)	Infusion (mg/kg/h)	Bolus <6 months (mg/kg/h)
Levobupivacaine	2.5	1.25	0.4	0.25
Ropivacaine	3.0	1.5	0.4	0.25
Bupivacaine	2.5	1.25	0.4	0.25
Lidocaine	3.0–7.0	1.5		
Prilocaine	6–10	3–5		

- Maximum concentrations seen 30–115 min after injection, perhaps owing to local vasoconstriction by ropivacaine.
- This potential for vasoconstriction makes ropivacaine unsuitable for blocks involving end-arterial blood supply.
- Maximum dose 2.5 mg/kg.

Prilocaine

- Avoided in infants <3 months of age owing to risk of methaemoglobinaemia (reduced activity of the enzyme methaemoglobin reductase).

Further reading

Bissonnette B, Anderson B, Bosenberg A, et al (eds). Pediatric Anesthesia: Basic Principles—State-of-the-Art—Future. PMPH-USA, 2012.

Absalom A, Struys M. *An Overview of TCI and TIVA*. Academia Press, 2007.

Section 2

Perioperative care

Preoperative assessment

Barry Lambert

Communication

- Good communication is key to effective enquiry and assessment of a child's fitness.
- The assessment takes place in conjunction with the parent. For younger children, there is a reliance on the parent or carer to provide the medical history, and, even for older children, clarification from parents and carers is important.
- Communication of risk is an important aspect and often guides decisions made.
  - Assume all patients and parents wish to know as much as possible about risks, side effects, and alternatives.
  - Body language can provide important non-verbal clues to enhance communication and trust.
  - Describe risk in terms that make sense to the patient or parent. For example, rather than percentages, use analogies such as 'this is the same risk as travelling in a bus across town'.
- Allow time for questions.
- Document plans made at the consultation.
- Provide age-appropriate written information (including approved websites) for patient and parent, so they can remind themselves and read in more detail about the issues discussed.
- Preoperative assessment is increasingly performed before the day of surgery. This requires robust processes to ensure effective communication between anaesthetist and other medical teams.

Preoperative assessment

- Preparation is key to a successful anaesthetic. Careful history, examination, and appropriate investigation are essential to effectively identify and manage risk.
- A structured approach is important to ↓ errors, especially in nurse-led preoperative assessment services. The anaesthetist is still ultimately responsible and they must satisfy themselves the patient is adequately prepared.
- History:
  - Access to previous medical notes and anaesthetic charts is invaluable to access vital information and identify previous anaesthetic complications. Digitization of electronic records provides improved access.
  - Previous anaesthetic history:
    —Identifying issues, e.g. anxiety, difficult airway, or venous access, PONV, and allergy, assist future anaesthetic plans.
  - Family history:
    —Anaesthetic-related, e.g. MH and pseudocholinesterase deficiency.
    —Significant inherited diseases:
      ○ Muscular dystrophies
      ○ Metabolic disease
      ○ Sickle cell disease and haemoglobinopathies
      ○ Bleeding diathesis
  - Prematurity (➲ Chapter 13):
    —Prematurity is a risk factor for postoperative apnoea. Ex-prem infants should be admitted to hospital overnight for monitoring if they are anaemic, <56 weeks postgestational age, or have a history of apnoea or neurological disease.
    —Current O_2 requirements, history of ventilation, or chronic lung disease may influence operative or postoperative requirements.
  - Past medical history:
    —Congenital syndromes:
      ○ Enquiry should focus on the functional health of the child.
      ○ Trusted on-line resources, e.g. Orphanet, provide quick access to other risks associated with congenital syndromes.
      ○ Neuromuscular disorders.
    —Respiratory:
      ○ Current or recent respiratory tract infection
      ○ Specific disease conditions, e.g. asthma, OSA, cystic fibrosis
      ○ Stridor
      ○ Smoking history: passive and active.
    —Cardiovascular:
      ○ Previous cardiac lesions or surgery
      ○ History of murmur, arrhythmia, or pacemaker
      ○ Pacemaker checked within the last 6 months
      ○ History of cyanotic episodes
      ○ Exercise tolerance and activity
      ○ Failure to thrive.
    —Neurological:
      ○ History of developmental delay, autism, or behavioural issues
      ○ History of epilepsy.

      —Gastrointestinal:
        o Reflux
        o Nutritional health
        o NG, PEG, or parenteral feeding.
      —Drug history:
        o Including herbal medications.
      —Allergies:
        o Drugs
        o Latex
        o Significant food allergies, e.g. kiwi fruit (linked to latex allergy), peanuts (linked to propofol).
      —Infectious disease and immunization status.
      —Teenagers:
        o Smoking, drug, and alcohol history
        o Use of oral contraceptive pill.
      —Social, cultural, and religious issues:
        o Identify families with particular difficulties, e.g. other caring commitments, involved with social services, or transportation issues.
        o Identify religious beliefs that may impact on surgery, e.g. Jehovah's Witnesses.
- Examination:
  - Airway:
    —Mouth opening
    —Head and neck flexion
    —Micrognathia
    —Dentition
    —Macroglossia
    —Some syndromes have known airway implications, e.g. Pierre Robin.
  - Respiratory:
    —Signs of cough, wheeze, and consolidation
    —Spinal or chest deformity.
  - Cardiovascular:
    —Cyanosis
    —Perfusion
    —Murmurs and added heart sounds.
  - Neurological:
    —Muscle tone
    —Airway reflexes
    —Communication difficulties.
  - Weight.
  - Temperature.
  - BP, HR, and SpO_2.
- Investigations:
  - Blood tests, sleep studies, respiratory function tests, ECG, and echocardiogram guided by medical/drug history, or if the surgery requires it.
  - Routine blood tests and urine analysis are unnecessary for healthy children.
  - Children born in the UK from at-risk ethnic backgrounds will have had their sickle cell status established and recorded in their personal child record 'Red Book'; if not, then a sickle cell test should be performed.

Common preoperative issues

The child with a 'cold'

- The child presenting, often on the day of surgery, with an upper respiratory tract infection (URTI) or 'common cold' is a frequent problem, especially in the winter months. This dilemma is not taxing, but does require careful enquiry and examination of the patient.
- The concern is the increased risk of perioperative complications:
  - Coughing
  - Laryngospasm
  - Bronchospasm
  - Hypoxia
  - Atelectasis.
- Most respiratory infections are viral and self-limiting. Occasionally they are complicated by bacterial infection. Significant symptoms and signs include:
  - Pharyngitis or laryngitis
  - Malaise and lethargy
  - Pyrexia >37.5°C
  - Cough
  - Purulent nasal secretions or sputum
  - Abnormal breath sounds on chest auscultation
  - Concern from parents that their child is unwell.
- Aspects of the patient's history that, in combination with the symptoms of a respiratory tract infection, cause additional concern include:
  - Prematurity
  - Apnoeas
  - Infants
  - Asthma or chronic lung disease
  - Parental smoking
  - Additional treatment, e.g. paracetamol, inhalers, or antibiotics.
- Central to the decision is the balance of risk for the patient and what is in their best interests. Factors such as parental inconvenience if the patient is cancelled, although regrettable, should not contribute to the decision-making process.
- If the surgery is urgent or cancellation may adversely affect the child, then you should continue with the case. If this is so, then:
  - Explain the increased risks of respiratory complications.
  - Consider if the procedure can be performed under LA.
  - Preoperative optimization as appropriate, e.g. saline or beta-agonist nebulizers, antibiotics, and chest physiotherapy.
  - Prepare for the complications, e.g. laryngospasm or bronchospasm.
  - If surgery permits, consider a 'minimal interference technique' using facemask or LMA, with child self-ventilating.
  - Use a non-irritant anaesthetic agent, e.g. sevoflurane or propofol infusion.
  - If intubation is required, ventilate with supportive PEEP to prevent atelectasis.
  - Suction secretions via the ETT after induction and prior to extubation.
  - Consider awake extubation.

- If the surgery is elective and the symptoms are significant, postpone surgery for 2–4 weeks. Note that young children have on average 6–8 URTI/year.
- The area of uncertainty occurs in two common scenarios:
  - The child in the convalescent phase following an URTI not treated by antibiotics who now feels well but continues to have mild symptoms.
    —The decision to proceed will depend on the experience of the anaesthetist, parental attitude to risk, and the nature of the surgery. Often, surgery for minor procedures will continue in such scenarios.
  - The child who has suffered frequent cancellations because of recurrent infections or a chronic condition.
    —A joint discussion involving parents and surgeons will be required to establish the best time to proceed with surgery, avoiding the periods of severest symptoms.

The child with a heart murmur

- Known cardiac patients should have had a cardiology review, echocardiogram, and ECG within the last year. Patients with more serious disease, e.g. those with left-ventricular outflow tract obstruction, single-ventricle circulation or pulmonary hypertension should have been assessed within 3 months of their surgery.
- A previously undiagnosed heart murmur presents the anaesthetist with a challenge to discriminate between an innocent flow murmur (common in preschool children) and a more pathological murmur that poses a significant risk.
- Innocent or physiological murmurs are commonly soft, systolic, and accompanied with normal heart sounds. The child will be otherwise well and asymptomatic, with normal growth and exercise tolerance. A normal ECG gives further reassurance.
- Patients with a past medical history of a condition associated with cardiac disease, e.g. Down syndrome, should be investigated further.
- Symptomatic patients (failure to thrive, poor exercise tolerance, or cyanotic episodes) should be investigated to exclude a possible pathological condition.
- The decision to proceed with surgery depends on local policy and access to diagnostic services. If surgery proceeds, the child should still be referred for investigation postoperatively to allow classification and documentation of the murmur.
- Children with structural cardiac defects have an increased risk of developing infective endocarditis. However, evidence-based guidance from NICE in 2015 does not recommend routine antibiotic prophylaxis for dental or non-dental surgery at the following sites:
  - Upper and lower gastrointestinal tract
  - Urological, gynaecological
  - Upper and lower respiratory tract, including ear, nose, throat and bronchoscopy.
- A child who is at risk of endocarditis undergoing a gastrointestinal or genitourinary procedure at a site where there is suspected infection should receive antibiotic therapy that covers organisms that cause infective endocarditis.

Infectious diseases

- Management involves the protection of other patients and staff as well as the patient.
- Management of the child:
  - Postpone surgery until the child has recovered, except in urgent or emergency scenarios.
  - They are often unwell and have increased O_2 and fluid requirements.
  - The incubation period and infectious period (Table 3.1) are important in understanding if and for how long surgery should be delayed and how the patient should be managed whilst in hospital.
  - The incubation period is the time between contact with a person with the disease until the onset of the disease.
  - Anaesthetic agents may impair the ability to mount an effective immune response. This may ↑ the risk of developing severe complications of the disease
  - Secondary infections or pneumonia may complicate these conditions.
  - Myocarditis can occur in severe forms of many diseases, e.g. mumps.
  - Septicaemia and multi-organ failure (including thrombocytopaenia or encephalopathy) can occur.
- Protection of other patients:
  - The infected child should be isolated, preferably in a single room.
  - A minimum of visitors should be allowed.
  - There should be strict adherence to effective handwashing techniques, with soaps and alcoholic gels, together with the use of protective measures (gowns, gloves, and masks) as per local hospital policies.
- Protection of staff:
  - Up-to-date immunization of staff is essential.
  - At-risk staff groups, e.g. pregnant women, should be transferred to other duties.

Table 3.1 Incubation and infection periods for common childhood infections

Disease	Incubation period (days)	Infectious period
Diphtheria	2–5	**14** days after start of illness and malaise
Measles	7–18	From onset of symptoms until 5 days after appearance of rash
Mumps	12–25	Several days before and 9 days after start of parotitis
Pertussis	6–20	**21** days after coughing started or six days after start of antibiotic therapy
Rubella	14–23	**10** days before and days after appearance of rash
Varicella (chickenpox)	10–21	**2** days before spots appear until all lesions have dried and crusted

Immunization

- There are frequent concerns regarding the timing of vaccinations in relation to GA and surgery.
- There is no evidence for normal children that immunization just prior to surgery increases the risk of complications or affects the outcome of surgery and GA.
- Approximately 20% of children develop symptoms of fever, myalgia, and lethargy following immunization with inactivated vaccines. This is less likely following immunization with live attenuated vaccines such as MMR. For major surgery, it may be prudent to delay surgery 48 h to avoid any diagnostic uncertainty in the perioperative period.
- The optimum time to vaccinate a child post-procedure is when they have fully recovered.
- Delaying immunization before surgery increases the child's risk of infection and has been shown to result in increased non-compliance with the vaccination schedule. This results in further infection risks for the individual child and their 'herd' community. For this reason many anaesthetists prefer that the immunization schedule be unaffected by admission for surgery.

Pregnancy testing

- Consider the possibility of pregnancy in all female patients who have commenced menstruation or who are >12 years old, in order to protect the patient and fetus from the associated risks of GA, surgery, or ionizing radiation.
- Pregnancy testing is a delicate issue and is best approached by focusing on patient safety and adherence to a local policy that is conducted in a consistent, sensitive, and confidential manner.
  - Proceed if the last menstrual period (LMP) is within 10 days of surgery.
  - If the LMP is outside 10 days, a pregnancy test should be performed or surgery delayed.
  - If a pregnancy is detected, the risks and benefits should be fully discussed before proceeding.
  - In an emergency procedure, priority is given to the patient.
- Consider safeguarding issues in patients <16 years of age found to be pregnant.

DVT prophylaxis

- The incidence of thrombotic events is rare.
- Most patients remain ambulatory and have day-case procedures.
- Those most at risk are:
  - Infants and teenagers
  - Patients with central venous catheters.

90% of incidents occur when two or more risk factors are present (Table 3.2).

- General measures to ↓ venous thrombosis include:
  - Maintaining hydration
  - Early mobilization
  - Upper extremity site for central line preferred
  - Removal of central venous access as soon as possible.
- If two or more risk factors are present, consider:
  - Thromboembolic stockings
  - Intermittent pneumatic compression stockings intraoperatively
  - Low-molecular-weight heparin (after considering bleeding risk)
- National bodies currently have no agreement for recommended guidelines for children and there is little evidence on which to base protocols.
- Hospitals should develop local policies with clear guidance regarding who is responsible for evaluating risk and checking management instituted.

Table 3.2 Risk factors for thrombosis in children

Patient factors	Medical factors
Post pubertal	Central venous line in situ
Use of oral contraceptive pill	Active cancer or cancer treatment
Pregnancy or <6 weeks post partum	Significant medical comorbidity, e.g. nephrotic syndrome, sickle cell disease, inflammatory bowel disease, or CHD
Obesity	Major trauma
History of previous thrombosis	Major burns >20%
Known thrombophilia disorder	PICU admission
First-degree relative with history of thrombosis under the age of 40 years	Expected reduced mobility for 3 or more days

Source: Data from Birmingham Children's Hospital VTE protocol.

Premedication

- The commonest indications for pharmacological premedication are sedation, anxiolysis, or analgesia. It is important that patients should not wait in pain for their procedure: there is rarely a contraindication to preoperative analgesics.
- Medicines may be prescribed preoperatively in order to optimize a patient's condition, e.g. beta-2 agonists for asthmatics.
- Sedation and anxiolysis:
  - Midazolam:
    - —Most frequently used.
    - —Short-acting benzodiazepine.
    - —Anxiolytic, anterograde amnesia and sedation.
    - —PO 0.5 mg/kg (maximum dose 20 mg).
    - —Alternative routes: nasal, IV, or PR.
    - —Onset after 10 min; maximum effect 30 min; starts to wear off after 60 min.
    - —Note that IV formula can be given PO.
    - —It has a bitter taste and is best disguised by sweetening it with fruit squash or other medicines required, e.g. sweetened paracetamol.
    - —A minority suffer negative behavioural effects and dis-inhibition.
  - Temazepam:
    - —Short-acting benzodiazepine.
    - —Used for older children.
    - —PO 1 mg/kg (maximum 20 mg).
    - —Slower onset, give 1 h before desired effect.
  - Diazepam:
    - —Longer-acting benzodiazepine.
    - —PO 0.2–0.3 mg/kg (maximum dose 10 mg).
    - —Given orally or PR 1 hour before desired effect.
  - Clonidine:
    - —α_2-adrenoceptor agonist.
    - —First or second line choice, often used in conjunction with midazolam.
    - —Tasteless, small volume.
    - —PO dose 4 mcg/kg given 30–60 min before desired effect.
    - —Effective as midazolam at producing anxiolysis and sedation.
    - —Effective additional analgesic.
    - —May cause hypotension and prolong recovery.
  - Ketamine:
    - —Third-line sedative, often used where midazolam ± clonidine has failed.
    - —PO dose 3–6 mg/kg and can be used in conjunction with midazolam.
    - —IM administration can be used for very uncooperative children.
    - —Analgesic.
    - —May prolong recovery time.

- Analgesics:
  - Paracetamol:
    —PO loading dose 20 mg/kg.
    —Alternative intraoperative administration routes: IV or PR.
  - Ibuprofen:
    —PO loading dose 10 mg/kg.
  - Morphine:
    —Sedating analgesic.
    —Oral dose of 0.1–0.3 mg/kg.
  - Gabapentin:
    —Sedating analgesic.
    —Indicated if risk of developing neuropathic pain.
    —PO initial dose 10 mg/kg.
- Antacid:
  - Ranitidine:
    —H_2-receptor antagonists are preferred to particulate antacids.
    —Indicated if known gastro-oesophageal reflux.

PO 1 mg/kg 1 h preoperatively.

Preoperative preparation

Barry Lambert and Nuria Masip

Introduction

- The goal of preparing a child for GA, whether for surgery, treatment, or a diagnostic investigation, is to minimize the psychological stress endured whilst optimizing the child's physical health.
- The outcome is to maximize the safety for the child whilst fostering a relationship of trust and confidence with the anaesthetist, vital for any future treatment.
- Preoperative preparation involves the child and their parents or carers. This optimally starts in clinic. The clinical setting should allow familiarization with the medical environment whilst providing an opportunity for the family to learn, understand, and ask questions in a non-threatening space. A holistic and sensitive approach to the whole family's needs, not just the patient's, will facilitate a successful hospital visit.

Developmental stages and behaviour

- For an anaesthetist to optimally communicate and interact with a child in the anaesthetic room, they must first understand how the child's behavioural response to stress alters with their development.
- Birth–6 months old:
  - Infants tolerate separation from mother, as long as there is a surrogate mother.
  - The parents are more concerned than the child.
  - Anxiolytic premedication is not indicated.
- 6 months–3 years old:
  - Separation anxiety from parents is prominent.
  - New environments may be frightening.
  - Aware that something unusual is happening but are too young to understand explanations.
  - Comforted by soothing interventions and distraction from parents.
  - Anxiolytic premedication is occasionally helpful.
- 3–6 years old:
  - Communication and explanations are easier.
  - Explanations describing new sensory experience such as smell, taste, noise, taste, and feel can reassure.
  - Increased acceptance of separation from parents and used to adults other than parents from experience in nursery or school.
  - Fear of the unknown and misconceptions of the planned treatment or anaesthetic may be prominent.
  - Play therapy and preoperative preparation are important.
  - Anxiolytic premedication can be helpful.
- 6–13 years old:
  - Greater recognition of autonomy; interventions that promote a sense of control likely to be successful.
  - Play therapy and preoperative preparation are important.
  - Distraction, including play, story books, computer games, or videos, is useful.
  - May have fears about death, pain, or awareness.
  - Anxiolytic premedication can be helpful.
- Teenagers:
  - Increased personal identity and independence.
  - Need for privacy and awareness of body image.
  - May have a very adult approach or may behave seemingly child-like.
  - Benefit from interventions that ↑ self-control or involve participation in discussions about their own health.
  - May benefit from more advanced coping and relaxation strategies.
  - Anxiolytic premedication can be helpful.

Preoperative anxiety management

- A child's behaviour and interaction at the preoperative assessment may highlight potential challenges for the day of surgery; however, prediction of a child's behaviour is often unreliable and is subject to change.
- Obtaining a history of previous bad experiences with GA or other medical interventions, e.g. dental treatment or vaccinations, may predict perioperative anxiety. Asking the parent how they think their child will cope is also useful. High parental anxiety is also a predictor of ↑ risk of preoperative stress in their child.
- Sedative premedication is an effective adjunct to ↓ distress in children (➔ Chapter 4). It may be used separately or together with the non-pharmacological techniques described below:
  - Preoperative visit:
    —The preoperative clinic is an invaluable opportunity to ↓ anxiety by planning and explaining the GA with parent and child.
    —Provide age-appropriate explanatory leaflets.
    —The child and parent can familiarize themselves with the hospital environment through an explanatory video or actual visits to the ward or anaesthetic room. Greater understanding of the processes involved on the day of surgery can ↓ fears.
  - Parental presence at induction (➔ Chapter 6).
  - Play therapy:
    —Through play, specialist play therapists can allow children to learn, explore, and understand better the process of GA and the procedure.
    —Play therapy is more effective if started before the day of admission and can be used to develop coping strategies and trust with members of staff. This can be very effective if there is continuity of the play therapist being available to accompany the child to theatre.
    —Useful for children who have repeated distressing medical procedures.
  - Hypnosis:
    —Has been used to improve coping mechanisms and postoperative pain.
    —Children may more readily accept suggestion and disassociation; however, the language and imagery must be age-appropriate.
  - Environment:
    —A calm waiting area with an opportunity for the child to play is an important start to the anaesthetic journey.
    —The use of softer lighting, projected images, videos, toys, books, and headphones for favourite music in the anaesthetic room can calm or distract an anxious child.
  - Psychologists:
    —Children who have had a particularly distressing experience or multiple unpleasant experiences may suffer significant anticipatory anxiety and benefit from the expertise of a psychologist.
    —The psychologist will explore the underlying anxiety in greater depth and work on strategies such as relaxation, distraction, and desensitization.

Fasting

- Pulmonary aspiration is rare.
- Fasting is often the most difficult and distressing aspect of a surgical procedure.
- A prolonged fast may contribute to dehydration or hypoglycaemia in neonates or infants. More commonly, thirst and hunger are simply unpleasant.
- An irritable child is less likely to cooperate in the anaesthetic room, whilst dehydration can lead to difficulty in obtaining IV access and increased risk of haemodynamic instability during GA.
- Efforts should be made to minimize fasting. Starvation times should be audited.
- Clear advice to parents and carers is important and can ↓ starvation times when the timing of elective surgery is known. Encourage fluids up to a specific time.
- Table 4.1 gives the fasting guidelines accepted in UK practice.
- Clear fluids are non-particulate, non-carbonated and fat-free, e.g. water, glucose water, squash, and tea without milk. The maximum volume of clear fluids 1 hour before elective anaesthesia is 3mls/kg.
- Formula milks tend to take longer than breast milk to empty from the stomach of infants, the rate depending on protein and fat content. Current recommendations advise that formula milk should be treated the same as solid food.
- Many infants feed during the night and many children wake relatively early in the morning and are fed. For inpatients, fasting instructions should not be 'fast from midnight'.
- A fasting time related to the likely time of surgery is preferable. For day-case procedures, where timings are usually predictable, the written fasting instructions sent to parents usually encourage clear fluids until 06.30–07.00 for children on morning lists and breakfast at that time (07.00) with clear fluids until 11.00 for those on afternoon lists.
- There is evidence that preoperative carbohydrate drinks are associated with improved recovery.
- Despite these guidelines, children are consistently starved for long periods of time, particularly when on an emergency list.

Table 4.1 Fasting times for elective paediatric anaesthesia or sedation (aged 0–16 years)

	Hours before GA
Clear fluids	1
Breast milk (children <1 year old)	4
Formula milk (children <1 year old)	6
Formula milk (children >1 year old)	6
Solid foods	6

- Despite these guidelines, there are patients who still may be at risk of delayed gastric emptying and for whom conduct of GA should be managed as if they have a full stomach. These include children with:
  - Congenital abnormalities, e.g. pyloric stenosis
  - Chronic diseases, e.g. renal or liver failure and diabetes mellitus with gastroparesis
  - Gastro-oesophageal reflux, oesophageal strictures and some enteropathies.
  - Emergency conditions or trauma who have suffered pain
  - Drug treatment that may alter gastric emptying, e.g. opiates.
  - Specific surgical contra-indictations.

Consent

- This is discussed in relation to English law; other jurisdictions may vary.
- A formal written consent for GA or related procedures is not legally required in the UK; it is assumed if the patient or carer has signed a consent form for surgery. However, it is good practice to document on the anaesthetic record the conversation and any specific risks discussed.
- Obtaining valid consent is just as important for children and young persons as it is for adults, but there are important distinctions.
- Allow time for the child and parent to understand what is being described and ask questions. The opportunity provided by having this discussion in a preoperative clinic rather than quickly on the day of surgery greatly enhances this process.
- Consent for GA should include a discussion about the patient's individual risks with GA. This discussion should also include any risks of associated procedures that may be required, e.g. regional blocks, suppository, invasive monitoring, blood products, and/or cell salvage techniques.
- In 2015, the law on informed consent changed. The previous 'Bolam test', which asks if a doctor's conduct would be supported by a responsible body of medical opinion, no longer applies to consent. Rather, a doctor must now ensure that patient or parent are aware of any 'material risks' involved in a proposed treatment and of any reasonable alternatives. The test of materiality is now whether a reasonable person in the patient's or parent's position would likely attach significance to that risk.
- For most children <16 years of age, it is for those who have parental responsibility to consent to or refuse treatment. In an emergency where a parent is unavailable, the doctor should treat the child in the child's best interests, limiting the treatment to that which reasonably deals with the emergency.
- A child aged <16 years may be considered Gillick competent if they have the maturity to understand the treatment options together with the associated risks and benefits. The child may then consent to treatment, and this cannot be overruled by a parent.
- Children aged 16–17 years can consent to investigations or treatments.
- Once a person reaches 18 years, provided that they have capacity, they are a competent adult capable of consenting to or refusing treatment.

The day of surgery

- Modern healthcare demands minimize the time that patients spend in hospital. Children are frequently admitted to hospital not only on the day of surgery, but commonly just hours before their planned procedure.
- The anaesthetist should visit the child and parents preoperatively even if a preoperative assessment has occurred prior to admission. The anaesthetist should aim to establish a rapport and check and discuss the planned conduct of GA and analgesia, confirm any discussions about risk or consent, and provide an opportunity for any last-minute questions.

Topical cutaneous anaesthesia

EMLA™ (Eutectic Mixture of LA) cream

- A eutectic mixture of 2.5% lidocaine base and 2.5% prilocaine base in an emulsifier with a thickening agent.
- The emulsion has a concentration of LA in the droplets of 80%. This fact accounts for the efficacy of the preparation, since the effective concentration of LA in contact with the skin is 80%, despite an overall concentration of only 5% in the cream.
- Licensed from 1 year of age.
- Cover with an occlusive dressing.
- After application for 1 h, it is effective in 65% of children. It is more effective if left in place for 90–120 min.
- Duration of action 30–60 min after removal.
- Blanching of the skin at the site of application occurs in almost all applications. This is not a side effect but a predictable pharmacological effect of the compound. Both lidocaine and prilocaine have vasoconstrictor and vasodilator effects that are dependent on concentration. Constriction or blanching occurs at lower concentrations and dilatation at higher concentrations.
- EMLA™ has a biphasic action on the cutaneous blood vessels, with a vasoconstrictor effect that is maximal after 1.5 h, followed after 2–3 h by vasodilation and erythema.
- The initial vasoconstriction sometimes makes venepuncture difficult.
- Side effects
  - Erythema caused by the late vasodilator effect
  - Conjunctivitis if there is contact with the eyes
  - Methaemoglobinaemia from the oxidative effect of prilocaine This is not a problem in normal clinical use.

Ametop® (tetracaine) gel

- A 4% gel. It is more lipophilic than lidocaine and prilocaine, and therefore crosses the skin more easily.
- Licensed from 1 month of age.
- Cover with an occlusive dressing.
- Similar to or better efficacy than EMLA™.
- Has a more rapid onset time of 40 min and an ↑ duration of action of 4 h following removal.

- Forms a depot in the stratum corneum from which it slowly diffuses. This helps limit systemic uptake and accounts for its prolonged duration of action.
- Erythema at the site of application occurs in 30–40% of patients after 40 min (and in more after longer application times) and is secondary to local vasodilation.
- Side effects:
  - Pruritus 10%
  - Local oedema 5%.

Key checks before the patient is ready for surgery

- Completion of essential ward admission paperwork. Registration of the patient's arrival at the clinic or hospital. Confirmation of the patient's identifying information: name, date of birth, address, next of kin, unique hospital ID, and the medical team responsible.
- A unique patient identification bracelet is placed on the patient
- Consent for procedure is confirmed and any laterality for the procedure confirmed and marked on the patient
- Confirmation of allergies to medicines or significant other allergens.
- Confirmation of any alerts, e.g. difficult airway, latex allergy, or medical conditions that may alter perioperative care.
- Repeat observations, including SpO_2, HR, BP, and temperature. Any abnormal results are highlighted to the medical team.
- Weight, if no recent weight from preoperative assessment clinic.
- Starvation status established.
- If IV induction is planned, LA cream is applied to possible venepuncture sites.
- If anxiolytic premedication has been prescribed, it must be carefully timed to achieve the optimum result. Good communication between theatre team and admission ward is essential.
- Children who have been identified, or those newly displaying behaviour that would benefit from play therapy, should be referred to the play specialist.
- If practical, children should be allowed to wear suitable clothing of their own to theatre. If hospital theatre gowns are required, consideration should be given to dignity and warmth
- Parents should be invited to accompany their child to theatre and their role at induction discussed beforehand. A ward nurse should also be present at induction to escort the parent back to the ward.
- The child is usually best coming to theatre using the means by which they entered the hospital, e.g. on foot, in a wheelchair. The exception is if they have received premedication or require a hoist for transfer from wheelchair to trolley (best performed on the ward).

Safeguarding

- Safeguarding is the responsibility of the clinical team, including the anaesthetist.
- The anaesthetist has two main opportunities to recognize abuse: first, at the preoperative assessment, and, second, during anaesthesia.
- Recognition of maltreatment or neglect is complex and requires specific training that is beyond the scope of this chapter; however, there are some key features that should alert to the possibility of abuse:
  - Past or current safeguarding concerns highlighted in the medical notes
  - Unusual pattern of bruising, especially in the non-ambulant baby
  - Unexplained injury without adequate explanation
  - Unusual location of injury, e.g. buttocks, hands, feet, or ears
  - Unexplained intraoral or anogenital injury
  - Observed poor quality of parent–child relationship, e.g. witnessed verbal or physical abuse or lack of emotional connection.
- Any member of the anaesthetic or theatre team may raise the possibility of abuse. Where there is concern, this should be referred to the hospital's 'named' consultant paediatrician, on-call paediatrician, or safeguarding lead. Refer to local protocol.

Anaesthetic equipment

Richard Craig

Airway equipment

Face masks

- Teardrop-shaped, single-use, clear plastic face masks with a soft inflatable cuff are suitable for babies and children, and provide a good seal with an acceptable dead space even in neonates, e.g. the Ambu UltraSeal mask (sizes 00 to 6).
- Round silicone face masks also provide a good seal and low dead space for use with small babies. They are reusable and require sterilization in a steam autoclave or high-level disinfection with sodium hypochlorite or Cidex OPA. The available sizes are: Laerdal silicone infant mask 0/0; Laerdal silicone infant mask 0/1; Laerdal silicone infant mask 2; Laerdal silicone child mask 3–4; Laerdal silicone adult mask 4–5.
- Scented varieties are available, e.g. cherry, strawberry, and vanilla. Intersurgical manufacture a range from size 0 (neonates) to size 6 (extra-large adults).

Oropharyngeal airways (OPAs)

- Available in sizes 000 to 5.
- They are colour-coded; e.g. Intersurgical OPAs have the following colours: size 000 – pink; size 00 – blue; size 0 – grey; size 1 – white; size 1.5 – yellow; size 2 – green; size 3 – orange; size 4 – red; size 5 – purple.
- The tip and bite block are covered with a softer material than the rigid body to ↓ the risk of trauma to teeth and soft tissues. Take care to avoid trauma to the upper airway; consider inserting with the aid of a laryngoscope and with the concave side towards the tongue. This is in contrast to the standard method of insertion in adults.
- The correct size extends from the incisors to the angle of the mandible when measured against the child's face.
- Do not insert unless the airway reflexes (including gag reflex) are adequately suppressed. Laryngospasm or vomiting may be provoked if the GA depth is inadequate.
- Can help prevent gastric distention during mask ventilation, particularly in children with upper airway obstruction due to large adenoids and tonsils, micrognathia, or macroglossia.

Nasopharyngeal airways (NPAs)

- Can be fashioned from an uncuffed ETT. Use an ETT with the same inner diameter as an appropriately sized ETT, or estimate the size from the size of the child's little finger or the diameter of the nostril.
- The length is estimated by measuring the length from the tip of the nose to the tragus of the ear. Document the NPA size and depth of insertion.
- If the NPA is for prolonged use, it should not cause blanching of the nostril.
- Purpose-designed NPAs are available, e.g. Rusch (size 12–36 Fr). These are available as an adjustable-flange, latex-free, single-use airway or as a simple PVC airway.

Supraglottic airway devices

- Used in elective and emergency cases, as well as difficult airway management.

- First-generation devices do not have a gastric access channel. Second-generation devices do have this feature (which allows the stomach to vent and a gastric tube to be passed); this may ↓ the risk of pulmonary aspiration and may result in a higher airway leak pressure.
- The leak pressure is typically measured by closing the expiratory valve on the anaesthetic breathing system while delivering a FGF of 3 L/min. The leak pressure is the airway pressure at which equilibrium is reached or an audible leak is heard.

Laryngeal mask airway (LMAs)

- LMAs are manufactured in sizes 1–5 (➔ Chapter 6, Table 6.1).
- The LMA Classic (Intavent) is a reusable (40 uses) silicone device. It should be sterilized in an autoclave.
- Single-use devices may differ in their design from the classic LMA; e.g. the Ambu AuraOnce has an airway tube with a 70° curve and no aperture bars. The angulation of the airway tube improves the ease of insertion.
- The LMA Unique (Intavent) is a single-use version of the LMA Classic.

Flexible laryngeal masks

- Have a kink-free wire-reinforced airway tube that is very flexible and can be positioned away from the surgical field without compromising the seal of the cuff at the laryngeal inlet.
- An example is the Ambu AuraFlex, which is disposable, single-use, and available in sizes 2, 2½, 3, 4, 5, and 6.
- Useful for some ENT, ophthalmic, oral, and dental procedures.

LMA Pro-Seal (Intavent)

- Has a wire-reinforced airway tube and a gastric access channel. Available in sizes 1–5. Unlike the adult sizes, paediatric sizes (1–2½) do not have a double-cuff design (Table 5.1).
- The integral bite block prevents airway obstruction with biting.
- A median airway leak pressure of 25 cmH$_2$O has been reported (range 10–30 cmH$_2$O).

Table 5.1 LMA Pro-Seal sizes based on patient weight

LMA Pro-Seal size	Patient weight (kg)	Maximum cuff inflation volume (mL)	Maximum-size orogastric tube (Fr)
1	<5	4	8
1½	5–10	7	10
2	10–20	10	10
2½	20–30	14	14
3	30–50	30	16
4	50–70	40	16
5	>70	40	18

LMA Supreme (Teleflex Medical)
- Is a single-use second-generation supraglottic airway device. It has a rigid curved airway tube with the gastric drain tube positioned in the centre of the airway tube. The cuff is made of polyvinyl chloride and it is relatively large compared with the LMA Pro-Seal. Available in sizes 1–5.
- The performance of the size 2 LMA Supreme is similar to that of the LMA Pro-Seal in terms of median airway leak pressure, with a median leak pressure of 19 cmH$_2$O (range 12–30 cmH$_2$O).
- The incidence of gastric insufflation is reduced compared with the LMA Unique.

i-gel (Intersurgical)
- Has a soft, gel-like, non-inflatable cuff and has a gastric channel (except size 1). Available in sizes 1–5 (Table 5.2).
- Outward displacement of the i-gel may occur after insertion and can be countered by downward traction and fixation with adhesive tape.
- In smaller children, it is not unusual to have to make adjustments to the position to maintain a patent airway.
- A median leak pressure of 20 cmH$_2$O (range 8–30 cmH$_2$O) has been reported.

Air-Q Masked Laryngeal Airway (Mercury Medical)
- Has an oval-shaped laryngeal mask, a short, wide airway tube, a keyhole-shaped airway outlet designed to elevate the epiglottis, an elevation ramp built into the airway outlet designed to direct an ETT toward the laryngeal inlet, and a removable tethered connector that allows access for intubation with a standard ETT.
- Is designed to give good fibreoptic views of the larynx and to act as a conduit for fibreoptic intubation. The short, wide airway tube allows passage of a cuffed ETT with pilot balloon and removal of the Air-Q after intubation. A removal stylet is used to stabilize the ETT during removal.
- The mean airway leak pressure reported for size 1.5 and 2 Air-Q is 19 cmH$_2$O.
- Sizes: size 1.0 for patients weighing <7 kg; size 1.5 for patients weighing 7–17 kg; size 2.0 for patients weighing 17–30 kg; size 2.5 for patients weighing 30–50 kg; size 3.5 for patients weighing 50–70 kg; size 4.5 for patients weighing 70–100 kg.

Table 5.2 Selection of i-gel size according to patient weight

i-gel size	Patient weight (kg)
1	2–5
1½	5–12
2	10–25
2½	25–35
3	30–60
4	50–90
5	>90

Table 5.3 ETT sizes for intubation through the Ambu Aura-i

Ambu Aura-i size	Maximum ETT size that can pass through the Ambu Aura -i
1	3.5
1½	4
2	5
2½	5.5
3	6.5
4	7.5
5	8
6	8

Ambu Aura-i
- Specifically designed to facilitate fibreoptic intubation (Table 5.3). The airway tube has a 90° angle designed for easy insertion of the device.
- There are no aperture bars in the bowl of the laryngeal mask. A cuffed ETT cannot be passed through the Ambu Aura-i size 1.0 or 1.5. It is available in eight sizes.

Cobra Perilaryngeal Airway (Pulmodyne)
- This device has a distal end, the cobra head, with slotted openings that allow ventilation. The shape of the cobra head is designed to hold the epiglottis and at the soft tissues of the hypopharynx out of the way.
- There is a soft high-volume low-pressure cuff proximal to the cobra head. This seals the upper airway at the base of the tongue and allows positive-pressure ventilation
- Single-use device.
- With the cuff inflated to 60 cmH$_2$O, a mean airway leak pressure of 27 cmH$_2$O was reported in children ($n = 40$) using sizes 1.5, 2, and 3.
- *Sizes:* size ½ for neonates >2.5 kg; size 1 for infants >5 kg; size 1½ for infants >10 kg; size 2 for children >15 kg; size 3 for children/small adults >35 kg; size 4 for adults >70 kg; size 5 for large adults >100 kg; size 6 for extra-large adults >130 kg.

Endotracheal tubes (ETTs)
- May be cuffed or uncuffed.
- Traditionally, uncuffed tubes were used for prepubertal children, with the tube size selected to allow a small audible leak at an inspiratory pressure of 20 cmH$_2$O.
- The narrowest part of the airway in prepubertal children is the cricoid ring. A correctly sized uncuffed tube creates enough of a seal at the level of the cricoid ring to allow positive-pressure ventilation and protect the airway from aspiration, without exerting excessive pressure on the mucosa. This avoids mucosal ischaemia and mucosal oedema. Even a small reduction in airway diameter can ↑ airway resistance and cause stridor. The smaller the airway, the more critical is the impact.

- This principle can be conceptualized in terms of the Hagen–Poiseuille equation, which describes the laminar flow of an incompressible fluid in a cylindrical pipe of constant cross section; accordingly, resistance is inversely proportional to the fourth power of the radius.
- Historically, cuffed ETT use was limited owing to concern regarding the potential for mucosal ischaemia and oedema. This was secondary to excessive pressure from the low-volume high-pressure cuff. However, the Microcuff ETT (Halyard) has an ultrathin high-volume low-pressure cuff that provides an airway seal at pressures of 8–15 cmH$_2$O and is increasingly used in prepubertal children, including neonates and infants.
- For children > 1 year of age, the tube size is predicted by the following formula:

    Internal diameter (mm) of ETT = Age (years)/4 + 4.5

- The predicted internal diameter may be too large with no audible leak or too small with an excessive leak. Smaller and larger tubes must be immediately available.
- The depth of insertion is predicted using the following formulas:

    Centimetre marking at teeth with ETT in corner of mouth = Age (years)/2 + 12

    Centimetre marking at nostril = Age (years)/2 + 15

- The correct depth of insertion must be checked by auscultation and observation of chest movement and, if prolonged intubation is anticipated, a CXR.
- For children <1 year of age, **➜** Chapter 6, Table 6.2 for predicted tube size and depth of insertion.
- An ETT of a given internal diameter will vary in external diameter depending on the specific product and manufacturer.
- This variation can be useful in selecting a tube that provides the best possible airway seal, avoiding an excessive leak as well as mucosal damage.
- Table 5.4 compares the Portex Blue-Line clear PVC, Portex Ivory PVC, and Vygon ETTs. Note the difference in external diameter for a given

Table 5.4 Difference in outer diameter (OD) of various makes of ETT for a given internal diameter (ID)

ID	Blue Line OD	Ivory OD	Vygon OD
2.5	3.5	3.7	4.1
3	4.2	4.4	4.6
3.5	4.8	5.1	5.2
4	5.5	5.9	5.7
4.5	6.2	6.6	6.2
5	6.9	7.3	7.0
5.5	7.6	8.0	8.0
6	8.2	8.8	8.5

internal diameter. The increasing use of the Microcuff ETT (Halyard) has largely circumvented the need for a range of uncuffed ETTs with different external diameters.
- Uncuffed ETTs may be plain or preformed. Preformed ETTs may be south-facing oral or north-facing oral (not to be confused with north-facing nasal preformed ETTs). The use of a preformed ETT is useful to direct the tube and breathing system away from the site of surgery, and avoids the need for a catheter mount, which ↑ dead space. They may also ↓ the likelihood of the tube kinking.

Microcuff Pediatric ETT (Halyard)
- The correct size is selected from the Microcuff sizing chart (Table 5.5).
- The Microcuff ETT has well-defined intubation depth markings (Fig. 5.1). The black line needs to be placed between the vocal cords.

Table 5.5 Microcuff ETT sizing chart

Tube size: ID (mm)	Age or weight
3.0	term ≥3 kg to <8 months
3.5	8 months to <2 years
4.0	2 to <4 years
4.5	4 to <6 years
5.0	6 to <8 years
5.5	8 to <10 years
6.0	10 to <12 years
6.5	12 to <14 years
7.0	14 to <16 years

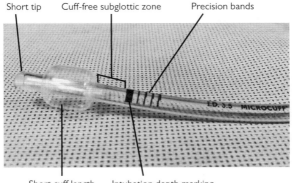

Fig. 5.1 Microcuff ETT depth markings.

- Before cuff inflation, there should be an audible leak at an airway pressure <20 cmH$_2$O. If there is no leak, then downsize the ETT.
- The cuff is inflated using the minimum occluding volume, which is the volume required to create an effective seal at the relevant inflation pressure for positive-pressure ventilation.
- Cuff pressure should not exceed 20 cmH$_2$O. Continuous monitoring of the cuff pressure is advised. In practice this is difficult to achieve.
- Cuff pressure can be monitored intermittently using a manual cuff pressure gauge, e.g. the VBM cuff pressure gauge or the Tracoe cuff pressure monitor, or continuously using an automatic cuff pressure gauge, e.g. the VBM cuff controller or Tracoe pressure controller.
- Microcuff ETTs are also available as south-facing preformed tubes.

Laser oral tracheal tubes
- Are available as cuffed or uncuffed tubes; the former have a dual cuff (Table 5.6).
- They are flexible stainless steel tubes that are laser-resistant and non-flammable. Should the laser beam hit the tube, the reflected beam is defocused.

Reinforced tubes
- These are kink-resistant, with a relatively large outer diameter for a given internal diameter (Table 5.7). They cannot be cut shorter. They may be cuffed or uncuffed.

Accessories

Bougies
- Come in three sizes.
- The 5 Fr bougie has a diameter of 1.7 mm and is used in combination with ETTs of internal diameter 2.0–3.5 mm, e.g. the Proact Pro-Breathe Premium ETT Introducer 5 Fr/470 mm.
- The 5 Fr bougie is straight, without a coudé angled tip; however, it has some memory retention to allow an angled tip to be temporarily created.
- With the 5 Fr bougie, load the ETT onto the bougie before inserting the bougie into the airway. Note the depth marking on the bougie with the tip of the ETT aligned with the end of the bougie.

Table 5.6 Paediatric sizes of laser ETTs

Mallinckrodt Laser Oral Tracheal Tube	ID (mm)	OD (mm)
Uncuffed	3.5	5.7
Uncuffed	4.0	6.1
Dual cuffed	4.5	7.0
Dual cuffed	5.0	7.5
Dual cuffed	5.5	7.9
Dual cuffed	6.0	8.5

Table 5.7 Paediatric reinforced ETT

PRO-Breathe Armourflex Oral/Nasal Endotracheal Tube	ID (mm)	OD (mm)
Uncuffed/cuffed	3.0	5.3
Uncuffed/cuffed	3.5	5.8
Uncuffed/cuffed	4.0	6.3
Uncuffed/cuffed	4.5	6.8
Uncuffed/cuffed	5.0	7.3
Uncuffed/cuffed	5.5	7.8
Uncuffed/cuffed	6.0	8.4
Uncuffed/cuffed	6.5	9.0
Uncuffed/cuffed	7.0	9.6
Uncuffed/cuffed	7.5	10.2

- With the 5 Fr bougie, there is a danger of tracheal or bronchial perforation. Take great care to insert the tip of the bougie only 1–2 cm beyond the glottis. Ensure that your assistant (ODP) does not inadvertently advance the bougie further. Do not look for 'hold-up' (resistance) as a means of confirming placement of the bougie in the airway.
- The 10 Fr bougie is 600 mm long with a diameter of 3.3 mm; it is used with ETTs of internal diameter 4.0–6.5 mm. It should have a coudé angled tip.
- The 15 Fr bougie is 600 mm long with a diameter of 5 mm, it is used with ETTs of internal diameter 7.0 and greater. It should have a coudé angled tip.

Suction catheters
- Soft graduated suction catheters with a side port for suction control are used to suction the ETT. The correct size in French gauge (Fr) may be selected by multiplying the ID (mm) of the ETT by 2 (up to a maximum catheter size of 12 Fr).
- The depth of insertion is ETT length plus 3 cm.
- The catheter is inserted gently until resistance is felt and then withdrawn as suction is applied.
- Suction pressure with suction applied and the suction catheter occluded should be −12 to −20 kPa.
- Suction can produce a vagal response, bronchospasm, or atelectasis.

Deflating the stomach
- This is necessary should the stomach become distended during bag-mask ventilation.
- The Tyco Kendall Argyle green O_2 catheter is ideal: it is quick and easy to insert and has multiple side holes plus an end hole that allows rapid deflation.
- The tip is rounded and atraumatic. The length may be a limiting factor in larger children where a standard NGT may be required.

Heat and moisture exchange filter (HMEF)
- Selected according to patient weight so as to limit the ↑ in dead space and minimize airway resistance, whilst providing passive humidification and warming of inspired gases. A range of sizes are available (Table 5.8).
- Adding a HMEF to the circuit will ↑ the MV required to maintain normocarbia in patients <2 years of age.
- Most HMEFs provide a connection for gas sampling. The larger HMEFs (Clear Therm Micro, Clear Therm Mini, and Clear Therm 3) are often connected to an elbow connector (angle piece), which will further ↑ the dead space.
- Avoid catheter mounts, so as to limit the dead space. The use of a preformed ETT helps avoid the need for an angle piece or catheter mount.

Laryngoscopes
- Classified into two groups: those that are designed to allow a direct view of the larynx (direct visualization) and those that use fibre-optic or video camera technology to allow the operator to see around corners (indirect visualization).

Direct visualization
Straight-blade laryngoscopes
- Likely to afford a better view of the larynx than a curved blade, given the high anterior larynx, relatively large tongue, and omega-shaped floppy epiglottis that projects over the glottic opening at an angle of 45° that are features of the infant airway.
- Preferred in infants since they elevate the tongue better, and the tip of the blade can be used to elevate the epiglottis directly rather than indirectly elevating it with the tip of the blade in the vallecula.

Table 5.8 HMEF characteristics

Model	Weight (kg)	Volume (mL)	Resistance	V_T (mL)
Humid-vent micro +3.0 (blue)	<3	2.7	1.1 cmH$_2$O at 5 L/min	10– 50
Humid-Vent micro 3.5 (red)	<3	2.7	1.8 cmH$_2$O at 5 L/min	10– 50
Humidstar 2 HME with the Smiths Medical Airway Adaptor	<3	2	0.5 cmH$_2$O at 5 L/min	
Twinstar 10A filter/HME	<3	10	0.4 cmH$_2$O at 5 L/min	
Clear Therm Micro	3–8	11	1.8 cmH$_2$O at 7 L/min	30
Clear Therm Mini	8–30	25	1 cmH$_2$O at 15 L/min	75
Clear Them 3	>30	48	1.1 cmH$_2$O at 30 L/min	150

- There are numerous options:
  - Miller blade: C-shaped cross section, flat flange, and curved tip. The light bulb protrudes into the channel and may be obscured by the base of the tongue. Introduction of the tube easily obstructs the view.
  - Wisconsin blade: C-shaped cross section similar to the Miller.
  - Seward blade: Reverse Z cross section. Adult-sized light bulb to improve illumination.
  - Robertshaw blade: Flat incomplete C-shaped cross section and small flange. Designed to allow binocular vision of the larynx.
  - Oxford blade: Curved tip intended for indirect elevation of the epiglottis.
  - Cardiff blade: Intended as a universal paediatric blade, suitable for neonates through to teenagers; its design combines elements of both curved and straight blades. The aim is to indirectly lift the epiglottis.
    —The original design was a 10 cm blade with the proximal 6 cm being straight. This avoids the problem encountered with the smallest Macintosh blades, where the curve on the blade obscures the line of sight.
    —The light bulb is mounted in the web of the blade. This avoids the problem encountered with the Miller blade, where the light may be obscured by the tongue.
    —The cross section is a reverse Z shape. This creates more room in the mouth and helps maintain a good view of the glottis as the ETT is introduced. The tip of the blade has a thickened transverse bead that is designed to minimise mucosal damage.
    —The blade forms an angle of 85° with the handle. It may be used to directly or indirectly elevate the epiglottis. Single-use Cardiff blades are manufactured by Proact in a range of sizes: 00, 0, and 1.

Curved-blade laryngoscopes
- Macintosh blade: Available in sizes 1–4. The size 1 blade is of little use, since the curve is such that the blade itself may obstruct a direct view of the larynx; a straight blade is generally preferred for infants <6 months of age. However, a size 2 blade is generally suitable for infants aged >6 months.
- McCoy blade: Available in sizes 1–4, with the smaller sizes based on a Seward straight blade.

Other devices
- Diaz laryngoscope: A tubular laryngoscope with an intraluminal fibreoptic light source. The tubular blade is dismantled for removal.
- Storz rigid ventilating bronchoscope: Can also be used for direct visualization of the larynx.

Indirect visualization
- These devices use fibreoptic bundles, a video camera, or glass rod-lens optics to bypass the need for a direct line of sight to the larynx.

Flexible optical scopes
- May be flexible fibreoptic bronchoscopes or videoscopes.
- Flexible fibreoptic bronchoscopes are available in a range of sizes.

- Examples of ultrathin bronchoscopes include:
  - Olympus BF-N2O bronchofibrescope, which has a 2.2 mm diameter
  - Pentax FI-7BS, which has a 2.4 mm insertion tube.
- The ultrathin scopes do not have a working channel to suction, pass a guidewire, or spray LA.
- The Storz 11301 AB1 intubation fibrescope has a 2.8 mm diameter and a 1.2 mm diameter instrument channel.
- The Olympus LF-DP tracheal intubation fibrescope has a 3.1 mm diameter and a 1.2 mm diameter instrument channel.
- The Pentax FI-10RBS has a diameter of 3.5 mm and a 1.31 mm diameter instrument channel. The instrument channel is used to deliver topical LA to the airway, pass a guide wire, and suction secretions. It will pass down a size 1 LMA.
- The Ambu aScope 3 Slim is a single-use flexible videoscope. It has a diameter of 3.8 mm and a 1.2 mm diameter instrument channel. It is used in conjunction with the Ambu aView monitor. It will pass through a size 1 LMA or greater. A size 4.5 ETT can be loaded directly onto the scope. It can be used with bronchus blockers size 5–9 and double-lumen ETT 37 Fr and greater.

Rigid optical stylets
- Brambrink and Bonfils retromolar intubation endoscopes:
  - Have a metal stylet with a fixed anterior curvature of 40°, a fibreoptic bundle, and an adjustable eyepiece (Fig. 5.2).
  - The Brambrink has an outer diameter of 2.2 mm and can be used with a 2.5 mm ETT.
  - The Bonfils 10332B scope has an outer diameter of 3.5 mm.
  - There is no instrument channel.
  - The ETT is loaded onto the scope so the tip of the scope is just within the bevel of the ETT. This coaxial arrangement is a great advantage; once a view through the glottis is obtained, the ETT is ready to deploy

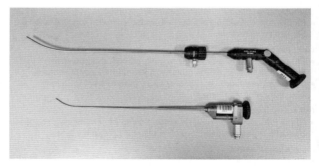

Fig. 5.2 The Paediatric Bonfils scope (top) and Brambrink scope (bottom).

- Unlike the Glidescope and Macintosh style videolaryngoscopes; there is no need to negotiate a separate path for the ETT to bring it into view (less risk of traumatizing the upper airway). Also, the view is not limited to the glottis: the tip of the scope is advanced into the subglottic space, affording the operator excellent views of the subglottis and upper trachea. This, together with the rigidity of the scope, can be most advantageous when dealing with supraglottic, glottic, or subglottic pathology.
- Hopkins rod-lens telescopes:
  - Storz manufacture a series of rod-lens telescopes that vary in diameter (2.7, 3, and 4 mm), length (11, 14, and 18 cm), and direction of view (0° = straight ahead, 30°, 45°, 70°, 90°, and 120°) (Fig. 5.3). An ETT can be loaded onto the telescope and then used in a similar fashion to the Bonfils and Brambrink scopes
- Shikani Seeing Optical Stylet:
  - Has a malleable (to 90°) stainless steel sheath containing a fibreoptic bundle.
  - The adult model is 37.9 cm long with a diameter of 5.01 mm and will accommodate ETTs from size 5.5 to 9.0 mm.
  - The paediatric model is 26.9 cm long and has a diameter of 2.4 mm. It will accommodate ETTs from size 3.0 to 5.0 mm.
- The Shuttle Fiberlightview Lighted Stilette:
  - Another malleable optical stylet. The paediatric model is 21 cm long and can be used with 3.5 and 4.0 mm ETTs. The adult model is 33 cm long and fits ETTs of 4.5 mm and greater.
- Video-optical intubation stylet:
  - The paediatric video-optical intubation stylet is a 1.5 m long video-endoscope with a diameter of 2.8 mm and an oxygen channel. The distal end forms a malleable stylet that is inserted into the ETT. A stylet connector attaches to the 15 mm ETT adapter. It can be used with ETTs of size 3.0 mm and greater.

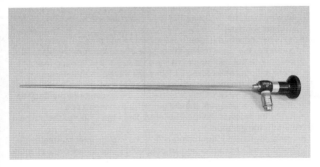

Fig. 5.3 Hopkins rod-lens telescope.

Videolaryngoscopes
- C-MAC Videolaryngoscope:
  - Quick and easy to set up and the laryngoscope blade design is familiar to anaesthetists. It does not have a steep learning curve, and the effect of laryngeal manipulation, applied by laryngoscopist or assistant, can be assessed.
  - It is manufactured by Storz, and has the following components:
    —Blades in a range of sizes: Miller #0 and #1 (both available as single-use blades); Macintosh #0, #2, #3, and #4; and the D-BLADE Ped
    —An electronics module that connects the videolaryngoscope blade to the monitor
    —A 7 inch TFT monitor (white balance performed automatically).
  - Disadvantages:
    —A good laryngeal view does not necessarily equate to successful intubation (the ETT still has to be negotiated into the field of vision displayed on the monitor and then into the larynx; cf. the Bonfils scope).
    —Risk of trauma to the lips, mouth and pharynx as the ETT is manipulated (blindly).
    —Not useful with supraglottic, glottic, or subglottic level pathology (cf. the Bonfils scope).
    —Limited mouth opening or neck movement may make insertion impossible.
- Glidescope
  - The GlideScope AVL preterm/small child videolaryngoscope has a blade angle that is designed to follow the natural anatomy of the airway, allowing a view of the larynx with little manipulation of the head, neck, and pharynx.
  - It is used in conjunction with a 6.4 inch colour monitor and either a reusable blade or single use 'stat' disposable blade.
  - The 'stats' are used over a reusable video baton and are available in four paediatric sizes: GVL 0 for babies <1.5 kg; GVL 1 for babies weighing 1.5–3.6 kg; GVL 2 for babies weighing 1.8–10 kg; GVL 2.5 for small children weighing 10–28 kg. The reusable blade GVL 2 is for patients weighing 4–20 kg.
  - It is inserted into the mouth in the midline and the ETT is inserted parallel to the blade to hug the tongue. Avoid inserting the blade too deep, since this may result in a poor view of the larynx and make it more difficult to direct the ETT through the glottis. It is important to look into the mouth and not at the screen when first inserting the ETT into the mouth. Only look back at the screen once the distal tip of the ETT is alongside the distal tip of the laryngoscope.
  - It may be necessary to use a stylet to direct the ETT into the trachea.
- McGrath laryngoscope:
  - Has a disposable Macintosh-profile blade with an internal steel reinforced CameraStick and an integrated video screen on the handle. It can be used for direct or indirect laryngoscopy
  - Disposable blades in sizes 1–4 and an acutely curved X blade are available. The size 1 blade can be used in neonates weighing <1 kg.

- Pentax airway scope:
  - Has an integrated LCD screen. It is used in conjunction with a disposable introducer blade called the PBLADE, which has a tube channel and a suction channel. The Neonate PBLADE accommodates ETTs with an *outer diameter* of <5 mm. The Pediatric PBLADE fits ETTs with an *outer diameter of* 5.5–7.6 mm.
- Angulated video-intubating laryngoscope
  - Has a disposable laryngoscope blade with a shape similar to an activated McCoy laryngoscope. There is a 3 mm channel running from the handle of the laryngoscope to the tip of the blade. This channel carries a fibreoptic endoscope that is 1.8m long and has a 2. 8mm diameter.
  - A camera is attached to the endoscope and the image is displayed on a screen.
  - It has been used in children <1 year of age.
- Bullard laryngoscope
  - A rigid indirect fibreoptic laryngoscope. It has an L-shaped blade with a 90° curve. The blade is 0.64 cm thick and 1.3 cm wide.
  - It is available in three sizes: paediatric, for use in newborn babies and children up to the age of 2 years; paediatric long, for use in children between the ages of 2 and 10; and adult.
- Airtraq
  - Uses an LED light and a combination of lenses, prisms, and mirrors to transmit the image to the eye piece. The image may be viewed directly through the eye piece, or displayed on a screen using a WiFi camera attachment, a phone adaptor (which allows video intubation using a smart phone), or the Endo cam connection (which allows an endoscopy camera to be attached).
  - It has a guiding channel through which the ETT is passed. It is inserted in the midline over the tongue.
  - The Airtraq SP is disposable and available in four sizes (Table 5.9).

Table 5.9 Airtraq sizes and associated ETT sizes

Size	ETT	Mouth opening (mm)
Infant Size 0	2.5–3.5	11
Pediatric Size 1	4.0–5.5	12
Small Size 2	6.0–7.5	15
Regular Size 3	7.0–8.5	16

Breathing systems

- With small tidal volumes (V_T), apparatus dead space needs to be minimal to avoid significant rebreathing of CO_2.
- Resistance to gas flow needs to be as low as possible to avoid fatigue of the diaphragm in spontaneously breathing infants and small children. This requires either an absence of valves or valves with very low resistance.
- Given that the closing capacity may exceed functional residual capacity in babies and small children, CPAP and PEEP may be required.
- Two breathing systems are in common use:

The Jackson Rees modification of Ayre's T-piece

- This has an open-ended 500 mL bag on the end of the expiratory limb of a T-piece circuit (Mapleson F).
- It has no valves, low resistance, and low dead space.
- It is lightweight.
- It can be used for spontaneous or controlled ventilation.
- CPAP can be applied by partially occluding the opening of the bag.
- Fresh gas flow (FGF) for spontaneous ventilation = 3 × predicted MV (and at least 4 L/min). This is relatively inefficient and pollution is the main disadvantage of the system.
- FGF for controlled ventilation = 1000 mL + 200ml/kg
- Monitor end tidal CO_2 and adjust the FGF to avoid rebreathing of CO_2.
- It is best suited for children weighing <20 kg: the volume of the open-ended reservoir bag will limit V_T in larger children who are breathing spontaneously.
- The same circuit can be converted into a Mapelson D circuit by removing the open-ended bag and replacing it with an APL valve and a standard (closed) reservoir bag. This reservoir bag can be a 1 L bag, which will accommodate the larger V_T of bigger children (>20 kg).
- Suggested FGF values for the Mapleson D system are: 2–3 × MV for spontaneous ventilation and 70 mL/kg/min for controlled ventilation.

Circle system

- This incorporates CO_2 absorption using soda lime.
- Paediatric circle systems use narrow 15 mm tubing to ↓ the compression volume and system compliance. However, compared with the T-piece, the relatively large compression volume and high system compliance make assessment of lung compliance with manual ventilation (squeezing the bag) more difficult.
- The resistance to spontaneous ventilation is too great for babies <5 kg. However, the system can be used in conjunction with modern anaesthesia ventilators to ventilate neonates, including preterm babies (see the following section on ventilators).

Ventilators

- These can be powered pneumatically (e.g. the classic bellows design of the Avance anaesthesia system by GE Healthcare) or electrically (e.g. the turbine design of the Perseus A500 anaesthesia workstation by Dräger, which uses the Turbovent 2).
- Modern technology compensates for the compliance of the circle breathing system and FGF to accurately deliver small TV.
- The measured V_T is also corrected for the sampling flow of the patient-gas measurement module.
- Breathing system compliance depends on the distensibility of the circuit tubing and the internal volume of the circuit (gas composition, altitude, temperature, and peak inspiratory pressure have a smaller role to play).
- A pre-use leak and compliance test with the end of the breathing system occluded must be performed to enable compliance compensation and ensure accurate delivery of small V_T during volume-controlled ventilation (VCV).
- Most modern ventilators have a minimum V_T specification of 20 mL, suitable for a 3 kg baby using VCV.
- Using pressure-controlled ventilation (PCV) modes, volumes as low as 5 mL can be measured. The Drager Perseus A500 can measure a V_T in the range of 0–2500 mL with an accuracy of ±8% of the measured value or ±15 mL. For V_T < 60 mL, the accuracy of the Avance is better than 10 mL for both volume delivery and measurement.
- The RR can be set within a range of 3–100 breaths/min for Perseus A500), and 4–100 breaths/min for Avance. The inspiratory time can be set within the range of 0.2–10 s for Perseus A500 and 0.2–5 s for Avance.
- A variety of ventilation modes can be selected. Controlled mandatory ventilation may be pressure-controlled or volume-controlled. Synchronized mandatory ventilation may be in conjunction with PCV or VCV. Pressure-supported ventilation delivers pressure-supported breaths triggered by the patient's spontaneous breathing efforts.

Pressure-controlled ventilation

- Historically, anaesthesia ventilators were unable to accurately deliver small V_T because of the impact of circuit compliance and variable FGF. This made PCV a popular choice for paediatric anaesthetists, because circuit compliance, FGF rate, and small leaks around an uncuffed tube do not influence the delivered V_T. The latter is dependent on the inspiratory pressure and the patient's lung–thorax compliance. V_T is not guaranteed. It will change with changes in the patient's lung–thorax compliance.
- The anaesthetist sets the inspiratory pressure (Pinsp), the inspiratory time (i-time or Ti) and the RR. The ventilator delivers a constant pressure for the duration of the i-time, resulting in a square-wave pressure waveform. This enables the ventilator to rapidly overcome airway resistance, with more of the area under the pressure time curve dedicated to overcoming the elastic forces of the lung when compared with VCV. Peak and plateau pressures are identical.

- The ventilator delivers mandatory breaths according to the set RR. These may be either machine-triggered or synchronized with the patient's breathing efforts. In the absence of synchronization, this mode of ventilation may be called *pressure control–controlled mandatory ventilation (PC-CMV)* or simply *PCV*, while with synchronization, it may be called *pressure control–BiPAP (biphasic positive airway pressure)* or *synchronized intermittent mandatory ventilation, pressure control (SIMV-PC)*. In *pressure control–BiPAP*, there is an inspiratory trigger window at the end of expiration. If a spontaneous breathing effort is detected within the inspiratory trigger window, it will trigger a mandatory breath. The patient can breathe spontaneously at any time, but only spontaneous breaths during the trigger window will trigger the ventilator. However, it is also possible to support spontaneous breaths during the expiratory phase that occur outside the trigger window by adding pressure-supported ventilation (*pressure control–BiPAP/PS*). In addition to setting the Pinsp for mandatory breaths (machine-triggered or patient-triggered) the operator enters ΔPsupp to set the inspiratory pressure for a pressure-supported breath (Fig. 5.4).

Volume-controlled ventilation

- The anaesthetist sets the desired V_T, the i-time (I:E ratio), and RR. The ventilator delivers a constant flow for the duration of the i-time, resulting in a square-wave flow waveform. The flow rate depends on the ratio of the set V_T to the i-time. There is an inspiratory pause

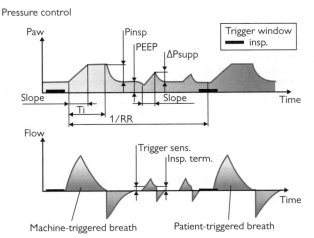

Fig. 5.4 Pressure–time and flow–time curves for pressure control–BiPAP/PS ventilation. Reproduced with permission from Drägerwerk AG & Co. (2015) Instructions for use Perseus A500. Edition: 3 – 2015-01. Copyright © Drägerwerk AG & Co. KGaA.

Volume control

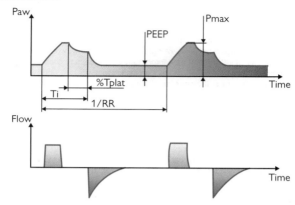

Fig. 5.5 Pressure–time and flow–time curves for volume-control ventilation.
Reproduced with permission from Drägerwerk AG & Co. (2015) Instructions for use Perseus A500. Edition: 3 – 2015-01. Copyright © Drägerwerk AG & Co. KGaA.

during which flow ceases and the airway pressure falls slightly from the peak pressure to a plateau pressure (Fig. 5.5). This pause improves gas distribution within the lungs. V_T is guaranteed, but the pressure will vary with changes in lung–thorax compliance. A maximum pressure limit is set to prevent barotrauma.

Best-of-both ventilation

- Modern ventilators can measure the patient's lung–thorax compliance from breath to breath to determine the inspiratory pressure required for a set i-time to deliver a set V_T. The ventilator delivers a square-wave pressure waveform like PCV but a constant V_T like VCV; it has been called 'best-of-both ventilation'. GE Healthcare call this mode *pressure control ventilation–volume guaranteed (PCV-VG)*. Dräger call it *volume control AutoFlow*.
- The mandatory breaths may be machine triggered or synchronized with the patient's inspiratory efforts. If there is no synchronization (synchronization turned off) the mode is called *volume control–controlled mandatory ventilation/AutoFlow*. With synchronization, it is called *volume control–synchronized intermittent mandatory ventilation/AutoFlow*, and a spontaneous breath detected during the inspiratory trigger window at the end of the expiration will trigger a mandatory breath. The patient can breathe spontaneously throughout the respiratory cycle, but only an inspiratory effort during the trigger window will trigger the ventilator. However, it is also possible to support spontaneous breaths

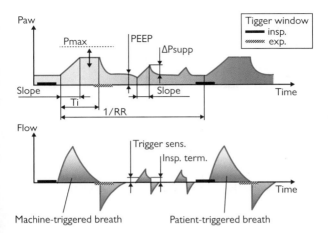

Fig. 5.6 Volume control–SIMV/AutoFlow/PS.
Reproduced with permission from Drägerwerk AG & Co. (2015) Instructions for use Perseus A500. Edition: 3 – 2015-01. Copyright © Drägerwerk AG & Co. KGaA.

during the expiratory phase that occur outside the trigger window by adding pressure-supported ventilation: *volume control–SIMV/AutoFlow/ PS* (Fig. 5.6). ΔPsupp is set to determine the inspiratory pressure for a pressure-supported breath.
• The use of a cuffed ETT will help achieve a constant V_T using volume control/AutoFlow ventilation.

Pressure-supported ventilation (PSV)
• The patient's spontaneous inspiratory efforts trigger a pressure supported breath. ΔPsupp is set by the operator and is the pressure difference between PEEP and the inspiratory pressure for a pressure-supported breath (Fig. 5.7). The patient-triggered breath is terminated once the flow falls below a set percentage of the measured peak flow; this is set as Insp. term. The trigger sensitivity is the flow that must be generated by the patient's inspiratory effort to trigger a supported breath; it can be set between 0.3 and 15 L/min. A trigger sensitivity of 1 L/min is suitable for infants. A minimum RR is set (RRapn) such that if no inspiratory effort is detected, machine-triggered breaths are delivered at this rate with the inspiratory pressure as set by ΔPsupp.

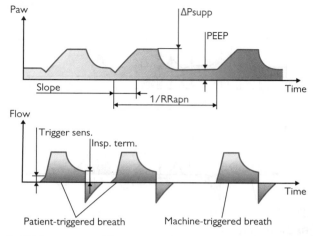

Fig. 5.7 Pressure–time and flow–time curves for pressure-supported ventilation.
Reproduced with permission from Drägerwerk AG & Co. (2015) Instructions for use Perseus A500.
Edition: 3 – 2015-01. Copyright © Drägerwerk AG & Co. KGaA.

Monitoring

Pulse oximetry

- Fetal haemoglobin and jaundice have no effect on SpO_2.
- Calibration is accurate down to an SpO_2 of 75%.
- A standard pulse oximeter probe placed on a small digit may be inaccurate because the two different wavelengths of light may have very different path lengths through the tissues of the digit.
- Prolonged use of standard pulse oximeter probes can cause pressure sores and burns.
- Wraparound probes for paediatric use, e.g. the Nellcor Neonatal-Adult SpO_2 sensor, can be placed on the fingers, toes, or palm of the hand or across the dorsum of the foot.
- Advances in pulse oximetry include the Masimo SET Measure Through Motion and Low Perfusion pulse oximeter. This uses a set of four adaptive filters, each with a unique algorithm, in addition to the conventional red over infrared algorithm, with parallel signal processing that identifies the venous blood signal, isolates it, and cancels the noise to extract the arterial signal. It performs better with low perfusion and motion. The wraparound adhesive sensors are available in a range of sizes, including neonatal, infant, and paediatric.
- The Masimo Rainbow Pulse CO-Oximeter uses more than seven wavelengths of light to continuously and non-invasively measure a number of blood constituents and physiological parameters. These include total haemoglobin concentration (SpHb), oxyhaemoglobin (SpO_2), carboxyhaemoglobin, methaemoglobin, HR, O_2 content, perfusion index and pleth variability index.
  - The perfusion index is the ratio of non-pulsatile to pulsatile blood flow through the capillary bed. The pleth variability index is the change in the perfusion index during the respiratory cycle. The pleth variability index can be used to predict the fluid responsiveness of mechanically ventilated patients.

Capnography

- As the ratio of dead space to V_T increases, the gradient between end-tidal and arterial CO_2 increases. This is particularly pertinent in small neonates, where V_T are small and dead space may be increased by the length of ETT, HMEF, gas sampling connector, and an angle piece. Under these circumstances, hypercarbia may go undetected.

Airway pressure, exhaled tidal volume, and lung compliance

- Modern ventilators have electronic pressure manometers that measure airway pressure. A flow sensor adjacent to the expiratory valve on the breathing system is used to measure volume. The ratio of exhaled volume to inspiratory pressure is displayed as the lung compliance.
- A reference loop can be saved and constantly displayed, making subsequent changes apparent. The impact of PEEP and recruitment manoeuvres can be assessed.

Non-invasive blood pressure measurement

- Suitable cuffs are available for all ages.
- The cuff should cover two-thirds of the upper arm length and the width of the cuff bladder should be 40% of the mid-circumference of the upper arm.
- The middle of the cuff bladder is placed over the brachial artery.
- If the cuff is too small for the patient, it will overestimate the BP.
- Modern patient monitors have multi-measurement modules with a number of profiles, such as neonatal, paediatric, and adult. The profiles influence measurement settings, monitor properties, alarm limits, and screen configuration. It is important to select the appropriate profile.

Bispectral index (BIS) monitor

- The bispectral index is derived from adult encephalographic data. It correlates with depth of sedation in adults.
- The same equipment and method of electroencephalogram analysis are used in infants and children.
- A four-electrode sensor is applied to the forehead. It is available in a paediatric size.
- A study investigating the use of the BIS monitor in infants and children found no difference in the BIS values before induction, during maintenance, and on emergence compared with adult values.
- There was also no difference in BIS values between infants and children at similar clinical levels of GA.
- The end-tidal sevoflurane concentration for a BIS of 50 was 1.55% (95% confidence interval 1.40–1.70%) for infants aged 0–2 years, and 1.25% (95% confidence interval 1.12–1.37%) for children aged 2–12 years.
- BIS has also been validated for measuring the depth of sedation in children.
- The use of BIS to guide closed-loop titration of propofol and remifentanil has been shown to be feasible in paediatric anaesthesia.
- There is, however, large inter-individual variability in BIS values at different depths of GA as assessed using clinical signs of inhalation anaesthesia, motor response to surgical anaesthesia, and signs of arousal. A BIS value >50 had a positive predictive value of 25% for distinguishing responders from non-responders to surgical incision.
- BIS values for intellectually disabled children are significantly lower than those for controls when awake, intraoperatively during stable GA, and on return of consciousness (Table 5.10).

Near-infrared spectroscopy (NIRS)

- Organ-specific perfusion monitoring that is continuous and non-invasive.
- An example of a NIRS monitor is the INVOS 5100C cerebral/somatic oximeter manufactured by Covidien.
- NIRS measures regional tissue oxygen saturation (rSO_2) of the brain, kidney, liver, intestines, and skeletal muscle.
- rSO_2 is an approximation of regional venous saturation (75–90% of the blood in tissue is post-arteriolar).
- The regional arteriovenous difference is derived as follows: $\Delta arSO_2 = SaO_2 - rSO_2$.

Table 5.10 Comparison of BIS values between intellectually disabled patients and controls.

| | BIS values: median (interquartile range) | |
	Intellectually disabled group	Control group
Awake	72(48–77)	97(84–98)
Stable intraoperative anaesthesia	34(21–45)	43(33–52)
Return of consciousness	59(36–68)	73(64–78)

- The fractional oxygen extraction is calculated as follows:
  $fOE = (SaO_2 - rSO_2)/SaO_2$
- $\Delta arSO_2$ and fOE are proportional to blood flow when haemoglobin concentration and metabolism are constant.
- Multisite monitoring (cerebral and somatic) provides an estimate of global as well as regional oxygen extraction and helps detect low CO.
- Near-infrared light passes through skin and bone with little absorption.
- Haemoglobin, myoglobin, cytochrome oxidase, bilirubin, and other chromophores absorb near-infrared light.
- In blood, it is oxyhaemoglobin and deoxyhaemoglobin that absorb near-infrared light.
- Hyperbilirubinaemia may be a source of error, causing a reduction in rSO_2.
- The NIRS device uses laser or light-emitting diodes to emit multiple wavelengths of near-infrared light (700–1000 nm).
- Oxyhaemoglobin and deoxyhaemoglobin have different absorption spectra. Measurement of light intensity at different wavelengths and application of the Beer–Lambert law provides estimates of the ratio of oxyhaemoglobin concentration to total haemoglobin concentration. This is displayed as regional saturation (rSO_2) or tissue oxygen index (TOI).
- The tissue field that is monitored is 2-3 cm deep.
- The average photon light path is an ellipse extending from the light source to the detector. The depth of the light path is about half the distance between the light source and the detector.
- A distance of 4–5 cm between light source and detector optimizes the depth of tissue interrogation and photon recovery.
- A second nearby light path may be used to enable subtraction algorithms to reject measures from superficial tissues.
- Measurement does not depend on pulsatile flow: it can be used during cardiopulmonary bypass and cardiac arrest.
- Normal cerebral regional saturation (rSO_2C) is 60–80%; it is 77% $\pm$ 8% in neonates in the first week of life.
- A rSO_2C of 35–45% corresponds to a 50% reduction in cerebral blood flow and the risk of injury.
- Cerebral oximetry can measure subcortical tissue oxygenation.
- When changes in BP parallel changes in rSO_2C, the limit of cerebral autoregulation can be detected. This is particularly useful during

cardiopulmonary bypass, which is associated with impaired cerebral autoregulation and the risk of neurological injury.
- The resting somatic–renal regional saturation (rSO_2S) in newborns in the first week of life is 86% ± 8%.

Temperature monitoring
- Continuous intraoperative monitoring should be used for procedures >30 minutes, neonates, and when an active warming device is used.

Core temperature monitoring
- A 9 Fr soft-tip temperature probe incorporating a thermistor is suitable for paediatric patients. It may be inserted via the nose, mouth, or rectum.
- The thermistor is a thermally sensitive resistor composed of a mixed metal oxide semiconductor with a negative temperature coefficient of resistance. The electrical resistance drops steeply with increasing in temperature. It is accurate to within 0.1°C from 25°C to 45°C.
- Oesophageal temperature should be measured with the tip of the probe in the lower third of the oesophagus. Inserting the probe via the mouth is preferable to the nose, because the latter insertion may be associated with bleeding from the adenoids.
- Rectal temperature is associated with a prolonged lag time because of insulation provided by faeces.
- Nasopharyngeal temperature can be used to estimate brain temperature, but a large leak around the ETT will cause a false low reading.
- Urinary catheters incorporating a thermistor are available in sizes from 8 to 18 Fr.
- Infrared thermometers incorporating a thermopile are used to intermittently measure tympanic membrane temperature.

Skin temperature monitoring
- Skin temperature probes have an adhesive pad and incorporate a thermistor. They have a reflective back to insulate the probe from theatre lights and overhead radiant heaters.
- Skin temperature monitoring should always be done in conjunction with overhead radiant heaters.
- The combined use of skin and core temperature measurement gives the core–peripheral temperature gradient. This is an indicator of peripheral perfusion and CO.
- The axilla is the best site for muscle temperature measurement and the early detection of MH.

Warming
- Theatre temperature: For neonates and infants, an ambient temperature of 26–28°C is required. This is essential as the baby arrives in theatre and during induction. Once the baby is draped for surgery and on a forced warm air blanket, the ambient temperature is less critical.
- Preventing exposure: Exposed areas should be covered to ↓ heat loss through radiation and convection. It is particularly important to cover the head. Cotton Gamgee can be used for this purpose.

- Forced warm air blanket: A variety of blankets are available for forced air warming. These include paediatric underbody blankets, full-body blankets, lower-body blankets, and surgical-access blankets. Clear plastic drapes combined with an underbody blanket create a warm air microclimate.
- Heating mattress: e.g. the Inditherm mattress, which uses a flexible polymer to create a uniform sheet of soft conductive material that is heated by an electrical current. The mattress moulds to the shape of the patient, giving a large contact area. A pressure relief pad is integrated into the mattress under the heating surface.
- Overhead infrared heaters are useful during induction and at the end of surgery when the infant is exposed.
- Fluid warmers: A variety of systems are available. These include dry warming systems, countercurrent heat exchangers, water baths, convective air systems, and insulated IV tubing. At low flow rates, there may be considerable heat loss between the warmer and the patient. A countercurrent water heat exchanger incorporated into the delivery tubing performs best at low flow rates. Limiting the length of tubing between the warmer and the patient is also important.

Further reading

Jagannathan N, Ramsey MA, White MC, Sohn L. An update on newer pediatric supraglottic airways with recommendations for clinical use. *Pediatr Anesth* 2015;25:334–45.

Kelly F, Sale S, Bayley G, et al. A cohort evaluation of the pediatric ProSeal laryngeal mask airway in 100 children. *Pediatr Anesth* 2008;18:947–51.

Jagannathan N, Sohn LE, Sawardekar A, et al. A randomised comparison of the LMA Supreme and LMA ProSeal in children. *Anaesthesia* 2012;67:632–9.

Beringer RM, Kelly F, Cook TM, et al. A cohort evaluation of the paediatric i-gel. *Anaesthesia* 2011;66:1121–6.

Theiler LG, Kleine-Brueggeney M, Luepold B, et al. Performance of the paediatric sized i-gel compared with the Ambu AuraOnce laryngeal mask in anaesthetised and ventilated children. *Anesthesiology* 2011;115:102–10.

Jagannathan N, Sohn LE, Mankoo R, et al. A randomised crossover comparison between the Laryngeal Mask Airway-Unique and the air-Q intubation laryngeal airway in children. *Paediatr Anesth* 2012;22:161–7.

Gaitini L, Carmi N, Yanovski B, et al. Comparison of the CobraPLA (Cobra Perilaryngeal Airway) and the Laryngeal Mask Airway Unique in children under pressure controlled ventilation. *Pediatr Anesth* 2008;18:313–19.

Chau A, Kobe J, Kalyanaraman R, et al. Beware the airway filter: dead space effect in children under 2 years. *Pediatr Anesth* 2006;16:932–8.

Doherty JS, Froom SR, Gildersleve CD. Pediatric laryngoscopes and intubation aids old and new. *Pediatr Anesth* 2009;19(Suppl 1):30–7.

Feldman JM. Optimal ventilation of the anesthetized pediatric patient. *Anesth Analg* 2015;120:165–75.

Denman WT, Swanson EL, Rosow D, et al. Paediatric evaluation of the bispectral index (BIS) monitor and correlation of BIS with end-tidal sevoflurane concentration in infants and children. *Anesth Analg* 2000;90:872–7.

Sadhasivam S, Ganesh A, Robison A, et al. Validation of the bispectral index monitor for measuring the depth of sedation in children. *Anesth Analg* 2006;102:383–8.

Orliaguet GA, Benabbes Lambert F, et al. Feasibility of closed-loop titration of propofol and remifentanil guided by the bispectral monitor in pediatric and adolescent patients: a prospective randomized study. *Anesthesiology* 2015;122:759–67.

Rodriguez RA, Hall LE, Duggan S, Splinter WM. The bispectral index does not correlate with clinical signs of inhalation anaesthesia during sevoflurane induction and arousal in children. *Can J Anaesth* 2004;51:472–80.

Valkenburg AJ, de Leeuw TG, Tibboel D, Weber F. Lower spectral index values in children who are intellectually disabled. *Anesth Analg* 2009;109:1428–33.

Scott JP, Hoffmann GM. Near-infrared spectroscopy: exposing the dark (venous)side of the circulation. *Pediatr Anesth* 2014;24:74–88.

Bernal NP, Hoffman GM, Ghanayem NS, Arca MJ. Cerebral and somatic near-infrared spectroscopy in normal newborns. *J Paediatr Surg* 2010;45:1306–10.

Induction

Nuria Masip and Barry Lambert

Managing the Anaesthetic Room

- A paediatric anaesthetist must be flexible in their approach to providing anaesthesia. They must exude confidence and control their anaesthetic room, since they are performing in front of a potentially critical audience!
- The approach will vary depending on age group (➲ Chapter 3).
- Create a quiet and relaxed anaesthetic room, preferably with friendly decorations on the walls and ceiling, and with distractions, e.g. bubbles.
- Huddle or team-brief with all the staff (including the surgeon) to discuss the patients and to agree the list order.
- Communication with the anaesthetic assistant about the agreed plan is fundamental.
- The anaesthetic machine and monitoring equipment should be checked and prepared in advance.
- Parental presence is beneficial and recommended.
- In some cases, especially in neonates, induction may be conducted in the theatre, with a warmer ambient temperature and warming device. In these cases, parents will not be allowed in for the induction (explain this at the preop visit; remember this age group does not suffer separation anxiety).
- There should be available a variety of sizes of masks, oral airways, laryngoscope blades, ETTs, LMAs, and functioning wall suction.
- Drugs should be drawn up prior to the child arriving.
- Do not draw up drugs in front of children.
- Be prepared for both an IV and inhalational induction. Situations change quickly.
- If the child is young enough to sit on their parents' knee, have a stool ready and positioned next to the theatre trolley.

Parental presence at induction

- Most UK paediatric anaesthetists allow one or both parents into the anaesthetic room.
- It is not suitable for all patients (e.g. some emergencies, or neonates) or all parents.
- The aim is to ↓ a child's anxiety. High anxiety is associated with emergence delirium and postoperative behavioural changes.
- RCTs have not shown an improvement in distress or postoperative behavioural problems with parental presence at induction. However, most parents who have been present at induction feel their presence was of benefit to the child, and would choose to be present again. Having both parents present allows them to support one another.
- A calm parent will help a child to be less anxious, while an anxious parent will often exacerbate a child's fears. Providing written and verbal information to parents regarding their role at induction and what happens to a child as they are anaesthetized (the child may have involuntary movements, have noisy breathing, or go limp) are useful to ↓ parental anxiety. They need to know that once their child is asleep they need to leave promptly to allow the safe management of their child.
- Parent(s) should arrive in the anaesthetic room understanding the proposed plan for induction of GA (e.g. IV or gas induction, fall-back plan, preoxygenation if indicated, and the possible need for restraint of the child).
- A member of staff must be designated to look after the parent(s) and promptly escort them from the theatre once the child is anaesthetized. The parent(s) may require further support once out of the anaesthetic room.

The uncooperative child

- Despite adequate preparation, a small number of children will be unexpectedly uncooperative in the anaesthetic room.
- These situations can be unpleasant and stressful for child, parent, and anaesthetist alike.
- Strategies to deal with this situation should be planned for and will depend on the urgency of the procedure.
- Positive persuasion and reward is more effective that threat.
- Offer a sense of re-establishing control for the patient whilst at the same time progressing towards successful induction. For example, offer a choice of smell to the patient requiring a gas induction. The child who chooses to breathe in the strawberry-smelling gas is also subconsciously accepting to breathe in the anaesthetic vapour.
- Re-establish a rapport with the patient by asking simple questions about their likes and dislikes, school, or hobbies.
- One voice should speak to the child rather than several people all speaking at once. The person with the greatest trust or rapport with the child should take this lead, whether that be the parent, play therapist, ward nurse, or anaesthetist.
- Careful consideration of verbal language can build and maintain trust. Well-meaning or ill-judged language can have the opposite effect. For example, suggesting to a child with LA cream before undergoing an IV cannulation that they will feel a sharp scratch is likely to result in the child withdrawing their hand and their questioning the truth about what they were told regarding the LA cream.
- Awareness of body language will help improve compliance. Approaching the patient at eye level is much less threatening.
- It may be necessary to de-escalate and give the child space for 5 minutes and leave them alone with their parents to calm down. Alternatively, returning to the ward and attempting again following premedication may be required.
- In some circumstances, the parents may agree that mild restraint is in the child's best interest in order for the procedure to be undertaken—in which case, this should be conducted with the parents' full cooperation, quickly, and with the minimum force necessary. Parental consent must be documented in the notes.
- It may be that the best course of action is to cancel the procedure and refer the child and parents for play therapy or psychology. The advantage in this scenario is that you may have an opportunity to build a trusting relationship for the next time.
- Where there has been a difficult induction, clear instructions should be made on the anaesthetic record for any future anaesthetic plan.

- Children with known behavioural or communication problems, such as those with learning difficulties, can be expected to be uncooperative. Such patients benefit from play therapy and psychological input with a joint plan agreed with the anaesthetist. The anaesthetist may have to be more flexible than usual, e.g. by avoiding triggers for uncooperative behaviour, such as by maintaining the patient's usual day clothes or providing IV sedation on the ward away from the anaesthetic room. Restraint may not be appropriate in the larger child and may cause injury to the child or staff.

Inhalational induction

- As core technique, this may be:
  - Requested by the patient (or parents), especially in patients undergoing repeat procedures
  - Anaesthetic preference because of poor venous access, e.g. a chubby toddler or an ex-prem child cannulated many times previously
  - Clinically indicated, e.g. difficult airway.
- Relative contraindications: MH and specific myopathies.
- Inhalational induction may be inappropriate in a child with limited cardiovascular reserve as in severe hypovolaemia, cardiac failure, right-to-left shunts and fixed CO states. Myocardial depression and vasodilation may cause profound hypoperfusion and cardiac arrest in these patients.
- At the preoperative visit, explain to the parent and child how you will perform the induction. With young children (<6 years of age), explain to the parent what will happen if the child becomes very upset during the induction, i.e. the anaesthetist will ↑ the sevoflurane to maximum, whilst the parent ensures that the child is held in a tight hug (this ensures the distress is as short as possible and prevents the child dismantling the breathing circuit and mask).
- Ensure the components of the breathing circuit, including face mask and angle piece, are pushed firmly together. A T-piece has the advantage of being more mobile than a circle circuit, especially where you expect a difficult induction, e.g. an autistic teenager (use a large reservoir bag).
- Scented face masks or scented lip balm rubbed onto the face mask may disguise the smell of volatile agent. The benefit, if any, is probably more in the ritual and sense of control it gives the child rather, than its efficacy in disguising the smell of anaesthetic agent.
- The child or parent may hold the mask, or the anaesthetist may hold the tubing in a cupped hand close to the child's face. As the child becomes more sedated, the mask can be applied to the face and a gentle chin lift performed if required. It does not matter who holds the mask, as long as it is kept on.
- Use sevoflurane in O_2 or an O_2/N_2O mixture [1:2].
- In neonates or where problems are anticipated (e.g. inhaled FB), induce with O_2 and volatile alone so that the child is well oxygenated.
- Sevoflurane is a non-irritant gas and therefore can be given in a high concentration quickly or even from the beginning of induction.
- An alternative is to relax the child with an O_2/N_2O mix, followed by a gradual introduction of sevoflurane.
- Induction takes 1–2 min.
- Patience is important. Avoid stimulating the child too early, e.g. by placing an OPA (Guedel airway), since this may result in breath-holding, coughing, or laryngospasm.
- During the 2nd stage of GA (the excitement phase), the child might experience an episode of agitation with involuntary movements, coughing, and/or snoring.
- Reassure the parent, and ask them to give the child a kiss and then leave.

- An IV cannula is sited after induction, preferably before any airway instrumentation or surgical intervention.
- It is important to ↓ the inspired concentration of volatile agent once the child is adequately anaesthetized, because of their depressant effects on cardiovascular (and to a lesser extent respiratory) function. In particular, 'bagging' the child with a high concentration must be avoided.
- A difficult inhalational induction may be remembered as an unpleasant experience. In these cases, discuss with the child and parent whether anxiolytic premedication should be considered next time. Document this in the anaesthetic chart.
- Atmospheric pollution is a feature of inhalational induction and many anaesthetists report increased fatigue.

Top tips

- Inform parents in the preoperative assessment about the excitement phase during induction, since this can frighten them.
- It may be worth giving a child the mask to play with preoperatively so they can act out the process with their parents—especially with asthmatic children who have spacers.
- Sit the child on their parent's knees with their back to the trolley and with the child's arm that is closest to the parent tucked under their parent's axilla. This makes the child feel secure, aids restraint, and helps with safe transfer onto the trolley once they are anaesthetized. Assist the parent during transfer by supporting the child's head whilst the anaesthetic assistant helps the parent support the body.
- Talk to the child through the whole process. Tell them to breathe through their mouth. Encourage them to 'blow the balloon up', 'blow the candles out', and 'make the bag whistle'.
- Many anaesthetists start with O_2/N_2O for 30 s–1 min (its smell is better tolerated and the breathing circuit can be primed with it); this allows the child to get used to the mask and at the same time will have some sedative effect (because of this, it is important to keep talking to the patient during this technique; e.g. ask them if they feel dizzy/funny and reassure them that is normal, since they can get scared owing to the feeling of loss of control). Then gradually introduce the sevoflurane.
- For a faster gas induction technique ensure the reservoir limb of the T-piece is pre-filled with 8% sevoflurane and nitrous oxide/oxygen mix. The amount of gaseous anaesthetic agent first inhaled by the child will be greater and speed induction.

Intravenous induction

- It may be:
  - Patient request, especially older patients
  - Best option if there is established IV access
  - Necessary to conduct a rapid-sequence induction (RSI)
  - Recommended if there is possible cardiovascular instability
  - Indicated for MH or certain myopathies.
- Often difficult in the following circumstances:
  - Chubby 1-year-old
  - Neonates, where scalp veins might be the only remaining option
  - Uncooperative child
  - If the first attempt fails there are a limited number of chances before the situation becomes very distressing for child, parents, and staff
  - Vasoconstriction due to hypovolaemia or hypothermia.
- Common insertion sites:
  - dorsum of the hands
  - dorsolateral aspect of the foot
  - long saphenous vein
  - antecubital fossa
  - radial aspect of the wrist
  - In young children, the small veins on the palmar aspect of the wrist may be the most prominent.
  - In infants, scalp veins can be used.
- Have a couple of cannulas of varying gauge ready. In smaller cannulas (22–24 G), the backflow of blood may be slow and the cannula mistakenly removed owing to lack of backflow into the hub; some anaesthetists find it helpful to flush their cannula with saline prior to cannulation, looking for the saline movement as an early indication that the vein has been entered.
- Using topical LA creams, hiding the cannulation from view, and distraction techniques frequently allow cannulation without the child noticing.
- When there is no time to wait for a LA cream to be effective and an IV is preferable, use ethyl chloride spray ("cold spray") and/or N_2O.
- A skilled assistant is required to hold the child's hand still; they must have tape readily at hand to immediately secure the cannula.
- Propofol is generally the induction agent of choice.
- Safety cannulas have the potential to ↓ sharps injuries and are generally felt to be easy to insert in most circumstances. However, the current devices are less easy to insert in difficult veins and moving patients; therefore standard cannulas should also be stocked.

Top tips

- Assess for the most promising veins preoperatively.
- Avoid using the word 'needle'; use more neutral words, e.g. 'plastic tube', 'straw', or even 'Spiderman web shooter'.
- Apply EMLA™ (lidocaine/prilocaine)cream (1–2 h before) or Ametop® (tetracaine) cream (30–40 min before) to two or more of the most promising veins.

- Keep the cannula out of sight.
- Distract the child during insertion. Parents and/or play specialists can be helpful.
- Younger children can be sat on their parent's knees, with the intended arm immobilized behind the parent's back.
- Have anaesthetic drugs and sharps bin close by.
- Remove the LA cream and get assistance to immobilize the limb and provide venous congestion.
- Identify the intended vein and cannulate as in adults.
- Rapidly secure the cannula before the child moves their hand or arm.
- Test patency with saline flush to avoid subcutaneous injection; then promptly administer induction agents.
- Either the anaesthetist or assistant must be holding the cannulated hand at all times until the child is asleep; otherwise, as the drug is injected, the child may withdraw their arm owing to discomfort and dislodge the cannula.
- Command the anaesthetic room, asking the parent politely but firmly to leave. Ensure you have access to head and airway despite the presence of parents, since the child may desaturate rapidly once anaesthetized.

Basic airway management

- Much of the morbidity associated with GA is due to airway problems. The same basic principles in managing adult airways apply to children:
  - Positioning
  - Oxygenation
  - Recognizing airway obstruction
  - Simple manoeuvres
  - Airway adjuncts.

Positioning

- The airway in neonates and infants obstructs easily because of the large head, short neck, large tongue, and lack of space in the airway.
- Anatomical changes with age group require different positioning.
- Neonates and small infants have relatively large head and prominent occiput creating a degree of flexion—predisposing to airway obstruction. A small roll underneath the shoulders is often required to open up the airway.
- For children, a neutral position of the neck with the eye in line with the ear canal is required. Further neck extension may obstruct the airway.
- As the child gets older, positioning changes towards the adult 'sniffing the morning air position'. A pillow to flex the neck is often useful in teenagers.

Oxygen supplementation

- O_2 consumption in the neonate approximates 7 mL/kg/min, decreasing gradually during childhood to the adult value of 3.5 mL/kg/min.
- There is rapid onset of hypoxia in the event of airway obstruction or apnoea.
- Effective preoxygenation is often distressing and is usually omitted, but it is essential that O_2 (preferably 100%) be given as soon as possible after induction.

Recognizing airway obstruction

- Remember to place your fingers onto the mandible when adjusting the face mask. Avoid applying pressure with the fingertips to the underside of the jaw, since this may obstruct the airway.
- A similar situation may occur with too much hyperextension of the neck, resulting in compression of the oropharynx.
- Any noisy breathing, e.g. stridor, wheeze, or grunting, may indicate partial obstruction. Quiet breathing is an indicator of airway patency.
- Paradoxical abdominal movement is an indicator of airway obstruction.

Simple manoeuvres

- Continual assessment of airway patency is required and repeated adjustment may be necessary.
- Correct positioning and clearing the airway is frequently all that is required (with nasal obstruction, ensure the mouth is held slightly open).
- Some infants may require CPAP. The positive pressure aids alveolar recruitment and prevents airway collapse due to tracheomalacia.
- Consider an OPA (Guedel airway) (➔ Chapter 5).

Advanced airway management

Insertion of the laryngeal mask airway

- Indications:
  - Airway maintenance during spontaneous ventilation
  - Airway maintenance during IPPV
  - Conduit for fibreoptic endotracheal intubation.
- Contraindications are mostly relative and include:
  - Patients at risk of regurgitation and aspiration (absolute unless used to deal with severe airway obstruction)
  - Limited mouth opening
  - Long procedures
  - Neonates
  - Infants other than for brief procedures
  - Many head and neck procedures.
- An appropriately sized LMA is selected (Table 6.1); note that the maximum intracuff pressure is 60 cmH$_2$O for all sizes.
- Many anaesthetists maintain the child with volatile agent in 100% O$_2$ for a period before insertion so that, in the event of airway obstruction caused by attempted insertion, there is an O$_2$ reserve to provide time for remedial measures. Others prefer to give a generous dose of propofol and place the LMA immediately.
- Adequate depth of GA is required to prevent laryngospasm on insertion. In healthy children, a dose of 4–6 mg/kg of propofol will usually allow relatively immediate insertion of the LMA. With an inhalational induction, be patient or administer 1–2 mg/kg of propofol to assist insertion.
- Lack of movement to jaw thrust is a useful indicator of adequate depth of GA (note that jaw thrust in a superficial anaesthetic plane may cause laryngospasm).
- The head is positioned in sniffing position; the mouth is opened and an assistant provides a jaw thrust to aid insertion.
- The technique of insertion is the same as for adults.

Table 6.1 Suggested LMA sizes

Patient weight (kg)	Mask size	Maximum cuff volume (mL)	ETT (mm) that will pass through LMA
<5	1	4	3.5
5–10	1 1/2	7	4.0
10–20	2	10	4.5
20–30	2 1/2	14	5.0
>30	3	20	5.5

- LMA position is assessed by observing for evidence of partial or complete obstruction and the ability to manually ventilate through the LMA.
- If the position is not satisfactory, the LMA is removed and a period of ventilation with volatile agent in 100% O_2 is provided before further attempts are made.
- The younger the patient, the more likely it is that the LMA will sit unsatisfactorily; some anaesthetists therefore prefer to place an ETT in children aged <6 months.
  - Removal of the LMA is carried out either deep or awake. Personal preference is usually the deciding factor. Where there have been airway difficulties or there is a risk of tracheal contamination, e.g. post tonsillectomy, it is often best to remove the LMA when the child is awake. Laryngospasm is a risk with both techniques, especially in younger children.

Endotracheal intubation

- Decide which route (oral or nasal) and which type of ETT is indicated (cuffed or uncuffed, north- or south-facing, cut or uncut, or armoured). Microcuff paediatric ETTs with ultrathin polyurethane cuffs (achieving high volume at low pressure) are available and can be used if the cuff pressure is checked regularly.
- Cuff tubes may be indicated in specific surgeries, e.g. laparoscopy, and when there is an ↑ risk of aspiration.
- For children <4 years old, Table 6.2 provides a guide to the appropriate choice of ETT internal diameter (ID).
- For children >4 years the formula is size = (age/4) + 4.5 mm, but pre-existing medical conditions may influence size.
- With uncuffed tubes, it is advisable to have available ETTs respectively 0.5 mm larger and smaller than the initial choice.
- Beware preformed ETTs in syndromic children whose tracheal diameter may be age-appropriate but whose tracheal length may be shorter than normal, thus predisposing to an endobronchial intubation.
- Anatomical differences require different approaches at various ages:
  - Relatively large tongue in infants
  - Cephalad larynx (C4–5 in adults vs. C2–3 in infants)
  - Anterior larynx compared with adults
  - Epiglottis shape and position (long, narrow, floppy, and angled over the larynx at 45°)
  - The subglottic area and the cricoid ring are the narrowest parts of upper airway in children. (Recent studies challenge the view that the larynx is cone-shaped in infants and children, with the apex of the cone positioned at the level of the cricoid ring. Instead, the most likely area of resistance to the passage of an ETT is the subglottic area owing to its smallest transverse diameter.)
- Intubation can be facilitated using muscle relaxant, deep inhalational GA, or a bolus of opioid, e.g. alfentanil 15 mcg/kg or remifentanil (1–2 mcg/kg).

Table 6.2 Suggested ETT sizes

Age	Plain ETT ID (mm)	Length, oral (cm)	Length, nasal (cm at nose)	Microcuff ID (mm)
Preterm < 2kg	2.0. 2.5	6–7	7.5–9	—
Preterm 2–4 kg	3.0, 3.5	7–8.5	9–10.5	3.0(if >3 kg)
Term–3 months	3.5	8.5–10	10.5–12	3.0
3 months–1 year	3.5, 4.0	10–11	12–14	3.0, 3.5
1 year	4.0, 4.5	11–12	14–15	3.5
2 years	4.5, 5.0	12–13	15–16	4.0
3 years	5.0	13–14	16–17	4.0
4–6 years	5.0, 5.5	14–15	17–19	4.5
6–8 years	6.0, 6.5	15–16	19–21	5.0
>8 years	6.5, 7.0, 7.5	16–20	20–23	5.5

Oral endotracheal intubation

- Straight-bladed laryngoscopes (e.g. Miller) are preferred in infants (bigger tongue).
- Curved-bladed laryngoscopes (e.g. Macintosh) are used for toddlers and older children.
- Straight blades can be used in the same way as curved blades, with the tip placed in the vallecula and used to elevate the base of the tongue and attached epiglottis.
- The classic technique of straight-bladed laryngoscopy involves advancing the blade until the tip is in the upper oesophagus. The blade is then withdrawn slowly until the tip comes out of the oesophagus and lies against the laryngeal surface of the epiglottis. In this position, the epiglottis is lifted out of the field of view and the laryngeal inlet is exposed.
- The little finger of the left hand holding the laryngoscope can be used to apply external laryngeal pressure to help bring the vocal cords into view.
- The laryngeal surface of the epiglottis is innervated by the vagus nerve, and the straight-bladed technique sometimes causes a transient bradycardia (rarely clinically significant).
- Vocal cords are identified and, under direct vision, the ETT inserted to an appropriate length.
- Check diameter by confirming that a small audible leak can be heard at an inspiratory pressure of 20 cmH$_2$O. It is essential to ensure that there is a small leak around the tube in order to prevent excess tracheal mucosal pressure and subsequent tracheal stenosis.
- Tube length must be confirmed clinically by observing the length of the tube through the vocal cords and checking for equal bilateral chest movement and breath sounds
- The formula to estimate the length of the ETT at the lips is

$$length = (age / 2) + 12 \ cm$$

- Many ETTs have a solid black mark at the distal end to provide an indication of the length of ETT that should be passed through the cords.
- Secure fixation is essential, since movement may lead to extubation or endobronchial migration.

Nasal endotracheal intubation

- Usually more difficult than the oral route.
- Preferred for long-term intubation since it is more secure and facilitates oral hygiene.
- Consider whether the situation warrants securing the airway by oral intubation followed by nasal intubation. This also allows sizing of the ETT.
- Warn parents at the preoperative visit of possible epistaxis.
- Technique:
  - Vasoconstrictor (oxymetazoline 0.05%, xylometazoline 0.1%, phenylephrine 0.5%) is applied in the nasal mucosa to ↓ the risk of epistaxis.
  - Pass the ETT through the preferred nostril (prior lubrication) until the tip is lying in the posterior pharynx.
  - Visualize the vocal cords as described for oral intubation and pass the ETT through the cords under direct vision with the help of Magill

forceps. This can be difficult owing to the acute angle and limited space available.
- Once the tube tip has passed through the cords, it often impinges anteriorly at the cricoid ring (because of the acute angle of approach from the nasopharynx to the trachea).
  —Use the Magill forceps to push the tip of the tube down towards the floor and away from the anaesthetist, since the plane of the trachea runs down and away.
  —An alternative is to rotate the ETT 180° anticlockwise so that the curvature follows the plane of the trachea. Pressure on the cricoid may help.
- Confirm ETT length, checking for equal bilateral chest movement and breath sounds.
- The formula to estimate the length of the ETT at the nostril is

$$\text{length} = (\text{age} / 2) + 14 \, \text{cm}$$

- Secure fixation is extremely important.

Rapid sequence induction

- Indications are the same as in adults.
- RSI requires a reasonable amount of cooperation and understanding from the child and therefore presents a number of challenges to the anaesthetist, their assistant, and the parents. There is no ideal solution to these problems and a degree of adaptability is necessary. Good communication with all parties beforehand helps.
- RSI is not always possible owing to limiting factors:
  - Difficulty in securing IV access
  - Application of monitoring pre-induction
  - Difficulty in preoxygenation and denitrogenation if the child is struggling and distressed
  - Discomfort associated with cricoid pressure
  - Distortion of the view of the laryngeal inlet by cricoid pressure
  - Parental presence and anxiety.
- In practice, RSI is usually limited to older (>5 years) cooperative children whose anatomy and physiology are adult-like. In younger children, many paediatric anaesthetists prefer an inhalational or IV induction followed by the administration of a neuromuscular blocking agent (suxamethonium or 1 mg/kg rocuronium) and then gentle face-mask ventilation, providing optimal conditions for endotracheal intubation in a fully oxygenated patient.
- Extubate when wide awake.

Intraoperative care

Nuria Masip

Maintenance of anaesthesia

- The basic choice is between volatile agents or total intravenous anaesthesia (TIVA).
- However, a combination of both could be used, e.g. volatile agent plus remifentanil.

Volatile anaesthesia

- Isoflurane is low cost compared to other agents, but it is an airway irritant.
- Sevoflurane has a fast onset/offset, and protects against airway reactivity.
- Desflurane has an ideal profile in terms of low blood/gas solubility and fast action, but it is an airway irritant.
- Differences between agents are more significant after prolonged GA. This has relevance in the neonate, where maintenance with desflurane as compared with sevoflurane provides faster emergence from GA.

Total intravenous anaesthesia

- Commonest drugs are propofol and remifentanil.
- Caution in paediatrics, because pharmacokinetics in the adult are not applicable in children (➔ Chapter 2).
- They can be administered using:
  - Manually controlled infusion schemes:
    —Propofol: The '10-8-6' scheme described by Roberts is not applicable in children. There are complex schemes adapted to paediatric practice, e.g. the McFarlan scheme.
    —Remifentanil: maintenance dose 0.05–0.5 mcg/kg/min
  - Target controlled infusion (TCI), using preprogrammed pumps with a selection of PK models:
    —Propofol: Marsh modified model (or Paedfusor), Kataria model
    —Remifentanil: the Minto model is not applicable in paediatrics; age limit >12 years and weight >30 kg.
- Indications:
  - Absolute:
    —Risk of MH
  - Relative:
    —Difficult locations or during transfers
    —Long procedures, to avoid side effects of volatiles and N_2O
    —To facilitate somatosensory- and motor- evoked potential monitoring, e.g. scoliosis surgery
    —Increased risk of PONV, e.g. middle-ear surgery
    —During neurological procedures to control ICP and for cerebral metabolic protection
    —Airway surgery, e.g. bronchoscopy
    —Porphyria

Fluid management and blood transfusion

- Normovolaemia is the goal of perioperative fluid management.
- Water, electrolyte, and glucose requirements are essential considerations.
- Ensure optimal fluid status preoperatively through minimal fasting times and IV fluid administration in emergency patients.
- Ensure adequate replacement, assess clinically using HR, BP (hypotension a late sign, often only after >30% total blood volume loss), capillary refill time, oliguria, ↑ core–periphery temperature gradient, sunken fontanelle, and ↓ LOC.
- Assess fluid balance and check electrolytes, especially in those patients on IV maintenance for more than 24–48 h.

Intraoperative fluid management

- There are three main components:
  - Replacement of deficits (secondary to GIT losses, sepsis, burns, or haemorrhage)
  - Maintenance
  - Replacement of additional losses.

Deficits

- A well child undergoing minor elective surgery has only a minor deficit, which does not need correcting, unless excessively fasted.
- For most major elective surgery, a 10 mL/kg IV bolus of isotonic solution (Hartmann's solution, Plasma-Lyte, or 0.9% saline) over the first hour will compensate for standard deficits.
- Further fluid is required to correct pre-existing hypovolaemia secondary to, e.g., GIT losses.
- Additional losses are replaced as appropriate with an isotonic solution containing potassium:
  - Nasogastric losses: volume for volume
  - Stoma losses: 50–75% of losses

Maintenance

- Maintenance fluids should be administered through a volumetric pump with a pressure limit set.
- Daily fluid intake in the neonate gradually increases from 75 mL/kg in the newborn on the first day of life to 150 mL/kg by the third day, and is maintained until 3 weeks of age.
- > 4 weeks of age: Holliday and Segar formula or '4–2–1 Rule' (Table 7.1) should be used as a baseline. This is likely to give an overestimate, but consistently prevents perioperative fluid and electrolyte abnormalities.
- Generally, in unwell hydrated children, two-thirds of the maintenance rate should be used, because they are likely to be secreting antidiuretic hormone as part of their 'stress response' (this is a physiological response since the body thinks it will need to retain fluid—do not confuse this with SIADH).
- An isotonic solution should be used, e.g. Hartmann's solution, Plasma-Lyte, or 0.9% saline.

Table 7.1 Maintenance fluid requirements in children: '4-2-1 Rule'

Weight	Daily fluid requirements
0–10 kg	4 mL/kg/h
11–20 kg	40 mL + 2 mL/kg/h for each kg over 10 kg
21–70 kg	60 mL + 1 mL/kg/h for each kg over 20 kg

- Most children maintain their blood glucose intraoperatively, but some are at risk of hypoglycaemia:
  - Neonates (in whom hypoglycaemia can cause brain damage) lack the glycogen stores of adults
  - Preterms and infants receiving glucose (simplest to continue intraoperatively)
  - Children on parenteral nutrition (simplest to continue intraoperatively)
  - Prolonged surgery
  - Children with sepsis
  - Children <3rd centile.
- Use a glucose-containing solution, e.g. Hartmann's/Plasma-Lyte with 1% glucose, or 0.9% saline with 5% glucose. Although neonates may require 10% glucose solution for maintenance; 20% glucose solution may be needed if septic or fluid restricted.
- Where there is a risk of hypoglycaemia, check blood glucose regularly.
- On the other extreme, perioperative hyperglycaemia may result in increased neurological deficits after surgery.
- Hypotonic fluid administration risks hypoNa$^+$, resulting in avoidable morbidity and mortality.
- Glucose-containing solutions effectively result in the administration of free water; therefore, there is a risk of hypoNa$^+$. In addition increased ADH secretion during the perioperative period (stress response, pain, hypovolaemia, drugs) further reduces plasma Na$^+$ concentration.
- Children develop hypoNa$^+$ more readily than adults and are more susceptible to CNS complications.

Additional losses
- Can be due to blood loss, evaporative losses from the wound, and third-space sequestration. They are replaced with isotonic solutions (Hartmann's solution, Plasma-Lyte, or 0.9% saline) or blood products. There is no evidence to suggest albumin is better.
- Evaporative and third-space losses are difficult to quantify, but are estimated as 2 mL/kg/h for superficial surgery, 4–7 mL/kg/h for thoracotomy, 5–10 mL/kg/h for open abdominal surgery.
- Children with cyanotic CHD and neonates may need a higher haematocrit to maintain oxygenation.

Blood transfusion
- Indication for blood transfusion depends on the child's age and health, and the clinical situation.

- There are no agreed haemoglobin transfusion triggers, but, as a rough guide:
  - 12 g/dL in a neonate
  - 10 g/dL in a child with severe sepsis
  - 10 g/dL in a child with a cyanotic CHD
  - 7 g/dL in an acutely ill child.
- Recommended volumes of blood components to be administered are calculated according to body weight:
  - Packed red cell concentrate: 4 mL/kg will ↑ Hb by 1 g/dL
  - Platelets: 10 - 20 mL/kg
  - Fresh frozen plasma: 10 - 15 mL/kg
  - Cryoprecipitate: 5 - 10 mL/kg.
- For neonatal blood transfusion, some centres provide 'paedipacks' or 'minipacks' of packed red cells from the same donor, thus allowing transfusion over a prolonged time and limiting the exposure to multiple donors, i.e. 1 adult bag (300 mL) is divided into 6 paedipacks (≈50 mL each).
- In the UK, all blood components (except granulocytes) are leucodepleted as a precaution against variant Creutzfeldt–Jakob disease. However, a standard sterile blood administration set with an integral filter ('blood giving set') is used to transfuse any blood component.
- All neonates should receive CMV-negative red cell and platelet components (despite the theoretical risk of CMV transmission, plasma components have not been shown to transmit CMV). Leucodepleted blood is enough protection (CMV IgG-negative is not required) in immunocompromised children who have not been infected with CMV.
- All children <1 year should receive HEV-negative blood components. Unlike CMV, this recommendation applies to both cellular components (red cells, platelets, and granulocytes) and plasma components (fresh frozen plasma and cryoprecipitate). It applies also for immunocompromised children, common indications being:
  - Patients awaiting/received solid organ transplant
  - Indefinitely for acute leukaemia
  - Allogeneic stem cell transplant recipients from 3 months pre-transplant to 6 months following transplant, or for as long as the patient is immunosuppressed
- Irradiated blood (this applies to cellular components: red cells, platelets, and granulocytes) prevents the proliferation of T-lymphocytes, which is the immediate cause of the fatal transfusion-associated graft-versus-host disease (TA-GVHD). Prestorage leucodepletion has significantly reduced the risk of TA-GVHD, but irradiation is needed to inactivate residual lymphocytes. It is not necessary to irradiate plasma components, since freezing causes lysis of lymphocytes. Some common indications are:
  - Patients with confirmed or possible congenital T-cell deficiencies, e.g. DiGeorge syndrome (triad of conotruncal cardiac anomalies, hypoplastic thymus, and hypoCa^{2+})
  - Indefinitely for Hodgkin's lymphoma
  - Bone marrow and stem cell transplant recipients from 2 weeks pre-transplant to 3 months after autologous transplant, and 6 months after allogeneic transplant
  - Indefinitely for patients taking purine analogues, e.g. fludarabine
  - All transfusions from first- or second-degree relatives should be irradiated, even if the patient is immunocompetent.

Intraoperative problems

- The morbidity and mortality of critical incidents can be reduced by:
  - Asking promptly for help
  - Good communication
  - Designating a team leader
  - Delegating tasks to named individuals
  - Working together as a team.
- Follow the ABC of resuscitation to help identify underlying problems.

Hypoxia

- Defined as a reduced availability of O_2 for tissue consumption.

Causes

- Hypoxaemia:
  - Hypoxic gas mixture:
    —Incorrect or inadequate flow
    —Second-gas effect
    —O_2 failure
    —Equipment or anaesthetic machine malfunction.
  - Hypoventilation which may be due to a ↓ RR or TV:
    —ETT or other equipment displacement/disconnection
    —Incorrect mode of ventilation or settings
    —Drugs: opioids, anaesthetic agents
    —Underlying medical conditions: metabolic disturbances, intracranial pathology, sleep apnoea syndromes, or hypothermia
    —Airway obstruction: ↑ airway obstruction and/or ↓ FRC
  - Shunt:
    —Intrapulmonary: atelectasis, secretions, or aspiration
    —Extrapulmonary: CHD.
- Anaemic hypoxia:
  - Consider especially in the neonate, when there is intraoperative bleeding, even a small quantity (remember the blood volume in a neonate is 90 mL/kg).
- Inadequate O_2 delivery:
  - Hypoperfusion, e.g. sepsis
  - Embolus
  - Local problem, e.g. limb ischaemia, hypothermia.
- ↑ O_2 requirement:
  - Sepsis
  - MH
- Use the Pneumonic 'DOPES' to check the most common causes:
  —D: Displacement of tube
  —O: Obstruction of tube/circuit
  —P: Pneumothorax
  —E: Equipment failure
  —S: Stacked breaths (auto-PEEP especially in the asthmatic child).

Management

- ↑ FiO_2 to 100%.
- Measure FiO_2 near patient end of the circuit.
- Observe RR and breathing pattern, look for signs of obstruction, e.g. tracheal tug, use of accessory muscles, paradoxical respiration, and noisy breathing.
- Hand-ventilate with 3–4 big breaths, this allows assessment of airway patency and airway resistance.
- If there is doubt whether it is a patient or a circuit problem, give manual ventilation breaths with a simple bag and valve plus a reservoir attached to an external O_2 source.
- If resistance is high at the patient end:
  - Suction down airway device to check patency.
  - Pull back ETT a short distance or adjust other airway devices while auscultating and observing chest movements.
  - If any doubt, remove airway device and revert to a face mask and manual ventilation.
- If further deterioration, call for help.
- Alert theatre team if not already aware.
- Determine and treat underlying cause.

Points to note

- Infants and neonates have a ↓ FRC, therefore less physiological reserve.
- Neonates and infants have ↑ O_2 consumption.
- Neonates and infants have fewer alveoli (at birth ~10% adult number) compared with adults.
- At birth, neonates are unresponsive to the CO_2 stimulus for respiration.
- Neonates (especially ex-prem) are more prone to apnoea secondary to opioids, sedatives, and GA.
- CV > FRC until 6 years of age. Use of CPAP during spontaneous ventilation, and PEEP during mechanical ventilation, prevent alveolar collapse during expiration by increasing FRC above closing capacity.
- Narrow airways have a high resistance to flow, and any small reduction in circumference due to secretions produces a marked ↑ in resistance.
- Smaller ETTs are more likely to kink and obstruct.
- Smaller LMAs are more likely to twist, displace, and dislodge.
- The work of breathing is high in a neonate, and many anaesthetists feel that LMAs are inappropriate for all but the shortest of cases.
- If the hypoxia does not improve with 100% O_2 and adequate ventilation, the cause is likely to be a shunt.
- Although a PDA usually closes within the first week of life, it can re-open in neonates during severe hypoxia.
- Atelectasis:
  - May occur with a high FiO_2 due to nitrogen absorption (required to splint the alveoli open).
  - Occurs in dependent parts of the lung during GA, it may occur with endobronchial intubation.
  - May persist postoperatively in those with poor lung function and difficulty clearing secretions.

Airway obstruction
- May occur in the mouth, pharynx, larynx, trachea, or large bronchi.
- Leads to hypoventilation and ↑ work of breathing.
- During spontaneous ventilation, it may present as:
  - Noisy respiration
  - Stridor
  - Use of accessory muscles
  - Tracheal tug, chest recession, and paradoxical respiration.
- Tachypnoea, tachycardia, hypoxia, hypercapnia, and poor movement of the reservoir bag may all be indicative of obstruction.
- Pulmonary oedema may occur if intrathoracic pressures are excessive and prolonged.
- During IPPV, warning signs include:
  - ↑ airway pressures with ↓ chest movement
  - Noisy respiration or wheeze
  - Hypoxia
  - Hypercapnia.

Causes:
- Anatomical:
  - Poor face-mask technique
  - Tongue
  - Inadequate head positioning
  - Large adenoids, tonsils, obesity
  - Pathology: stricture, tumour, oedema, infection
  - Foreign body, gastric content, blood
  - Overinflated stomach
  - Mechanical obstruction within breathing circuit.
- Functional
  - Upper airway:
    —Inadequate anaesthesia
    —Laryngospasm
    —Hypotonia of oropharyngeal muscles
    —Opioid-induced glottic closure.
  - Lower airway:
    —Muscle rigidity
    —Bronchospasm
    —Tracheomalacia
    —Alveolar collapse.

Management
- In spontaneous ventilation:
  - ↑ FiO_2 to 100% and ↓ FGF.
  - Airway opening manoeuvres: mouth opening, head tilt and chin lift, check patency and position of airway device.
  - Remove secretions.
  - CPAP.
  - It may be easier to maintain airway in recovery position.
  - ETT.

- In IPPV:
  - $\uparrow$ FiO$_2$ to 100%.
  - Ventilate by hand.
  - Check ventilator tubing for obstruction.
  - Pass suction catheter down ETT.
  - Auscultate chest to exclude bronchospasm or pneumothorax.
  - Withdraw ETT slightly; if there is no improvement, remove and use face mask.
  - Consider inadequate neuromuscular blockade.
- Treat any underlying cause.

Laryngospasm

- Defined as the reflex closure of the upper respiratory airway caused by adduction of the vocal cords due to a glottis muscular spasm. It may cause partial or complete obstruction.
- More common problem (up to 3% of infants) due to a more reactive upper airway compared with adults.
- Inverse correlation with age: young children at greatest risk.
- Severe episodes with profound hypoxia and bradycardia are more likely in infants <12 months of age.
- It can occur at any point during GA, although it is more frequent at induction and emergence.

Causes

- Local stimulation of the larynx by:
  - Blood (adeno- and/or tonsillectomy patients have up to 25% incidence of laryngospasm)
  - Saliva
  - Vomit
  - FB, including laryngoscope, LMA, suction catheters, or ETT (after its immediate removal, because while the ETT is in place, the cords cannot close).
- Irritant volatile agents, e.g. desflurane.
- Inadequate depth of GA plus response to stimulation: surgery (especially anal and cervical stimulation), movement (transferring the patient: from bed/trolley to operating table, and vice versa).
- Tracheal extubation (or LMA removal) at a light plane of GA.
- Ten times more common with an active or recent URTI (within past 4 weeks).
- Patient risk factors: asthma, passive smoking, obesity with OSA, GOR, pre-existing airway anomalies.

Presentation

- Inspiratory stridor (high-pitched noise) with partial laryngospasm. There is no stridor with complete laryngospasm, which is therefore more difficult to recognize.
- Use of accessory muscles, tracheal tug, intercostal and subcostal recession.
- Paradoxical respiration.
- Difficulty in ventilating through face mask or LMA.
- Desaturation, cyanosis.
- Bradycardia.

Management

- Stop or remove stimulus (e.g. if there is an LMA present, remove it to take over control of the airway).
- ↑ FiO$_2$ to 100%.
- Open the airway and deliver CPAP through face mask:
  - By closing the APL valve from the anaesthetic circuit.
  - By partially occluding the reservoir bag opening on the T-piece (Mapleson F-circuit).
- Try gentle bag-mask ventilation. There is a risk of gastric distension if the vocal cords are closed (once the laryngospasm is resolved, consider decompressing the stomach of air).
- Deepen GA with volatile or propofol 0.5–1 mg/kg.
- If laryngospasm persists, give suxamethonium (2 mg/kg IV, or 4 mg/kg IM if there is no IV access).
- Endotracheal intubation if not recovering or deteriorating, and then extubate when fully awake.
- Postobstructive pulmonary oedema can develop.
- Use of suxamethonium in severe hypoxia may lead to profound bradycardia and/or cardiac arrest.

Prevention

- Use sevoflurane (non-irritant) for gas inductions.
- When using LMA, ensure child is deep prior to initial surgical stimulus. Surgeon should ask prior to starting operation.
- Suction pharynx prior to extubation/LMA removal.
- Then extubate/remove LMA either in a deep plane of GA or fully awake, never in-between.

Bronchospasm

- Defined as a reversible narrowing of the medium and small airways due to smooth muscle contraction.
- Presents as:
  - ↑ airway pressures
  - ↑ expiratory time and rising EtCO$_2$
  - ↓ TV
  - Desaturation
  - Wheeze.
- It is more frequent where there is a history of asthma, allergy, active or recent respiratory infection, or a light plane of GA.

Causes

- Surgical stimulation.
- Airway stimulation: oropharyngeal airway, LMA, ETT, or suction.
- Pharyngeal, laryngeal, bronchial secretions or blood.
- FB inhalation.
- Aspiration of gastric contents.
- Anaphylactic or anaphylactoid reactions.
- Pulmonary oedema.
- Histamine-releasing drugs.
- Exclude differential diagnoses:
  - Pneumothorax
  - Mechanical obstruction within the circuit or ETT

- Laryngospasm
- Oesophageal intubation or displacement of ETT
- Pulmonary oedema.

Management
- ↑ FiO_2 to 100%.
- ↑ inspired concentration of sevoflurane.
- Treat primary cause.
- Nebulized salbutamol 2.5 mg (or 5 mg if >5 years).
- Nebulized ipratropium bromide 250 mcg (or 500 mcg if >12 years).
- Salbutamol 5–15 mcg/kg IV over 10 min, then infusion of 1–5 mcg/kg/min.
- Magnesium sulfate 40 mg/kg (max. 2 g) IV over 20 min.
- Aminophylline 5 mg/kg over 20 min, then infusion 0.5–1 mg/kg/h (if no recent doses).
- Hydrocortisone 4 mg/kg IV.
- If unresponsive to treatment, escalate to adrenaline (epinephrine) 1 mcg/kg IV (or 10 mcg/kg IM), followed by an adrenaline infusion of 0.01–0.1 mcg/kg/min.
- Consider ketamine 2 mg/kg IV.

Hypotension
- When working out the causes, remember:

$$MAP = CO \times SVR$$

$$CO = HR \times SV$$

- Neonates have a relatively fixed SV and are dependent on HR to maintain CO (➲ Chapter 1).
- Neonates have little or no ability to constrict capacitance vessels.
- The baroreceptor reflexes of infants, especially those born prematurely, are immature and limit the response to hypovolaemia.
- Systolic BP in an infant is closely related to the circulating volume.

Causes
- ↓ CO:
  - ↓HR:
    —Vagal reflexes
    —Drugs, e.g. halothane, remifentanil, and neostigmine
    —Dysrhythmias.
  - ↓ SV:
    —Reduction in venous return: hypovolaemia, head up position, aortocaval compression, tension pneumothorax, cardiac tamponade, or PEEP.
    —Dysrhythmias.
    —↑ afterload: Aortic stenosis, pulmonary embolus, tension pneumothorax, cardiac tamponade.
    —↓ myocardial contractility: drugs, hypoxia, hypercapnia, acidosis, hypothermia, cardiomyopathy, myocarditis, or cardiac failure.
- ↓ SVR:
  - Drugs, e.g. anaesthetic agents
  - Adverse drug reactions
  - Sepsis.

Management
- ↑ FiO_2 to 100%.
- Treat underlying cause.
- Hypovolaemia is a reduction in circulating blood volume. This may be a result of:
  - Blood loss
  - Plasma loss, e.g. burns
  - Extracellular and/or intracellular fluid loss, e.g. dehydration, third-space loss during surgery, or sepsis
  - Evaporative loss during surgery or pyrexia
  - Relative hypovolaemia occurs when there is vasodilation, e.g. sepsis or anaphylaxis.
- Treatment consists of replacement of appropriate fluid.
- Use crystalloids (0.9% saline, Hartmann's solution, Plasma-Lyte) as standard resuscitation fluid; bolus 20 mL/kg then reassess.
- Escalate therapy as dictated by clinical situation and seek advice if >40–60 mL/kg IV fluid is required as part of initial fluid resuscitation.

Massive haemorrhage
- Definition:
  - Loss of 1 blood volume within 24 h, or
  - Loss of 50% of blood volume within 3 h, or
  - Loss of ≥ 2–3mL/kg/min.
  - The context may be trauma, major surgery, or an underlying coagulopathy.
  - Estimate the total blood volume (TBV):
    —Preterm neonate 100mL/kg
    —Term neonate 90mL/kg
    —Infant 85mL/kg
    —Children 80mL/kg
    —Adult 70mL/kg.

Management
- Recognize and activate pathway for management of massive haemorrhage; assemble the emergency response team.
- Allocate team roles:
  - Communication lead—dedicated person for communication with other teams, especially transfusion laboratory.
  - Sample-taker to assist with testing (e.g. ABGs and thromboelastography/thromboelastometry), which is fundamental to guide transfusion strategy.
  - Documenter
  - Transporter—usually the theatre porter (ensure they carry a bleep), to transport specimens from the scene of the massive haemorrhage situation to the laboratory and to transport blood products from the laboratory to the scene of the massive haemorrhage situation.
- Consider cell salvage.
- Complete request forms, take blood samples, label samples correctly, and recheck labelling.
- Communicate stand-down of pathway and let lab know which products have been used.

- Ensure documentation is complete:
  - Vital signs, timings of blood samples and communications with transfusion laboratory, transfusion documentation.
- Repeat laboratory blood investigations (PT, APTT, fibrinogen, and FBC):
  - At least every hour if bleeding is ongoing
  - After replacement of one-third of the TBV.
  - And after giving blood products.
- Anticipate the need for blood products:
  - Acute loss of 10% of TBV in a neonate → transfuse red cells.
  - Acute loss of one-third of TBV in any other child → red cell transfusion is likely.
  - Consider FFP after loss of 50% of TBV.
  - Consider platelets after loss of 100% of TBV.
  - Consider fibrinogen after replacement of 150% of TBV.
- Anticipate the time delay between requesting and receiving blood products:
  - Red cells:
    —O Rh-negative red cells should be immediately available in theatre fridge.
    —Group-specific red cells should be rapidly made available by the transfusion laboratory: 30 min from time sample is received.
    —Fully cross-matched: 90 min from time sample is received.
  - Platelets, FFP, and cryoprecipitate may need 10–20 min to thaw, depending on each transfusion laboratory
  - Some products may be stocked on site, or may need to come from offsite blood bank.
- Based on the CRASH-2 adult study, tranexamic acid should be given to children after major trauma: bolus of 15mg/kg IV, followed by 2 mg/kg/h until bleeding controlled.

Points to note
- Blood products usually come in the following volumes:
  - Red cells (adult unit) 250–300 mL
  - Red cells (paediatric unit) ~50 mL
  - Octaplas 200 mL
  - FFP neonatal unit ~50 mL
  - Cryoprecipitate (single-donor unit) ~40 mL
  - Platelets (1 adult therapeutic dose) 200–300 mL
  - Platelets (single paediatric pack) ~50 mL.

Dysrhythmias
- Bradycardia, junctional rhythm, and ventricular ectopics are common during GA but are usually benign.
- Certain conditions are associated with an ↑ incidence of dysrhythmia:
  - Pre-existing cardiac disease
  - Hypoxia
  - Hypercarbia
  - Acid–base disturbance
  - Electrolyte abnormalities especially K^+, Ca^{2+}, and Mg^{2+}

- Some drugs, e.g. high concentrations of halothane combined with hypercarbia or catecholamines, suxamethonium
- Insertion of CVP lines into the cardiac chambers
- Activation of reflex pathways, e.g. dental surgery, neurosurgery, oculocardiac reflex, visceral manipulation, tracheobronchial suction

Management
- ↑ FiO$_2$ to 100%.
- Correction of any underlying cause.
- Drug therapy and cardioversion are discussed in the context of resuscitation (➔ Chapter 29).

Anaphylaxis
- A systemic type I hypersensitivity reaction.
- Risk factors include:
  - Known allergy or previous allergic reaction
  - History of atopy or asthma
  - Cross-sensitivity, e.g. latex and some food (kiwi fruit, melon and bananas); penicillin and cephalosporin; aspirin and NSAIDs
  - Some drugs, e.g. radiographic contrast media, penicillin, and arachis oil (purified peanut oil).
- Common anaesthetic-agent triggers:
  - Muscle relaxants (60% of GA-related anaphylaxis cases), e.g. suxamethonium and vecuronium
  - Latex (up to 20% of cases)
  - Antibiotics (15% of cases)
  - Colloids (5% of cases), e.g. gelatins, and dextrans
  - Anaphylactic reactions to LA drugs are very uncommon (esters > amides)
  - Chlorhexidine
  - Aprotinin, protamine.
- The use of propofol in patients with simple egg/soya allergy is likely to be safe; however, previous egg/soya anaphylaxis is a contraindication.
  - Propofol contains purified egg phosphatide (from egg yolk) and soya-bean oil. The manufacturing process removes the proteins responsible for most egg allergy (ovoalbumin, contained in the egg white) and soya allergy (soya-bean protein).
  - Most children grow out of their allergy to eggs, soya, milk, and wheat.
- Most patients with a history of a penicillin-related rash are not allergic to cephalosporins. However, if there is a convincing history of penicillin-related anaphylaxis, consider avoiding first-generation cephalosporins.
- Signs usually consist of a mixture of cardiovascular collapse, dysrhythmia, stridor, bronchospasm, erythema, angioedema, and urticarial rash.

Management
- Follow departmental protocol to guide treatment and prevent omissions.
- Initiate ABC of resuscitation.
- Remove trigger agent if possible.
- ↑ FiO$_2$ to 100%.

- Secure airway with ETT.
- Adrenaline (epinephrine):
  - 1 mcg/kg IV (1 mcg/kg is 0.01 mL/kg of a 1:10,000 solution).
  - 10 mcg/kg IM (10 mcg/kg is 0.1 mL/kg of a 1:10,000 solution).
  - Repeat every 5 min as necessary.
  - Severe reactions will need an infusion of 0.01–0.5 mcg/kg/min:
    —Prepare 0.3 mg of adrenaline/kg in 50 mL 0.9% saline.
    —1 mL/h = 0.1 mcg/kg/min.
    —Infusion rate 0.1–5 mL/h (0.01–0.5 mcg/kg/min).
- Administer 20 mL/kg of crystalloid, repeat as necessary.
- Ensure adequate IV access; if the reaction is severe, establish invasive monitoring.
- In a severe reaction where adrenaline is not maintaining BP, add noradrenaline (norepinephrine) (use similar dose range and solution to adrenaline).
- Bronchospasm will be alleviated by adrenaline, although bronchodilator therapy may also be necessary:
  - Salbutamol 2.5 mg nebulized
  - Aminophylline 5 mg/kg IV over 20 min followed by infusion of 0.5–1.0 mg/kg/h.
- Antihistamines (chlorphenamine 250 mcg/kg) and hydrocortisone 4 mg/kg have little or no effect in the acute phase, but should be given as they may ↓ the incidence of late relapse.
- Blood samples:
  - ABG
  - Clotting screen
  - For diagnosis: three blood samples for serum tryptase (the sample should be stored and shipped in ice). Ideally: first sample immediately, second sample after 1 h, and third sample 6–24 h after the event.
- Exclude the following differential diagnoses:
  - Tension pneumothorax
  - Septic shock
  - Acute severe asthma
  - Drug-induced histamine release, e.g. opioids, atracurium
  - Flushing syndrome (red man syndrome secondary to vancomycin).
- HDU/PICU admission.
- It is the anaesthetist's responsibility to refer the patient to the Allergy Department for further investigation.

Hypothermia

- Core temperature <36°C.
- Usually due to heat loss during GA.
- Prevention is important, especially in neonates owing to their reduced reserves.
- Some of the adverse effects are:
  - ↑ postoperative O_2 consumption caused by shivering
  - ↑ duration of action of neuromuscular blockers
  - Delayed drug excretion.

Causes
- Prolonged surgery.
- ↑ heat loss through radiation (patient uncovered, vasodilated), convection (uncovered), evaporation (open body cavity, low environmental humidity, unhumidified inspired gases), and conduction (cold irrigating fluids).
- Reduced heat production.
- Impaired temperature regulation through peripheral mechanisms (vasodilation, shivering, impaired piloerection) or central mechanisms (drug effects).

Prevention
- Identify groups at high risk:
  - Neonates
  - Patients with cerebral palsy
  - Surgery requiring a large body surface area exposed
  - Undergoing combined general and regional anaesthesia (especially epidural or LA catheter)
  - Major haemorrhage
- Temperature monitoring for all procedures >30 min.
- Multimodal approach is essential:
  - Cover during transfer from anaesthetic room to operating theatre
  - Maintenance ambient temperature of 22–24°C (26–28°C for neonates) and humidity about 50%.
  - Forced air warming blanket or warming mattress.
  - Avoid unnecessary exposure. Cover patient with drapes, blanket, and hats in neonates.
  - Warm solutions for skin cleaning or irrigation.
  - Warm IV fluids.
  - Circle system and HME; passive humidification is more effective than in adults owing to higher MV per kg body weight.
  - Active warming and humidification of inspired gases.
  - Warming of bed for recovery period.
- Use an overhead radiant heater or a forced air warming blanket while neonates and infant are exposed for cannulation, intubation, and other preoperative procedures. It should also be used at the end of surgery when the patient is uncovered for extubation.

Management
- If hypothermia does occur, treatment methods are the same as for prevention.

Hyperthermia
- Core temperature >38°C.
- When >41.6°C, this implies an impaired thermoregulation mechanism.

Causes
- Hypothalamic lesions.
- ↑ heat production: drug-induced (MH, neuroleptic malignant syndrome, salicylate poisoning, cocaine poisoning), hyperthyroidism, phaeochromocytoma, tetanus, status epilepticus, or sepsis.

- Impaired heat loss: autonomic neuropathy, drug-induced (anticholinergics, phenothiazines, neuroleptic malignant syndrome), or dehydration.
- Iatrogenic excessive warming.

Management
- Remove or switch off warming devices.
- Cooling with tepid water.
- Irrigation of body cavity with cold fluid, e.g. peritoneal lavage.
- Paracetamol IV.
- Exclude MH.

Malignant hyperthermia

- A pharmacogenetic disease of skeletal muscle, which presents as a hypermetabolic response induced by exposure to suxamethonium or a volatile agent.
- Very rarely, it is triggered by stressors, e.g. vigorous exercise or heat.
- Inheritance is autosomal-dominant with variable penetrance and expressivity.
- In most cases, there is a mutation in the gene encoding the Ca^{2+} channel (the ryanodine receptor).
- Incidence is 1:10,000–1:50,000. Sex ratio 2M:1F.
- An episode involves the uncontrolled release of intracellular Ca^{2+} from skeletal muscle sarcoplasmic reticulum, activating muscle contraction, increasing O_2 consumption and CO_2 production, ATP hydrolysis, and heat production.
- A previous uneventful anaesthetic with triggering agents does not preclude MH (75% have had a previous GA). On average, patients require three GA before triggering an episode.
- Presentation is very variable: from a life-threatening classic fulminant episode, to elevation of end-tidal CO_2, tachycardia, or hyperthermia of unknown cause.
- Mortality (with prompt diagnosis and treatment) is 2–3%.

Risk factors
- Family history.
- Exposure to triggers.
- Central core disease (➔ Chapter 26).

Pathophysiology
- May occur at any time during GA as well as in the early postoperative period, but not after an hour of discontinuation of volatile agents
- The signs are all related to a hypermetabolic response:
  - Hyperthermia
  - Tachycardia
  - Tachypnoea (if spontaneous breathing)
  - ↑ CO_2 production
  - ↑ O_2 consumption
  - Metabolic acidosis (due to rapid consumption of energy stores and ATP)

- Muscle signs: masseter spasm after suxamethonium, generalized muscle rigidity
- HyperK$^+$ (due to myocyte death and rhabdomyolysis)
- ↑ creatine kinase
- Myoglobinuria (may lead to acute renal failure)
- Dysrhythmias
- DIC

Diagnosis
- Clinical presentation:
  - Masseter spasm after suxamethonium
  - Unexplained tachycardia
  - Unexplained ↑ in end-tidal CO_2 or minute volume
  - ↓ SpO_2 despite ↑ FiO_2
  - Cardiovascular instability, including peaked p waves
  - Generalized muscle rigidity
  - ↑ in core temperature >2°C/h
- Laboratory testing:
  - In vitro contracture test (IVCT), based on contracture of muscle fibres in the presence of halothane or caffeine
  - IVCT is expensive, confined to specialized testing centres, and requires a muscle biopsy

Management
- Follow departmental protocol to guide treatment and prevent omissions during the episode.
- ABC and ask for help.
- Discontinue volatile agent.
- Endotracheal intubation (if not already intubated).
- Hyperventilate with 100% O_2 using high fresh gas flow (2–3 times estimated minute volume).
- Dantrolene:
  - Ryanodine receptor antagonist; inhibits abnormal Ca^{2+} release.
  - Immediate bolus of 2.5 mg/kg IV.
  - Repeat 1 mg/kg IV every 10 min up to a total of 10 mg/kg
  - Mix 20 mg (one vial) of dantrolene with 60 mL of sterile water to make a solution of 1 mg in 3 mL. Initial bolus of 7.5mL/kg of the dantrolene solution (= 2.5 mg/kg). Repeat further doses of 3 mL/kg (= 1 mg/kg) up to a maximum of 30 mL/kg in total
  - Remember to include the dantrolene in the overall fluids given (especially in small children)
- Notice that falling HR and central temperature are evidence of a response.
- Depending on circumstances, stop surgery, convert to TIVA, and use a volatile-free machine.
- Not every department has a dedicated vapour-free anaesthetic machine. In this case, a 'contaminated' anaesthetic machine can be used once vaporizers have been removed, the full breathing circuit and soda lime cannister changed, and an activated charcoal filter inserted into the inspiratory port, and a high FGF of 10 L/min maintained for at least 90 min.

- ↓ body temperature: warming mattress or blanket set to cool, ice in groins and axillae, peritoneal lavage with cold fluids, cold IV fluids (but do not induce shivering). Fluids must be potassium-free.
- Institute invasive monitoring and urinary catheter.
- Tests:
  - ABG
  - Blood sample for creatine kinase
  - Urine sample for myoglobin.
- Supportive therapy:
  - Arrhythmias:
    —Mg^{2+} (slow administration 0.2 mmol/kg = 50 mg/kg).
    —Amiodarone (5 mg/kg over 20 min, then infusion at 300 mcg/kg/h).
    —Esmolol (loading dose of 500 mcg/kg over 1 min, then infusion at 50–200 mcg/kg/min).
    —Avoid Ca^{2+} channel blockers since they interact with dantrolene.
  - HyperK⁺:
    —Calcium gluconate 10% (0.5 mL/kg to a maximum of 20 mL).
    —5 mL/kg of 10% glucose + 0.1 units/kg of insulin administered over 20 min.
    —Monitor blood sugar.
  - Acidosis:
    —Sodium bicarbonate 0.5–1 mmol/kg (= 0.5–1 mL/kg of 8.4% $NaHCO_3$).
  - Low UO; if < 2mL/kg/h:
    —Mannitol 0.5–1 g/kg (= 2.5–5 mL/kg of 20% solution).
    —Furosemide 1 mg/kg IV.
  - DIC:
    —FFP 10 mL/kg.
    —Cryoprecipitate 5 mL/kg.
    —Platelets 10 mL/kg.
- PICU admission.

Postoperative care

Nuria Masip

Recovery area or post-anaesthetic care unit (PACU)

- All patients should be recovered in a specially designated area: the recovery area or PACU.
- The PACU should be adjacent to the operating theatres, and ideally have a separate access for patient transfer to the ward.
- It should be open-plan, allowing good observation of patients, but have curtains for patient privacy.
- The ratio of PACU bays to theatres should not be <2:1.
- Each bay should have:
  - Emergency call system (staff must understand the system and test it daily)
  - One O_2 and one air pipeline outlet
  - High-flow vacuum/suction
  - Monitoring equipment: ECG, NIBP, SpO_2, and capnography, with display screen
  - Adequate number of electrical sockets
  - Local lighting to assist clinical examination.
- There should be full and accessible supply of airway/IV access/resuscitation equipment, emergency drugs and fluids.
- There should be adequate ventilation (potential pollution by anaesthetic gases), and scavenging system when using an anaesthetic machine with volatile agents.
- Noise levels should be kept to a minimum.
- A good communication system is required, especially with the operating theatres and wards.
- Specific to paediatric recovery areas:
  - Child-friendly decoration
  - Cots and beds with padded side rails
  - Toys (recovery's or child's own) readily available
  - Extra chairs for parents
  - If a child uses a dummy, have it available.

PACU Staff

- Led by recovery nurses or registered PACU practitioners.
- Two staff must be present when there is a patient (one must be a recovery nurse).
- Nurse-to-patient ratio should be >1:1 (at least one nurse to each patient), and a health care assistant to help with difficult patients, e.g. autism, and to get help or equipment during an emergency.
- There should be an anaesthetist immediately available.

Transfer and Handover to PACU

- Monitoring during transfer to PACU is advised.
- All lines should be flushed prior to handover (to remove any residual anaesthetic drugs).
- The anaesthetist formally hands over the patient to a trained recovery nurse.

Management of patients in PACU

- Time spent in the recovery area varies from 15 min for healthy children after a short procedure to hours for more complex cases.
- Often patients will be handed over to the PACU nurse with a supraglottic airway device in place. The nurse must be specifically trained in the management of these patients and in the removal of the airway device.
- All patients with an LMA or ETT in place should have continuous capnography.
- Removal of the ETT is the responsibility of the anaesthetist.
- Assessment of airway patency, vital signs, and level of consciousness are the first priorities upon admission. Other important checks are:
  - Adequate circulation and organ perfusion (normal capillary refill time <2 s)
  - Temperature
  - Pain score
  - Patency and security of cannula, and rate of IV fluids
  - Surgical site and dressings
  - Circulation in extremities after orthopaedic surgery or cardiac catheterization
  - Paraesthesia after regional anaesthesia
  - Patency of drainage tubes/drains
  - Double-check PCA/NCA/epidural settings.
- Reunite parent with child as soon as it is safe to do so. They will help reassure their child and can make the management of any distress or disorientation easier.
- Encourage the use of comforters or favourite toys.
- Special considerations:
  - BP is not routine in paediatric recovery, therefore ensure it is performed where clinically indicated, e.g. epidural anaesthesia.
  - In a neonate, glucose blood level should be checked.
  - Cerebral palsy patients have an increased risk of hypothermia.
  - Children with learning difficulties or post ketamine may benefit from recovering in a designated area with lower levels of noise and lighting.

Discharge from PACU and handover to the ward

- It is mandatory that there be agreed and written criteria for patient discharge to the ward.
- If the physical layout is appropriate, parents should come to the recovery room with a ward nurse to collect the child.
- Thorough handover from recovery to ward staff is paramount.

Postoperative problems

Postoperative nausea and vomiting (PONV)

- Often little emphasis is placed on the management of PONV in children, since it is thought to be a rare occurrence.
- However, it is a common cause of unplanned hospital admission.
- Incidence varies, depending on patient, anaesthetic, and surgical factors.

Patient risk factors for PONV

- Age:
  - Children <2 years rarely suffer PONV.
  - The incidence of PONV rises with age.
- Previous PONV.
- Motion sickness.
- Female gender, especially those who have reached puberty.

Anaesthetic risk factors for PONV

- Volatile anaesthetic agents.
- There is no evidence for the benefits of avoiding N_2O.
- Opioids.
- Prolonged GA.
- Perioperative fluids:
  - Reducing fasting times may protect.
  - Intraoperatively: 30 mL/kg IV crystalloids has been shown to halve the incidence of PONV when compared with those receiving 10 mL/kg.
  - Postoperatively forcing children to drink who do not wish to is associated with increased PONV.

Surgical risk factors for PONV

- Strabismus surgery.
- Adenotonsillectomy.
- Otoplasty, tympanoplasty, mastoidectomy.
- Orchidopexy.

Prevention

- The emetic pathway is complicated and triggered by many different types of receptors. Patients who do not respond to a single antiemetic given regularly should be given a combination of drugs that act at different points of the pathway.
- Ensure intraoperative IV hydration; do not force oral fluids postoperatively.
- Consider TIVA.
- Ondansetron:
  - First-line choice.
  - $5-HT_3$ [5-hydroxytryptamine (serotonin)] receptor antagonist.
  - 0.1–0.15 mg/kg PO or IV 8-hourly (maximum 4 mg).
  - 0.15 mg/kg is more effective than 0.1 mg/kg.
  - PO or IV routes are equally effective.
  - There is no evidence demonstrating any benefit of dose timing.
  - Avoid rapid bolus administration.
  - Contraindicated in congenital long-QT syndrome. Caution when susceptibility to QT-interval prolongation.

- Dexamethasone:
  - First-line choice.
  - Corticosteroid.
  - 0.1–0.2 mg/kg IV 8-hourly (maximum 4 mg).
  - More effective than ondansetron at ↓ late PONV.
  - Avoid injection in an awake child, since it may cause disturbing perineal warmth.
  - There is no evidence for detrimental effects on the immune system or wound infection rates.
  - May induce acute tumour lysis syndrome. Avoid in patients with acute leukaemia and non-Hodgkin's lymphoma.
  - May destabilize blood sugars in diabetics.
- Other antiemetics:
  - Other 5-HT$_3$ receptor antagonists:
    —Tropisetron, granisetron, dolasetron, ramosetron, palonosetron.
    —Some may be effective, but are not yet licensed in children.
    —Granisetron is approved for chemotherapy-related nausea and vomiting.
    —Dolasetron is contraindicated in children (risk of changes in QT interval).
  - Metoclopramide:
    —Second-line option.
    —Dopamine receptor (D$_2$) antagonist, but at higher doses is a 5-HT$_3$ receptor antagonist.
    —100–150 mcg/kg PO, IV or IM 8-hourly (maximum 10 mg).
    —Proven efficacy in treating chemotherapy-induced nausea and vomiting, but less so in PONV.
    —Side effects: extrapyramidal effects and dystonic reactions (particularly facial ones), especially after IV administration, and more common in children.
  - Cyclizine:
    —Second-line option in our institution (Alder Hey), although APA PONV Guidelines 2016 do not recommend it.
    —Histamine receptor (H$_1$) antagonist, with anticholinergic properties.
    —1 mg/kg PO or IV 8-hourly (maximum 50 mg).
    —Painful IV injection (give over 3–5 min).
    —Rapid injection may cause tachycardia
    —Side effects: sedation; occasional dry mouth and blurred vision.
  - Droperidol:
    —Discontinued in the UK in 2001 because of QT-interval prolongation, but relicensed in 2009.
    —Second-line option in children >2 years old.
    —A butyrophenone (structurally related to haloperidol), it is a powerful dopamine receptor (D$_2$) antagonist.
    —20–50 mcg/kg IV 6-hourly (maximum 1.25 mg).
    —Contraindicated in patients with known or suspected QT-interval prolongation. Caution when concomitant administration of drugs that prolong the QT interval or are known to induce hypoK$^+$ or hypoMg^{2+} (may precipitate QT-interval prolongation).
- Non-pharmacological prophylaxis:
  - Acupressure/puncture at P6 point on the wrist.

Delirium

- Different to agitation, in which children are consolable and recognize their parents. Causes of agitation include:
  - Hypoxia
  - Pain
  - Full bladder
  - Disorientation
  - Hunger
  - Parental separation.
- Emergence delirium is a drug-induced disorientation; commonest in preschool children.
- The child cries/screams, may hallucinate, is uncooperative, inconsolable, and thrashes around.
- They do not recognize their parents.
- Rapid awakening seems to contribute (desflurane increases the risk).
- TIVA ↓ incidence.
- Midazolam can paradoxically cause delirium if given as premedication.
- Premedication with or intraoperative use of α_2-agonists (e.g. clonidine) ↓ incidence.
- Usually lasts <30 min, although it can last longer.

Management:

- Exclude causes of agitation, particularly hypoxia, hypercapnia, and pain.
- Observe, prevent self-injury, and allow time to settle.
- Reassure and explain situation to parents.
- At times, pharmacological intervention may be beneficial:
  - Propofol 0.5–1mg/kg, which will make the child remain still, and re-emerge gradually.
  - IV clonidine 1 mcg/kg.
  - IV fentanyl 0.5–1 mcg/kg.
  - Midazolam is NOT effective.
- Afterwards discuss with parents future options to avoid a recurrence, e.g. TIVA.

Pain

- Ensure adequate analgesia in the immediate postoperative period, but also think ahead about further pain control in the later postoperative period.
- Severe pain is rapidly managed with 0.5–1 mcg/kg of fentanyl; followed by a longer-acting opiate.

Postoperative critical care

- The Paediatric Intensive Care Society in the UK has established four clinically based levels of care and patient dependency.
- Level 1:
  - High-dependency care.
  - Requires a nurse-to-patient ratio of 0.5:1 (1:1 if in a cubicle).
  - May require single organ support (excluding intubated children).
- Level 2:
  - Intensive care.
  - Requires a nurse-to-patient ratio of 1:1.
  - Often patient is intubated and ventilated, or unstable non-intubated.
- Level 3:
  - Intensive care.
  - Requires a nurse-to-patient ratio of 1.5:1.
  - Patient is intubated, ventilated, requires inotropes, or has multiple organ failure.
- Level 4:
  - Intensive care.
  - Requires a nurse-to-patient ratio of 2:1.
  - Patient is on ECLS (ECMO), haemofiltration.

High-dependency unit (HDU)

- Usually used as step-up or step-down care area between general wards and ICU. Ideally, situated adjacent to PICU.
- Close monitoring and observation are required; there are no facilities for mechanical ventilation.
- Should be used to care for patients with, or likely to develop, single organ failure.
- Should not be used to manage patients with multiple organ failure.
- Referral and communication are with senior nurse in HDU.
- Medical staff responsible for patients should be clearly identified, including 'multidisciplinary care' where different staff may be responsible for various elements of care.
- PICU consultant should be aware of any potential multiple organ failure patients being treated in HDU, especially those with potential airway compromise.

Likely patient groups

- Acutely ill medical patients at risk of organ failure, requiring more detailed observation/monitoring than can safely be provided on a general ward.
- Step-down patients from PICU, not yet ready for ward-level care.
- Postoperative patients following major surgery, who need close monitoring for more than a few hours.
- Patients requiring single organ support (excluding mechanical ventilation).
  - Respiratory monitoring and support:
    —Need for non-invasive ventilation:
      ○ High-flow nasal O_2, e.g. Optiflow, AIRVO
      ○ Continuous positive airway pressure (CPAP)
      ○ Bilevel intermittent positive airway pressure (BiPAP).
    —Possibility of progressive deterioration to the point of needing advanced respiratory support.

—Need for physiotherapy to clear secretions at least 2-hourly.
—Patients recently extubated after a prolonged period of intubation.
—Patients with a NPA to protect the airway, who are otherwise stable, e.g. postoperative cleft palate patients.
—Children requiring long-term chronic ventilation (with tracheostomy) are included in this category.
• Circulatory support:
—Need for vasoactive or inotropic drugs.
• Neurological monitoring and support:
—CNS depression, sufficient to prejudice the airway and protective reflexes.
—Invasive neurological monitoring.
• Renal support:
—Haemodialysis, haemofiltration, or haemodiafiltration.

Paediatric intensive care unit (PICU)

• PICU beds are a very expensive and limited resource because they provide:
  • Specialized monitoring equipment
  • Mechanical ventilation and other organs support if needed
  • A high nurse-to-patient ratio ($\geq$ 1:1)
  • A high degree of medical expertise.
• Used to care for patients with or likely to develop multiple organ failure.
• Referral and communication are directly to PICU consultant.
• Joint care between PICU and referring clinicians.
  • Often multiple specialties are involved.
  • Medical staff responsible for the various aspects of the patients care should be clearly identified.
  • Care coordinated by PICU staff.
• PICU consultant retains overall responsibility for patient management until ready for discharge to ward or HDU.

Different patient population from adult ICU

• Diseases are skewed to infective and congenital problems, e.g. viral laryngotracheobronchitis, meningococcal sepsis, postoperative congenital anomalies, and metabolic diseases.
• Fewer intercurrent chronic medical problems.
• Physiological reserve is usually greater in children.
• Decompensation from pathological insults is rapid and severe once the physiological reserve is exhausted.
• Lower mortality rates in paediatric units compared with adult units.

The child's family in PICU

• Dealing with parents can be fraught, and care should be taken to be informative and realistic about the patient's prognosis and progress.
• Accurate communication and documentation are essential to preclude misunderstandings.
• A specific member of staff should be tasked with communicating with relatives:
  • This ensures consistency of approach and helps avoid misunderstandings.
  • The communicator should be a senior member of staff, able to relate to the relatives or carers, but also able to give objective information.
• On-site accommodation should be available to parents.

Further reading

Barry P, Morris K, and Ali T (eds). *Paediatric Intensive Care* (Oxford Specialist Handbooks in Paediatrics). Oxford University Press, 2010.

Section 3

Practical procedures

Advanced airway management

Richard Craig

Introduction

- Difficult airways are anticipated or unanticipated, and involve one or more of:
  - Difficulty maintaining a patent airway with adequate ventilation in a patient breathing spontaneously under GA (i.e. partial or complete airway obstruction)
  - Difficult face-mask ventilation
  - Difficult laryngoscopy
  - Difficulty passing a tube into the trachea and ventilating the lungs.
- Refer to Table 9.1 for sizes of airway equipment required.

Aetiology

- Commonest associated conditions are as follows.

Congenital
- Reduced neck mobility:
  - Klippel–Feil syndrome.
- Reduced mouth opening:
  - Arthrogryposis multiplex.
- Nasal obstruction:
  - Choanal atresia
  - Pyriform aperture stenosis
  - Congenital bony nasal stenosis
  - Post-nasal mass—teratoma.
- Oropharyngeal obstruction:
  - Micrognathia, retrognathia, mandibular hypoplasia, maxillary hypoplasia: Pierre Robin sequence, Treacher Collins syndrome, Goldenhar syndrome
  - Tongue base collapse secondary to hypotonia
  - Macroglossia: Beckwith–Wiedemann syndrome
  - Lymphatic malformations/congenital masses: cystic hygroma.
- Laryngeal pathology:
  - Laryngomalacia
  - Glottic webs
  - Bilateral vocal cord palsy
  - Subglottic stenosis
  - Laryngeal cleft.
- Tracheal pathology:
  - Tracheal stenosis
  - Tracheomalacia.

Acquired
- Reduced neck mobility/ stability:
  - Unstable cervical spine: trauma, Down syndrome, juvenile idiopathic arthritis.
- Reduced mouth opening:
  - Temporomandibular joint ankylosis: post septic arthritis or trauma, juvenile idiopathic arthritis.

- Upper airway soft tissue pathology:
  - Trauma: burns to the face and neck, or caustic substance ingestion
  - Infective: retropharyngeal abscess, dental abscess
  - Tumours: myofibroma, teratoma, or haemangioma
  - Inflammatory/immunological: angioedema
  - Hereditary connective tissue disease: epidermolysis bullosa.
- Laryngeal pathology:
  - Post intubation: intubation granulomas, acquired subglottic stenosis, or subglottic cysts
  - Infective: acute epiglottitis, croup, or recurrent respiratory papillomatosis.
- Tracheal/lower airway pathology:
  - Anterior and superior mediastinal masses with airway compression: lymphoma
  - Bacterial tracheitis.
- Multilevel pathology:
  - Mucopolysaccharidosis (● Chapter 26).

Table 9.1 Airway equipment sizing chart

Age/weight	ETT	LMA size	Bougie	Stylet	Wire	Airway exchange catheter	Flexible fibreoptic scope	Ambu aScope 3 Slim	Rigid fibreoptic stylet	Ravussin cannula	Tracheostomy surgical cricothyroidotomy
Neonates including preterm	2 2.5 3	1	5 Ch Proact Bougie 1.7 mm diameter	X Portex tracheal intubation stylet 2 mm OD × 225 mm	TSF 38–145 0.038 inch = 0.965 mm	X X CAE 8–45 8 Fr = 2.7 mm	Keymed 2.2 mm insertion tube No working channel	Flexible videoscope 3.8 mm insertion tube 1.2 mm working channel	Brambrink 2.2 mm OD	Ravussin 16 G	Tracheostomy 5mm vertical tracheal incision 11 blade on scalpel Shiley 3.5 neonatal tracheostomy tube
<5 kg	3.5										
Infant	4	1½	10 Ch Proact Bougie 3.3mm diameter	Portex tracheal intubation stylet 2 mm OD × 225 mm	TSF 38–145 0.038 inch = 0.965 mm	CAE 8–45 8 Fr = 2.7 mm	Pentax FI-7BS 2.4 mm insertion tube No working channel	Can be passed through size 1 LMA or greater. Can load size 4.5 ETT and greater	Bonfils 3.5 mm OD	Ravussin 16 G	Tracheostomy 5 mm vertical tracheal incision 11 blade on scalpel Shiley 3.5 neonatal tracheostomy tube
5–10 kg	4.5						—				
1–5 years	5	2	10 Ch Proact Bougie 3.3mm diameter	Portex tracheal intubation stylet 4 mm OD xx 335 mm	TSF 38–145 0.038 inch = 0.965 mm	CAE 11–83 11 Fr = 3.7mm	Keymed LF-DP 3.1 mm insertion tube 1.2 mm working channel	Can be used with bronchus blockers size 5–9		Ravussin 14 G	Scalpel cricothyroidotomy or tracheostomy 11 blade on scalpel Shiley 3.5 neonatal tracheostomy tube
10–20 kg	5.5										

Age/Weight	ETT			Bougie	Stylet	Guidewire	Catheter	Bronchoscope	Needle	Surgical
5–8 years 20–30 kg	6	2½	6.5	10 Ch Proact Bougie 3.3 mm diameter	Portex tracheal intubation stylet 4 mm OD × 335 mm	TSF 38-145 0.038 inch = 0.965 mm	CAE 11-83 11 Fr = 3.7 mm		Ravussin 14 G	Scalpel cricothyroidotomy 10 blade on scalpel 4 mm Microcuff ETT
9–16 years 30–50 kg	7	3	7.5	10 Ch Proact Bougie 3.3 mm diameter	Portex tracheal intubation stylet 4 mm OD × 335 mm	TSF 38-145 0.038 inch = 0.965 mm	Aintree catheter or CAE 19-83 19 Fr = 6.3 mm	Pentax FI-10RBS 3.5 mm insertion tube 1.4 mm working channel — Can be used with 37 Fr DLT and greater	X	Scalpel cricothyroidotomy 10 blade on scalpel 5 mm Microcuff ETT stab, twist, bougie, tube

Airway assessment

- Review history, previous anaesthetic records, and any awake nasendoscopy findings.
- On examination listen for stridor and stertor.
- Look for signs of increased work of breathing, note the RR, SpO_2 and the FiO_2.
- Look for dysmorphic features, e.g. maxillary/mandibular hypoplasia, retrognathia and micrognathia. Look at the child in profile.
- If the child is cooperative, assess mouth opening and range of movement at the atlanto-occipital joint.
- Other useful information may be available from imaging, e.g. CT scans and CXR.

Planning airway management

- If difficulty is anticipated, consider the following:
  - Is the procedure necessary?
  - Are the risks of GA balanced by the benefit of the procedure?
  - Can the procedure be done awake?
  - Is airway obstruction under GA likely to be a problem?
- If the anticipated difficulty relates to airway obstruction, then it is likely to become worse on induction of GA, since upper airway muscle tone is reduced. There may be potential for complete airway obstruction and it may prove impossible to ventilate the lungs using mask ventilation or via a supraglottic airway device. It may also be impossible to intubate the patient.
  - Have an ENT surgeon present and ready to perform front-of-neck access
  - If possible, induce GA in the operating theatre with two anaesthetists and an experienced assistant.
  - Consider placing an NPA prior to induction. This can be fashioned from a plain ETT with the 15 mm connector removed and the proximal end split lengthways. The proximal end is folded flat against the face to achieve a good face-mask seal. This is particularly useful in small babies with Pierre Robin sequence, where the obstruction is usually at the level of the base of the tongue; the NPA needs to be relatively long to overcome this.
  - A relatively new method of maintaining oxygenation during the management of a difficult airway is nasal high-flow oxygen. This has been shown to safely increase apnoea time in children—a technique known as Transnasal Humidified Rapid Insufflation Ventilatory Exchange (THRIVE). Preferably, it is started prior to induction. It cannot be used in conjunction with volatile anaesthesia. Total intravenous anaesthesia is required
  - Induce GA slowly and patiently. One option is to use sevoflurane in 100% O_2 with the child in position they are most comfortable. Gradually ↑ the percentage of sevoflurane. Use of CPAP will help overcome dynamic airway collapse and obstruction. Maintain spontaneous ventilation.
  - It is possible to induce GA and maintain spontaneous ventilation using TIVA.
  - If it is possible to maintain a patent airway with adequate ventilation throughout induction, do not instrument the airway until the eyes are centrally fixed with mid-sized pupils, the HR has settled, and the breathing pattern is regular.
  - If the child becomes apnoeic, but the airway is not completely obstructed and the SpO_2 is stable, maintain CPAP and jaw thrust, and await resumption of spontaneous ventilation.
  - If there is increasing airway obstruction or complete obstruction, use two hands to apply jaw thrust, slightly open the mouth, and get a good face-mask seal. A second person should apply CPAP.
  - Options for managing increasing airway obstruction:
    —NPA– reasonably tolerated even in a light plane of GA.
    —Turn the patient lateral or three-quarters prone.

—OPA–an adequate depth of GA is required.
—Use a supraglottic airway device.
—Attempt to wake the patient.
- If the above measures fail and there is complete obstruction with falling SpO_2, attempt laryngoscopy and intubation.
- If this fails proceed to 'front-of-neck access' (FONA; for details, see later in the chapter), preferably performed by an ENT surgeon.
- Alternatively, an ENT surgeon may attempt intubation with a rigid ventilating bronchoscope.
- If airway obstruction under GA is not a concern, e.g. a past history of difficult direct laryngoscopy but no difficulty with mask ventilation, then IV induction and the use of a neuromuscular blocking agent may be entirely appropriate. Just as for conventional direct laryngoscopy, when using a video-laryngoscope or rigid-optical stylet, the best intubating conditions are provided by a smooth induction and neuromuscular blockade.
  - Is intubation required? Many patients who would be difficult to intubate because of difficult laryngoscopy can be easily managed with an LMA.
  - If intubation is required and difficulty is anticipated obtaining a direct line of sight from the laryngoscopist's eye to the glottic opening, consider the following options:
    —Indirect laryngoscopy and intubation using a flexible bronchoscope
    —Indirect laryngoscopy and intubation using a videolaryngoscope
    —Indirect laryngoscopy and intubation using a rigid optical stylet
    —Tracheostomy.

Indirect laryngoscopy and intubation: flexible bronchoscope (fibreoptic or videobronchoscope)
- Decide whether to intubate orally or nasally (easiest).
- There may be surgical or patient factors that dictate the route chosen.
- Decide between having the ETT loaded directly onto the scope or using a guidewire/airway exchange catheter technique. The problem with having the ETT loaded directly onto the scope is selecting the correct ETT size: too small a tube and it will need changing because of a large leak (change via airway exchange catheter); too large a tube risks airway trauma and failure to intubate even with the bronchoscope in the trachea. Using a cuffed tube may help to avoid these problems.
- Consider oxygenation, ventilation, and maintenance of GA during airway endoscopy and intubation.
- Multiple techniques are possible; two examples are described in detail in Boxes 9.1 and 9.2.

Indirect laryngoscopy and intubation using a videolaryngoscope, e.g. C-MAC videolaryngoscope
- For equipment details, ➔ Chapter 5.
- If mask ventilation is adequate, the use of a neuromuscular blocking agent will make laryngoscopy and intubation easier.
- A common pitfall is to position the scope tip too close to the glottis—this provides an excellent view, but negotiating the ETT into the airway

Box 9.1 Asleep nasal intubation using a flexible bronchoscope with the ETT loaded directly onto the scope and the patient breathing spontaneously

Personnel
- Two anaesthetists: one to manage the anaesthetic; one to perform the airway endoscopy and intubation.
- One assistant experienced with the procedure.
- Team well-rehearsed with the technique.

Equipment preparation
- Select an appropriately sized ETT. A Microcuff tube has advantages in terms of sealing a leak whilst avoiding too large a tube to fit through the cricoid ring.
- Select an appropriate sized flexible bronchoscope (Table 9.1).
- Connect the bronchoscope to camera and light source. Display scope image on monitor; pay attention to image orientation, white balance and focus. Adjust the image size on the screen. Select an appropriate light intensity.
- Have an anti-fogging agent, e.g. Ultrastop, available.
- Load the ETT onto the scope, using tape to secure it to the proximal end of the scope's insertion tube. Place a small bead of lubricant (sterile aqueous gel) on the insertion tube about 10 cm from the distal end. This will ease deployment of the ETT over the scope. Avoiding the distal 10 cm of the scope prevents lubricant potentially obscuring the image and avoids making the scope slick and difficult to handle.
- At this point, do not place lubricant on the outside of the ETT;, it will make a mess and should be applied just prior to advancing the ETT into the airway.
- Prepare an uncuffed plain (not preformed) ETT for use as an NPA (⥁ Chapter 5).
- Administer topical vasoconstrictor, e.g. xylometazoline 0.05% paediatric nasal drops or lidocaine 5% and phenylephrine 0.5% spray. This reduces the risk of bleeding, which might obscure the view.
- Draw up 1 mL of lidocaine 2% in a 10 mL syringe with 9 mL of air. The air facilitates the spray of LA onto the laryngeal inlet. Connect syringe to working channel of bronchoscope.
- Stat doses of 4 mg/kg of lidocaine are safe (8.5 mg/kg is safe when administered over 15 min and the 2013 British Thoracic Society guidelines for flexible bronchoscopy in adults state that doses up to 15.4 mg/kg may be used without serious adverse events, but subjective symptoms of lidocaine toxicity have been reported in studies using ≥9.6 mg/kg lidocaine).
- In small patients, ensure that the total dose of topical LA is safe.

Induction of anaesthesia
- Gas induction using sevoflurane in O_2.
- Maintain spontaneous ventilation.
- Establish routine monitoring.
- Establish IV access.

Topical vasoconstrictors
- Apply topical vasoconstrictor to nasal mucosa.
- Xylometazoline 0.05% paediatric nasal drops, 1–2 drops per nostril.
- Lidocaine 5% and phenylephrine 0.5% spray. Caution: severe hypertension, acute left ventricular failure, pulmonary oedema, cardiac arrest, and death have followed the indiscriminate use of poorly quantified doses of topical phenylephrine. This spray delivers 0.65 mg of phenylephrine per spray. The product literature states that it is not recommended in children <12 years of age. A maximum of 8 sprays is recommended for adults.

Insert NPA
- Once an adequate depth of GA has been achieved, insert the uncuffed ETT as an NPA and connect the anaesthetic breathing system to the NPA via the standard 15 mm connector. Maintain jaw thrust to keep the airway open and create space for the airway endoscopy to follow.
- The patient breathes spontaneously through the NPA, which is connected to the anaesthetic breathing system, which delivers O_2 and volatile anaesthetic agent throughout the procedure.

Airway endoscopy
- Start at the anterior nares and follow the black air space. Avoid getting too close to the mucosa: red-out or white-out on the screen. If this happens, withdraw the scope until there is a black air space visible again.
- Keep the scope reasonably straight so that movements of the hand on the proximal controls are translated to the scope tip.
- The scope can be advanced, withdrawn, rotated left or right, and the tip can be deflected up or down. Start with the tip in neutral position.
- A good jaw thrust should create the necessary air space at the back of the tongue as the scope exits the nasopharynx and enters the oropharynx.
- Once the glottis is in view, spray the LA down the working channel of the scope onto the laryngeal inlet. If the depth of GA is adequate, this is well tolerated. If there is coughing, simply wait for it to subside.
- As the tip of the scope approaches the glottic opening, aim towards the anterior commissure. When the scope tip is at the anterior commissure, deflect it down and it will enter the trachea.
- Advance the scope into the trachea as far as the carina.
- At this point, hand the scope over to the trained assistant. Their job is to hold the scope without advancing or withdrawing it. This frees up the operator's hands to negotiate the ETT over the scope through the upper airway and into the trachea.

Lubricant
- Apply a generous amount of sterile aqueous lubricant to the outside of the ETT and the nostril.

Railroading the ETT
- Advance the ETT through the nose with the bevel facing the turbinates. In this fashion, the very tip of the ETT will be alongside the septum and less likely to cause 'hold-up' (resistance).
- Once the ETT tip passes through the nose, rotate it so the bevel is directed toward the posterior commissure of the glottis. The sharp leading tip will be directed towards the anterior commissure and resistance will be less likely.
- If resistance is encountered, withdraw the ETT slightly (remember to neither withdraw nor advance the bronchoscope). Sandwich the ETT between the palms of the hands and rotate the ETT anticlockwise as it is advanced.
- Be careful not to traumatize the airway.

Confirmation of tracheal intubation
- Once the ETT has been railroaded over the scope into the trachea, withdraw the bronchoscope confirming that the ETT tip is in the trachea.
- Connect the ETT to the anaesthetic breathing circuit and check capnography.
- Auscultate the chest to ensure there is bilateral air entry.

Measure the distance from the main carina to the tip of the ETT
- Connect a bronchoscopic angle piece to the end of the ETT and reconnect the anaesthetic breathing system.
- Insert the bronchoscope through the bronchoscopic angle piece port and advance through the ETT and into the trachea.
- Insert the scope until its tip is at the carina.
- The operator pinches the insertion tube of the scope at the point where it enters the bronchoscopic angle piece port. The fingers are kept in position as a marker.
- Withdraw the bronchoscope until its tip is at the tip of the ETT.
- The distance from where the operators' fingers are pinching the bronchoscope insertion tube to where it enters the angle piece port is the distance from the ETT tip to the carina.

may be more difficult. Withdraw the tip of the scope slightly if there is difficulty negotiating the ETT into the airway.
- When using the C-MAC, run the ETT along the laryngoscope blade to guide it into the trachea. Unlike conventional direct laryngoscopy, there is no need to insert the ETT from the right-hand side of the mouth. The ETT is not going to obstruct the line of sight, so run it along the blade. This helps avoid trauma to the pharynx.
- A bougie can be useful if there is a good view of the glottis, but directing the tube is proving difficult.

Box 9.2 Intubation through the LMA using a flexible bronchoscope and a guidewire/airway exchange catheter technique

Personnel
- Two anaesthetists: one to maintain GA and monitor the patient; one to instrument the airway.
- One ODP (assistant) experienced with the procedure.
- The team must be well-rehearsed in the technique.

Equipment preparation
- Select an appropriately sized LMA. A single-use device with a design similar to the LMA classic, e.g. P3 Medical LMA, is preferable.
- Bronchoscopic angle piece with a bronchoscopy port.
- Vascular guidewire, e.g. COOK TSF 38-145 wire (diameter 0.965 mm and length 145 cm).
- Flexible bronchoscope with a working channel. Examples are given in Table 9.1.
- Airway exchange catheter. Consult Table 9.1 for size.
- ETT.
- Lidocaine for topical anaesthesia of the airway. Draw up 1 mL of lidocaine 2% in a 10 mL syringe with 9 mL of air. The 9 mL of air facilitates spraying the LA onto the laryngeal inlet. 4 mg/kg of lidocaine can be safely administered.

Induction of anaesthesia
- A gas induction maintaining spontaneous ventilation may have some advantages if you anticipate difficult mask ventilation.
- Establish monitoring.
- Establish IV access.

Insert LMA and connect breathing system via a bronchoscopic angle piece
- Ensure that the airway is patent, spontaneous ventilation is adequate, and depth of GA is adequate.

Insert the flexible bronchoscope through the bronchoscope angle piece port
- Advance the bronchoscope to view the glottis.
- Spray LA on the vocal cords via the working channel.
- No need to advance scope beyond the vocal cords.

Insert the guidewire through the working channel of the scope
- Advance the guidewire until it appears at the distal end of the scope.
- Position the scope tip over the glottic opening to direct the guidewire into the trachea as it is advanced. Alternatively, in larger patients, the bronchoscope can simply be advanced into the trachea and then the guidewire advanced.
- Pay close attention to the length of the guidewire inserted into the trachea. The trachea is about 4 cm long in a neonate and 15 cm in an adult. Do not insert if there is resistance. Tracheal or bronchial injury is possible.

Withdraw the scope, leaving the wire in the airway
- The assistant (ODP) needs to pay close attention.
- Grasp the wire firmly between thumb and index finger about 5 cm proximal to where the wire enters the working channel at the proximal end of the bronchoscope. Without moving the fingers holding the wire, withdraw the scope over the wire until it meets finger and thumb. Repeat this manoeuvre about 4 times and the bronchoscope will have been withdrawn to the point where the distal tip is just free of the bronchoscopic angle piece. The assistant grasps the guidewire distal to the bronchoscope at the point where it enters the bronchoscopic angle piece. Holding the wire securely, completely remove the bronchoscope. This procedure must be performed meticulously and the assistant must be poised and ready to grasp the guidewire as the scope is withdrawn from the LMA and angle piece. The wire should not move relative to the airway.

Advance the airway exchange catheter over the guidewire
- To measure the likely depth of insertion of the airway exchange catheter place it over the patient's body and use your knowledge of the surface anatomy of the trachea. Estimate the depth of insertion required to have the exchange catheter comfortably beyond the glottis and in the trachea but not too deep risking bronchial injury.
- There may be slight resistance at the level of the glottis. Rotate the exchange catheter as it is advanced over the guidewire. Avoid excessive force - this will simply loop the guidewire out of the airway and push everything down the oesophagus. If necessary, withdraw the exchange catheter slightly and try again, rotating the catheter as it is advanced.

Remove the guidewire
- Confirm the position of the airway exchange catheter
- The exchange catheter comes packaged with an adaptor that clips on to the proximal end. The adaptor has a 15 mm tapered connector that can be connected to an anaesthetic circuit with waveform capnography (used to confirm that it is in the airway).

Remove the LMA and bronchoscopic angle piece over the airway exchange catheter
- Remove the bronchoscopic angle piece first and then the LMA. Do not remove both together.
- As the LMA is removed, grasp the airway exchange catheter within the patients' mouth at the earliest opportunity.
- The airway exchange catheter should not move relative to the airway.

Railroad the ETT over the airway exchange catheter
- This is similar to having a bougie in the trachea and railroading the tube. Use a conventional laryngoscope to lift the tongue and jaw out of the way. This reduces friction with the soft tissues of the upper airway and makes this step easier.

- The assistant must hold the proximal end of the exchange catheter and make sure that it does not move relative to the airway.
- There may be slight resistance at the level of the glottis. Withdraw the ETT slightly and try again, rotating anticlockwise as the ETT advances. Rotate the ETT so that the bevel is directed toward the posterior commissure of the glottis. The sharp leading tip will be directed towards the anterior commissure and resistance will be less likely.

Confirm correct position of ETT and bilateral lung ventilation
- Capnography

Use the bronchoscope to check the distance from the ETT tip to the carina

Indirect laryngoscopy and intubation using a rigid optical stylet, e.g. Brambrink or Bonfils retromolar scope

Equipment preparation
- It is best to display the image from the scope on a monitor, e.g. the TELE PACK X LED. manufactured by Karl Storz. This system includes a monitor, camera, and light source.
- Connect the camera and light cable to the Bonfils scope.
- Optimize the image, paying attention to image orientation (a vertical line in reality must be a vertical line on the screen, and 12 o'clock in reality must be 12 o'clock on the screen). White-balance and focus the image. Adjust the size of the image on the screen. Select an appropriate light intensity.
- Have anti-fogging agent, e.g. Ultrastop, available.
- Select an appropriately sized ETT and load it onto the scope so that the scope tip is just short of the ETT tip. The ETT tip will be visible as a thin crescent on the edge of the image on the monitor. Sometimes the light reflected off the ETT tip degrades the image. Advance the tip of the scope just a fraction further so that the crescent disappears—the scope tip is then aligned with the ETT tip. Fix the ETT in this position using the adjustable tube-holder. The position of the tube-holder is adjusted according to the length of ETT selected so as to position the scope tip as described above. The tube-holder is a tapered connector and, once fixed in position, the ETT can be deployed simply by sliding it out of the tapered connector. The tube-holder has a port for the insufflation of O_2. Preformed ETT can be used; just straighten the ETT to load it onto the scope. Lubricant gel is not required.

Induction of anaesthesia
- Establish IV access and monitoring.
- Administer a neuromuscular blocking agent, unless mask ventilation is likely to be difficult.

Insert a Mackintosh laryngoscope
- Use a conventional technique to lift the tongue and jaw and create an air space in the oro- and hypopharynx (this can also be done with the free hand lifting the tongue and jaw, but is less satisfactory).
- As for any fibreoptic technique, an air space is necessary to visualize the anatomy and advance the scope.
- Suction the pharynx under direct vision to clear any secretions.

Airway endoscopy
- Insert the Bonfils scope between the molars on the right-hand side of the mouth with the tip directed towards the tonsil bed on the left-hand side.
- Look at the patient's mouth, not at the screen. Make sure the scope is right over in the right-hand corner of the mouth. The scope should be almost vertical as it is inserted into the mouth.
- Look at the screen and identify the uvula, which acts as a depth marker. Keep the scope close to vertical as it is inserted into the mouth with the tip directed towards the left tonsil until the scope is almost touching the uvula. Go slowly.
- If misting occurs, gently touch the tip of the scope against the mucosa. Failing that, remove the scope and apply anti-fogging agent to the tip.
- Rotate the scope tip through 90°, directing it towards the base of the tongue and epiglottis.
- Identify the epiglottis.
- Negotiate the scope tip under the epiglottis to identify the glottic opening. As the scope tip advances toward the epiglottis, change the alignment of the proximal end of the scope, dropping from the nearly vertical starting position to a retromolar position. All of this is done whilst watching the screen.
- Go slowly. If the scope is too close to the mucosal surfaces, the image will red-out, in which case withdraw slightly. It is essential when advancing the scope to have an air space ahead.
- Advance the scope into the subglottis (just through the cords).

Intubation
- Have the assistant deploy the ETT. One of the advantages of the Bonfils scope is that once there is a view of the subglottis, the ETT is immediately ready to deploy. It does not need to be negotiated into that field of view as with a video laryngoscope, and there is no hold-up as you try to railroad the tube over the scope, as there may be with a flexible bronchoscope. The rigidity of the scope may also be of benefit when dealing with supraglottic, glottic, or subglottic pathology.

Withdraw the scope
- Whilst holding the ETT firmly in position.

Confirm position
- Use capnography and bilateral lung ventilation to assess.

Confirm correct depth of insertion
- Insert the Bonfils scope alongside the ETT to view the depth markers at the level of the glottis. This is particularly useful when using a Microcuff tube.

Tracheostomy

- The only way to get a tube into the trachea may be for an ENT surgeon to perform a tracheostomy while GA is maintained with either a face mask or LMA to manage the airway. This is an uncommon scenario, but the option should not be forgotten when planning for the anticipated difficult airway.

Planning extubation

- Dexamethasone 0.15 mg/kg intraoperatively.
- Ensure full reversal of residual block.
- Consider placing an NPA prior to extubation.
- Consider placing an airway exchange catheter—this can act as a guide to allow reintubation.
- Check for a leak around the ETT (with the cuff down for cuffed tubes).
- Prepare for reintubation: personnel (including ENT surgeon), equipment, location, drugs.
- Prepare equipment for the delivery of O_2 (it may be worth considering CPAP or non-invasive ventilation in selected cases).
- Reapplication of high-flow nasal oxygen postoperatively is a relatively new strategy.
- Consider preparing for admission to HDU or ICU.
- Extubate awake: the patient should have an adequate respiratory effort and a vigorous cough and be making purposeful movements.

Front-of-neck access (FONA)

- Indication: 'Can't intubate can't oxygenate' (CICO) scenario.
- Ensure complete neuromuscular block: do not attempt on a moving patient. Any attempt at waking the child has already failed and is no longer a viable option. For the same reason, sugammadex is not administered.
- The clinical course has been committed to.

If an ENT surgeon is available:

- Note that management is not age-dependent.
- Continue to attempt oxygenation with a face mask or LMA.
- Proceed to surgical tracheostomy.
- Rigid bronchoscopy is an alternative option if all the equipment is already set up; otherwise it takes too long to be a useful technique.

If no ENT surgeon is available:

- Other team members should continue to attempt oxygenation using a face mask (with Guedel airway and/or NPA) and utilizing a two-person bag-mask ventilation technique. Alternatively, an LMA can be tried.
- The patient should be supine with a small roll under the shoulders and the head and neck maximally extended. Tape the chin in a cephalad direction, thereby stretching the soft tissues and improving access to the neck.
- A right-handed operator should stand on the child's left-hand side. The operator palpates and stabilizes the airway with their non-dominant hand and operates with their dominant hand.
- There is no consensus on FONA for all age groups. The following is one option.
- Management options are divided into three age groups:

<1 year of age

- The neonatal cricothyroid membrane is only 2.5 mm long (sagittal plane) and 3 mm wide (transverse plane). The hyoid bone lies over the thyroid cartilage, making palpation and identification of the relevant anatomy difficult. The mandible gets in the way because of the cephalad position of the larynx; this influences the angle at which a needle can be inserted into the cricothyroid membrane.
- For these reasons, needle or surgical cricothyroidotomy do not work.
- Needle tracheostomy:
  - Use a kink-resistant transtracheal cannula, e.g. a 16 G VBM Ravusin or 16 G BD Insyte.
  - If US immediately available, it may be useful to guide needle insertion. Obtain a transverse view of the trachea and use an out-of-plane needling technique. Insert the needle tip so as to puncture the trachea at the 12 o'clock position.
  - Hold the hub of the needle: as the needle advances, a loss of resistance may be felt. The trachea is mobile and compressible, and it is therefore likely to collapse entirely during needle insertion.
  - A syringe with 1 mL of water is attached to the needle and aspirated slowly as the needle is withdrawn. It is likely that the posterior

tracheal wall will be hit initially, and the needle tip will only enter the tracheal lumen as it is withdrawn.
- If it is possible to aspirate air, advance the cannula over the needle, then remove the needle and recheck that air aspirates freely.
- Attach a high-pressure O_2 source: a Manujet III or a COOK Enk O_2 flow modulator. The latter connects to a wall-mounted O_2 flowmeter. It has a flute with 5 holes that one occludes to jet oxygenate in the same way that one would occlude a Y-connector:
  —The Manujet III is set to the lowest possible delivery pressure and then increased slowly if necessary.
  —The COOK Enk O_2 flow modulator is set at an O_2 flow rate of 1 L/min, ↑ in increments of 1 L/min if chest expansion is inadequate.
- Look for chest expansion when jetting.
- Look for adequate chest deflation before delivering the next jet; there is no fixed ratio for inspiratory and expiratory time. There is a risk of gas trapping and barotrauma. Passive expiration via the upper airway is essential. Maintain all efforts to open the upper airway.

- Surgical tracheostomy:
  - Indicated if needle tracheostomy fails.
  - Performed by anaesthetist or another member of the team, e.g. general surgeon.
  - Stay in the midline.
  - Vertical incision through the skin and soft tissues from the upper part of the larynx to the sternal notch.
  - Separate the strap muscles in the midline by blunt dissection. Use a **blunt but pointed scissors** to open the area in a vertical plane.
  - Get assistant to put **cat's paws** to hold apart the skin and soft tissue.
  - Ensure that you have correctly identified the trachea: insert a 23 G needle attached to a 10 mL syringe containing 2 mL saline into the presumed trachea and confirm aspiration of air. The common carotid artery and the anterior cervical vertebrae can be mistaken for the trachea.
  - Make a 5 mm vertical incision through the tracheal rings using a number 11 blade on a scalpel.
  - Insert a Shiley 3.5 mm neonatal tracheostomy tube.

1–8 years of age
- Needle cricothyroidotomy or tracheostomy:
  - 16 G or 14 G cannula (VBM Ravusin or BD Insyte).
  - Technique as for age <1 year for needle tracheostomy.
  - For the COOK Enk O_2 flow modulator, set the O_2 flow rate to 1 L/min/year of age; ↑ in increments of 1 L/min to achieve adequate chest expansion.
- Surgical cricothyroidotomy or tracheostomy:
  - Indicated if needle cricothyroidotomy or needle tracheostomy fails.

>8 years of age
- Scalpel cricothyroidotomy:
  - Palpable cricothyroid membrane:
    —Transverse stab incision through the cricothyroid membrane with a No. 10 scalpel blade on a suitable handle.
    —Turn the blade through 90° (sharp edge caudal).

—Slide the coudé tip of a 10 Ch bougie along the blade into the trachea.
—Railroad a lubricated age-appropriate Microcuff ETT (size 6.0 for adult-sized patients) over the bougie.
• Impalpable cricothyroid membrane:
—Make an 8 cm vertical skin incision from caudad to cephalad over the larynx.
—Use blunt dissection with the fingers of both hands to separate the tissues.
—Identify and stabilize the larynx.
—Make a transverse stab incision through the cricothyroid membrane and proceed as for a palpable cricothyroid membrane.

Further reading

Association of Paediatric Anaesthetists/Difficult Airway Society. APA/DAS Paediatric Difficult Airway Guidelines for the management of the unanticipated difficult airway in children aged 1 to 8 years. https://das.uk.com/guidelines/paediatric-difficult-airway-guidelines

Advanced vascular access

Richard Craig

Ultrasound guided of vessel cannulation

- Ultrasound (US) can facilitate arterial and peripheral/central venous cannulation either with a cannula-over-needle device or in combination with the Seldinger technique.
- Standardizing your technique is advantageous (Box 10.1)

Box 10.1 Equipment and preparation
- US machine with colour Doppler and zoom functions.
- High-frequency (10–5 MHz) Linear US probe with a 25 mm footprint.
- Sterile probe cover.
- Sterile gel.
- Suitable over-the-needle IV cannula, e.g. Jelco I.V. catheter (Smiths Medical). Flush with saline. This can be used for either direct cannulation or to pass a guidewire for the Seldinger technique. Start with this cannula irrespective of the type of line inserted: peripheral/central venous, arterial, or PICC line.
- Straight guidewire with a soft tip on both ends.

Positioning
- Exact positioning depends on the specific vessel and is discussed later.
- Ensure the US machine is positioned so there is a straight, comfortable line of sight: screen, patient, probe, and operator must be aligned.

Scanning
- Optimize the US image by selecting the appropriate preset, e.g. 'vascular' or 'small parts', adjusting the depth and gain.
- Clean skin with antiseptic, e.g. 2% chlorhexidine in 70% isopropyl alcohol (allow to dry).
- Cover probe with a sterile sheath.
- Use sterile gel as an acoustic couplant.
- The short-axis view of the vessel is most commonly used. In cross section, it appears as a round or oval anechoic structure. Use the probe to gently compress the vessel. Veins collapse easily. Arteries can be compressed with slightly greater pressure and pulsate. This is accentuated by gentle probe pressure over the artery.
- Use the colour Doppler function to examine the vessel for pulsatile flow. Always return to standard 2D scanning mode before needling.
- Scan up and down the vessel to assess vessel patency and map the course of the vessel before choosing a puncture site.
- Thrombus will appear iso- or hyperechoic.
- For very small vessels, the zoom function can be utilized to magnify the area of interest. Be sure the magnified area corresponds to the section of the image closest to the skin surface and is aligned with the middle of the probe.

Needling

- Hold the probe with the non-dominant hand, resting the little finger on the patient's body to provide extra stability and control.
- Use the dominant hand to hold the needle at the hub—like a dart. If it is decided to attach a syringe to the end of the needle, do not attempt to control the needle by holding the syringe plunger; this is too ungainly since it uses the proximal muscles of the elbow and shoulder to control the movement instead of the small muscles of the hand.
- The out-of-plane plane (OOP) approach is used most commonly in conjunction with a short-axis view of the vessel.
- The probe is placed so the target vessel is in the middle of the screen. Note the depth of the vessel.
- The needle insertion point is behind the middle of the probe.
- Scanning during needling is an active process. Do not work with a single static image. Constantly alter the probe position by tilting and sliding the probe back and forth to find the needle tip from the moment it pierces the skin until it enters the vessel.
- A relatively steep angle of approach is acceptable to pierce the skin, advancing the needle tip towards the 12 o'clock position above the vessel. But once the tip of the needle is positioned just above the vessel, flatten the angle to facilitate cannulation.
- Pierce the skin and find the needle tip on the screen. Gently agitate the needle tip without advancing the needle. This will create tissue deformation and aid tip location. Tilt the probe away from the needle and then back towards the needle. The needle tip will be the first part of the needle observed (hyperechoic dot).
- Remember that the shaft of the needle will also appear as a hyperechoic dot on the screen. The only way to differentiate the needle tip from the shaft is to tilt the probe away until no part of the needle is imaged and then tilt the probe back to regain sight of the hyperechoic dot. Agitating the needle tip without advancing it helps. As the needle is advanced, continue to repeat this manoeuvre.
- Assess your puncture site once the needle tip is identified. If the puncture site is not directly above the target vessel, take the needle out and make the necessary adjustment. Do not persist with a poor approach.
- Advance the needle towards the vessel, aiming for the 12 o'clock position (the vessel will be a roundish anechoic structure—think of it as a clock face). Use tilting and sliding movements of the probe to follow the needle tip as it is advanced.
- Do not apply constant pressure as you advance the needle—it distorts the anatomy on the screen. Instead, use short sharp jabbing movements to advance the needle, then release the pressure on the tissues—always reassess needle tip position after this manoeuvre.
- Once the needle tip is at the 12 o'clock position above the vessel, it tents the top of the vessel as the needle is agitated. To pierce the vessel, a precise jab is better than slow continuous pressure. The vessel wall can be quite elastic. A steep angle of approach may make cannulation of the vessel difficult, even though vessel puncture will be successful. This is particularly true for small peripheral vessels.

Continued

- The desired end point is to see the needle tip in the vessel lumen.
- The end point of needling is not a flashback or aspiration of blood. If you are trying to aspirate whilst manipulating the needle, you are holding the needle incorrectly (see above) and you will not have the necessary dexterity when working with very small vessels. Forget about the syringe and adopt a uniform technique irrespective of the size of the vessel.
- Once the needle tip is in the vessel, it is usually easier to see (due to the greater contrast with the anechoic blood). When needling larger veins, e.g. the internal jugular, it is not uncommon to have a thin layer of intima still covering the needle tip after it has punctured the vessel. This can usually be seen as very thin layer of tissue draped over the needle tip. Advancing the needle further to puncture this will result in a clear image of the needle tip as a single bright dot within the anechoic vessel. Even in very small vessels, you should aim to get a clear image of the needle tip within the vessel. Do not stop with vessel puncture: continue to advance the needle up the vessel under ultrasound guidance. Slide the probe to view the vessel 1–2 mm beyond the needle tip with the probe angled slightly towards the needle tip, then advance the needle up the vessel by 1–2 mm. In this way, you can guide it up the vessel step by step. Stop only once you have a good length of cannula within the vessel. If the cannula was flushed with saline, there will be a flashback on puncturing the vessel. This can be delayed or even absent with peripheral veins—remember the end point of needling is seeing the needle tip in the vessel Even with arterial puncture, do not expect pulsatile blood spurting out of the cannula. Ignore the flashback—look at the screen.

Cannulation

- Direct vessel cannulation. As with any over-the-needle cannula, it is insufficient to get the needle tip in the vessel. Once the needle has been advanced into the vessel far enough to ensure the cannula is within the lumen, put the US probe down. Withdraw the needle, leaving the cannula in situ. If the cannula immediately fills with blood as the needle is withdrawn, then advance the cannula into the vessel over the needle. If it does not, then you may have transected the vessel—see below.
- Seldinger technique with the cannula transecting the vessel. A straight guidewire is easier to handle. Take it completely out of any coiled packaging. The Babywire is a double-ended nitinol guidewire (0.012 inch/0.031mm diameter and 18 cm long). It is useful with 24 G cannulas. Slowly withdraw the cannula, keeping it fairly flat against the skin. When there is a steady drip of blood out of the cannula, insert the guidewire. With arterial cannulation, there will not necessarily be pulsatile blood flow as the cannula is withdrawn.
- At this point, there is either a cannula or guidewire in the required vessel: proceed to insert the necessary line.

Central lines

Short-term non-tunnelled central venous lines

- Variables to consider include the diameter (French Gauge), length, number of lumens, and entry site (femoral and internal jugular are commonly used).

Examples of central lines

- Vygon 4.5 Fr 6 cm triple-lumen central line: suitable for neonates; femoral or internal jugular placement. The guidewire fits through a 22 G IV cannula.
- Cook 5 Fr 5 cm triple-lumen central line: suitable for infants and internal jugular placement. The guidewire fits through a 20 G IV cannula.
- Cook 5 Fr 8 cm triple-lumen central line: suitable for infants and femoral placement, or older children and internal jugular placement. The tip must be extrapericardial and should not be advanced beyond the innominate vein or initial segment of the SVC.
- Cook 5 Fr 12 cm triple-lumen central line: suitable for toddlers and femoral placement, or adult-sized patients and internal jugular placement. The tip must be extrapericardial and should not be advanced beyond the innominate vein or initial segment of the SVC.
- Cook 5 Fr 15 cm triple-lumen central line: suitable for femoral placement in older children.
- Cook 7 Fr 15 cm triple-lumen central line: suitable for adult-sized patients and internal jugular placement. The tip must be extrapericardial and should not be advanced beyond the innominate vein or initial segment of the SVC.
- Cook 7 Fr 20 cm triple-lumen central line: suitable for adult-sized patients and femoral placement.

Entry site

Femoral central line

- Position patient supine with slight degree of head up.
- Insert a small support under the hips—a square of Gamgee folded double or a clean nappy folded into a small roll. In particularly chubby infants, it is useful to apply a strip of pink Elastoplast tape along the length of the thigh, continuing beyond the knee and onto the table top. This will stretch the skin and open out the skin crease at the groin.
- A right-handed operator will usually find it easiest to insert a right-sided femoral line.
- Prep and drape both sides at the start of the procedure.
- Place the US machine at the contralateral shoulder to create a straight line from screen to probe to operator's eye.
- On US imaging, the long saphenous vein can often be identified joining the femoral vein at about the level of the skin crease at the groin. The vessel puncture site should be above the skin crease.
- The vessel puncture site should also be below the inguinal ligament. There is a risk of severe haemorrhage should the vessel be lacerated within the pelvis, as well as a risk of visceral perforation.
- Take care to avoid air embolism, particularly if the child is breathing spontaneously.

Internal jugular central line
- Position patient supine in the Trendelenburg position.
- Insert a shoulder roll to extend the neck. Rotate the head slightly away from the insertion side. Do not rotate the head excessively as this makes line insertion more difficult.
- In chubby infants, it may be useful to apply pink Elastoplast tape across the top of the shoulder, continuing down to the table top. This will stretch the skin and improve access.
- Position the US machine to create a straight line of sight—either side of the table at the level of the patient's hips.

Long-term central venous access devices
- Indications: parenteral nutrition, chemotherapy, IV antibiotics, frequent blood/blood component transfusions, and frequent blood sampling. They can remain in situ for > a month.
- Skin-tunnelled cuffed central venous catheters, e.g. Hickman and Broviac lines:
  - Usually inserted by a surgeon or interventional radiologist.
  - Inserted via a venotomy or a percutaneous US-guided Seldinger technique.
  - X-ray control is essential.
- Peripherally inserted central venous catheters:
  - Inserted via peripheral veins in the limbs.
  - The Cook silicone PICC is one example; the 3 Fr 50 cm and 4 Fr 60 cm lines are commonly used.
  - The line is cut to the desired length and on-table X-ray imaging with a image intensifier is essential to ensure correct line tip placement— extrapericardial in a central vein.
  - The Cook PICC line insertion set includes a needle for venipuncture (although a standard 22 G IV cannula is preferable for initial vessel puncture and cannulation), a highly flexible and kink resistant guidewire, a Peel-Away introducer sheath with a Luer-locking dilator, the silicone PICC, and a hydrophilic-coated obturator that helps to stiffen the PICC as it is inserted through the Peel-Away sheath.
- Implanted port devices, e.g. portacath:
  - Have a subcutaneous reservoir (one or two) with a self-sealing septum attached to a central venous catheter. The port is accessed via a non-coring gripper needle.
  - Do not use needles that are not designed for port access—they will damage the septum, and the port will have to be removed.
  - Gripper needles are available in a variety of needle gauges and needle lengths (usually 20 G 3/4 inch needle). The length depends on depth of subcutaneous tissue overlying the port.
  - Topical LA cream is applied over port prior to needling.

Arterial lines

Equipment
- It is possible to use an over-the-needle IV cannula, e.g. a Jelco I.V. catheter; however, they are more difficult to secure and less reliable because of kinking.
- Specifically designed kit, e.g. ARROW arterial catheterization: 5 or 8 cm 22 G polyurethane catheter with a straight spring-wire guide that has a soft tip at both ends (0.021 inch/0.53 mm in diameter and 35 cm long).

Sites
- Usually the radial and femoral artery are used.
- Other sites include: posterior tibial, dorsalis pedis, axillary, and brachial arteries.
- The brachial artery has no collateral circulation and a relatively high risk of thrombotic sequelae.
- The radial artery has the advantage of good collateral circulation provided by the ulnar artery and palmar arch.
- The relatively large diameter and high flow rates in the femoral artery make thrombosis less likely. Complications, particularly thrombosis with distal ischaemia, are more common in children <5 years of age.

Technique
- US guidance is increasingly common.
- For femoral arterial line insertion, positioning, scanning, and line insertion are similar to those for femoral central line insertion.
- For radial arterial line insertion:
  - The arm is abducted and the forearm held in supination.
  - Place a small support under the wrist (a 50 mL syringe makes a good wrist support) with adhesive tape across the palm. Do not over-extend the wrist.
  - An US-guided approach (with the zoom function useful in neonates) is useful, particularly in neonates and infants.
  - Palpation of the arterial pulsation can also be used to identify the artery.
  - Using an aseptic technique, with either palpation or US guidance, an over-the-needle IV cannula (24 or 22 G) is used for cannulation. A 22 G cannula can then be exchanged, using the Seldinger technique, for a more kink-resistant and easy-to-secure arterial line.
  - Remove the plastic bung from the hub of the IV cannula needle. Flush the needle with sterile saline.
  - Insert the needle at an angle of 45° or less.
  - On puncturing the radial artery, a flashback is observed, but not necessarily pulsatile flow. Flatten the angle of insertion and advance the needle tip another 2–4 mm

- Withdraw the needle, leaving the cannula in situ. If the cannula immediately fills with blood as the needle is withdrawn, advance the cannula into the vessel over the needle. If not, hopefully the vessel is transected. Take a straight guide wire such as the soft tip spring-wire guide from the ARROW arterial catheterization set. Slowly withdraw the cannula, keeping it fairly flat against the skin. When there is a steady drip of blood out of the cannula, insert the guidewire. There will not necessarily be a pulsatile flow of blood as the cannula is withdrawn. Complete the line insertion over the guidewire and remove the wire
- Connect the transducer set; aspirate before flushing to ensure that there are no bubbles

Long lines

- Cannot be used for blood sampling (although they may bleed back, especially at the time of insertion). They are used for IV fluid and medication administration, e.g. antibiotics. They are not generally suitable for parenteral nutrition or chemotherapy.
- They last about a week. If the need for IV access is expected to be >1 week, consider a PICC line.
- Long lines are inserted via a peripheral vein using the Seldinger technique. As their name suggests, they are longer than a peripheral IV cannula, but they are not central catheters and, unlike PICCs, they are not cut to the desired length.
- Available in a range of sizes, e.g. 4 cm, 6 cm, 8 cm, and 20 cm Vygon 22 G Leaderflex catheters.
- A standard peripheral IV cannula is usually inserted first and then the guidewire is inserted via the cannula. The soft-tip flexible guidewire from the 22 G Leaderflex kit can be inserted via a 24 G peripheral IV cannula. If the guidewire meets an obstruction, try altering the position of the limb. It is also possible to create a small 'J' at the end of the wire with a finger and thumb and a pulling motion. Gently rotate the wire between finger and thumb to negotiate the tip past the obstruction.

Intraosseous vascular access

Equipment

- The ARROW EZ-IO interosseous (IO) vascular access system includes a battery operated hand-held driver (drill) with a magnetic tip that attaches to a 15 G IO needle. The ARROW EZ-IO is not used for IO access via the sternum.
- Selection of needle length is based on clinical judgement following an estimate of the depth of soft tissue overlying the insertion site.
- The needles are associated with the following patient weight ranges:
  - 15 mm, pink: 3-39 kg
  - 25 mm, blue: >3 kg
  - 45 mm, yellow: >40 kg.

Sites

- Proximal humerus: 1–2 cm above the surgical neck of the humerus over the most prominent part of the greater tubercle. Needle insertion 45° to the coronal plane directed posterior and medial.
- Proximal tibia: 1 cm medial to the tibial tuberosity. Needle insertion perpendicular to the surface of the bone.
- Distal tibia: 1–2 cm proximal to the medial malleolus. Needle insertion perpendicular to the surface of the bone.
- Distal femur: knee extended, the insertion point is just proximal to the patella and 1–2 cm medial to a line passing through the middle of the femoral shaft in the sagittal plane. Needle insertion perpendicular to the surface of the bone.

Contraindications

- Fracture of the target bone.
- Infection at the insertion site.
- IO access, or attempted access, in the target bone within the previous 48 h.
- Inability to identify the landmarks.
- Orthopaedic prosthesis, or orthopaedic procedures, near the insertion site.

Technique

- Aseptic non-touch technique.
- Skin preparation with 2% chlorhexidine in 70% isopropyl alcohol and allow to dry.
- Prime the EZ-Connect Extension Set with 1 mL of saline.
- Attach a needle of a suitable length to the driver—the driver has a magnetic tip that attaches to the needle hub.
- Insert the needle through the soft tissues and make contact with the bone. Check that the 5 mm black mark closest to the hub is visible above the skin. If it is not visible, select a longer needle.
- Squeeze the trigger on the driver and apply the minimum amount of pressure to advance the needle. This should be gentle allowing the driver and needle to do the work.
- Stop drilling when there is loss of resistance.

- Avoid any recoil movement when drilling is stopped.
- Hold the hub of the needle and remove the driver.
- Remove the stylet from the needle and discard into a sharps container.
- Apply the EZ-Stabilizer Dressing over the hub.
- Attach the EZ-Connect Extension Set.
- Aspirate bone marrow and blood. It may be necessary to flush the needle before aspiration is possible. The sample can be sent to the laboratory (label as an IO sample).
- A rapid flush of 2–5 mL saline is essential to facilitate fluid infusion.
- Fluid has to be infused under pressure: syringe by hand, infusion pump, or pressure bag.
- Any medication that can be given via a peripheral IV cannula can be given IO.
- Pain on infusion may be a problem in awake patients. It is treated with an initial dose of 0.5 mg/kg 2% lidocaine IO given over 2 min; systemic analgesic may also be required.
- The most common complication is infiltration and extravasation, with the risk of compartment syndrome. The infusion site needs to be closely monitored.

Regional anaesthesia

Steve Roberts

Overview and safety

- The advantages of excellent intra- and postoperative analgesia, and opioid-sparing effects should make the use of an LA technique mandatory unless there are specific contraindications.
- In the UK, virtually all blocks in children are performed under GA. The principle concern with this is the masking of signs and symptoms of intravascular and intraneural injection.
- Compared with central blocks, peripheral nerve blocks (PNBs) provide more profound and targeted analgesia, greater suppression of the stress response, a safer profile, and are more acceptable to patients and parents.
- Ultrasound (US) is a superior method of delivering effective and safer regional anaesthesia, allowing real-time needle guidance, ↑ success rates and ↓ doses of LA. US imaging in children is generally of higher quality than in adults, since nerves are more superficial, thus allowing the use of higher frequencies.
- When learning US techniques, initially use saline to confirm needle tip position.
- The main complication is a failed block. It is therefore prudent to take a balanced approach to analgesia, i.e. also administering paracetamol and an NSAID. Equally this will help postoperative pain due to non-surgical reasons, e.g. sore throat or headache.
- Preoperatively, a history is taken to elicit contraindications to LA techniques. If possible, the area where the block is to be sited should be examined. Note the patient's weight to calculate the maximum safe dose of LA.
- Absolute contraindications:
  - Patient or parent refusal
  - Local infection
  - Allergy to LA.
- Relative contraindications (block-dependent):
  - Anticoagulation
  - Neuromuscular disease
  - Risk of masking a compartment syndrome (discuss with surgeon)
  - Systemic sepsis.
- Verbal consent should be documented and recorded in the anaesthetic record, together with, where age-appropriate, assent from the patient. Common or serious complications/side effects should be discussed.
- Attempt to explain postoperative block sensations to the child, e.g. 'pins and needles', since they can find paraesthesias upsetting. Warn parents that their child may well find this initially upsetting when they emerge from the GA.
- Discuss a 'plan B' should the block fail.
- Safe nerve blockade requires a thorough knowledge of anatomy, IV access, standard monitoring, appropriate equipment, and aseptic precautions (this is assumed for all blocks described).
- Stop Before You Block—double-check operative site marking and consent form, just before the needle is inserted.

- Use a short-bevelled needle. It is helpful to first nick the skin to avoid missing the feel of the underlying fascia during the puncture. A 50 mm long 22 G needle is usually appropriate in most situations.
- Use the safest LA, e.g. levobupivacaine or ropivacaine.
- Adequate analgesia is usually achieved with a concentration of 0.25%.
- In infants, a lower LA concentration of 0.125% is as effective owing to the non-myelinated nervous system.
- 0.125% is used where there is a risk of compartment syndrome.
- Higher concentrations, e.g. 0.5%, can be used where postoperative muscle spasm is a major problem.
- The practice of incremental slow injection with repeated aspiration is mandatory.
- The calculated maximum LA dose should never be exceeded.
- Consider how GA maintenance is provided: N_2O and remifentanil can mask block failure.
- PNB are prolonged by the IV administration of dexamethasone and/or an α_2 agonist, e.g. clonidine, intraoperatively.
- A failed block should be readily recognized intraoperatively. Consider whether the surgery has extended into a non-blocked dermatome, requiring a rescue block, LA infiltration, or IV analgesia.
- In the recovery area, it can be difficult to differentiate between pain and agitation. If in doubt, assume the former.
- Awake regional techniques may be useful for ex-premature neonates undergoing hernia repair, or in older children with, e.g., difficult airway or MH. Patient, parents, and staff need briefing on what is expected from them. A soother dipped in sucrose may help a neonate. For older children, distraction by a play specialist or electronic device may help. Entonox or a mild sedative may also be useful.
- Continuous catheters are useful where prolonged blockade is desirable:
  - To facilitate physiotherapy regime
  - Major surgery
  - Chronic-pain patients.
- Catheter dislodgement is overcome by subcutaneous tunnelling and skin glue; this ↓ LA leak, which lifts the dressing off.
- Commonly 0.1–0.125% levobupivacaine is used for PNB infusions. For central blocks, an opiate or clonidine may be added to the LA solution.
- Provide verbal and written postoperative instructions.

LA toxicity

- Often presents as cardiovascular collapse.
- ECG may show T-wave morphology or ST-segment changes.
- Follow AAGBI guidelines:
  - Start CPR and follow resuscitation guidelines and Intralipid.
  - If there are signs of toxicity but no cardiac arrest, treat with standard drugs and consider use of Intralipid:
  - Intralipid® 20% 1.5 mL/kg over 1 min and an infusion of 15 mL/kg over 1 h.
  - After 5 min, if there is cardiovascular instability:
    —Give a maximum of two repeat boluses (same dose, 5 min apart).
    —And double the infusion rate.

Infiltration and field block

Indications
- Where a specific nerve or plexus block is contraindicated.

Contraindications
- General.

Anatomy
- LA is injected subcutaneously or intradermally.

Technique
- Infiltration involves injecting LA subcutaneously into the wound edges.
- A field block involves the injection of LA into the skin around the surgical site.
- After initial aspiration of the syringe, the needle is kept moving as LA is injected, thus minimizing the risk of intravascular injection.
- It is usually best performed preoperatively with the benefit of allowing a lighter plane of GA. However, this may distort the wound, e.g. the vermillion border of the lip.
- Alternatively, LA is injected or instilled into the incision prior to closure. If this technique is used, a gradual emergence from GA is preferred to allow the LA to take effect.
- In awake patients, injection can be painful. This is minimized by distraction techniques, application of a topical LA, e.g. EMLA (lidocaine/prilocaine) or LET (lidocaine, epinephrine (adrenaline), and tetracaine mix), warmed LA, use of a 27 G needle and slow injection.

Complications
- Intravascular injection
- LA toxicity
- Haematoma.

Ilioinguinal/iliohypogastric nerve block

Indications
- Herniotomy
- Orchidopexy (if a low scrotal incision is made, supplement with infiltration or pudendal nerve block)
- Varicocele ligation
- Hydrocele.

Contraindications
- General
- Relative: obstructed hernia.

Anatomy
- Both nerves originate from the primary ventral ramus of L1. The iliohypogastric runs superior to the ilioinguinal nerve.
- The nerves lie between the internal oblique muscle (IOM) and transversus abdominis muscle at the level of the anterior superior iliac spine (ASIS).
- At the level of the ASIS or more ventrally, the iliohypogastric nerve pierces the IOM to lie beneath the external oblique muscle (EOM).
- The distance between the ASIS and the nerves is not related to age or weight. Both cadaver and US studies show the nerves to be closer to the ASIS than traditional techniques assume.

Top tips
- Does not provide visceral analgesia; simple analgesics must be given preoperatively or intraoperatively.
- The numerous methods described and the 10–25% failure rate suggest that this is not a simple block to perform successfully. This is due to anatomical variation between patients.
- Patient supine.
- Note: to avoid laryngospasm, keep a deep plane of GA until peritoneal, spermatic cord, or testicular manipulation, is complete since the stimulation from these manoeuvres will not be blocked.

US technique
- Probe is placed on a line between the ASIS and the umbilicus, resting the lateral end of the probe on the ASIS. Either an out-of-plane (OOP) or an in-plane (IP) needle–probe alignment is effective.
- Similar doses as used for landmark technique can lead to higher plasma levels of LA. Therefore, use a smaller (but equally effective) volume of LA <0.2 mL/kg.

Landmark technique
- The needle is inserted perpendicular to the skin at a point 2.5 mm medial along a line between the ASIS and the umbilicus.
- A single fascial click is advised (50% of patients have only two muscles at the level of the ASIS). This ↓ the risk of intraperitoneal injection (average nerve–peritoneum distance is 3.3 mm).
- 0.25% levobupivacaine 0.3–0.5 mL/kg is injected slowly.

Complications
- Femoral nerve block (in up to 11% of patients). Test for prior to discharge. US may ↓ this risk.
- Intraperitoneal injection with possible bowel perforation.

Rectus sheath block

Indications
- Umbilical and periumbilical surgery, e.g. pyloromyotomy.

Contraindications
- General.

Anatomy
- The rectus muscles extend from the xiphisternum to the pubis. In infants, they are only a few mm thick.
- A fascial sheath encloses each rectus muscle. The sheath is formed by the combination of the aponeuroses of the lateral abdominal muscles (EOM, IOM, and transversus abdominis).
- The posterior wall of the sheath is loosely connected to the rectus muscle, allowing LA to spread.
- The rectus muscle is divided into three parts by intertendinous intersections. These are found at the level of the xiphisternum, at the umbilicus, and halfway between the two.
- The lateral border of the rectus muscle is called the semilunaris. In small infants, it may be difficult to define.
- The rectus muscles meet in the midline—the linea alba.
- The 9th–11th intercostal nerves penetrate the sheath to supply the periumbilical skin.

Technique:
- No visceral analgesia, simple analgesics must be given preoperatively or intraoperatively.
- Remember this is a bilateral block.
- Patient is supine.

US technique
- Recommended.
- Easier to perform the side closest to the operator first (Fig. 11.1).
- Using a flat trajectory the needle is guided IP (lateral to medial) so the tip is just anterior to the posterior sheath.
- A 'give' may not be felt: assess needle tip position with a small injection of LA—the posterior sheath should be seen to peel off the muscle.
- Use 0.1–0.3 mL/kg/side.

Landmark technique
- The needle is inserted just medial to the semilunaris at the umbilical level. The needle is inserted at an angle of 60°, aiming towards the umbilicus. If the semilunaris is not identifiable, then insert the needle 2–3 cm lateral to the umbilicus. The needle is felt to 'pop' as it passes through the anterior sheath into the rectus muscle.
- The needle tip needs to reach the space between the muscle and the posterior sheath, since this allows optimal spread of LA. This is felt as a 'scratch' by gently moving the needle from side to side.

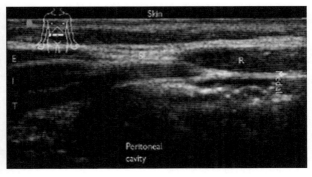

Fig. 11.1 Ultrasonographic appearance of the rectus sheath, external oblique muscle (E), internal oblique muscle (I), transversus abdominis muscle (T), rectus muscle (R) and semilunaris (SL).

- Volume of LA is 0.2–0.4 mL/kg/side.
- The depth of insertion is not related to age or weight, in children <10 years of age, the needle should not be inserted perpendicularly beyond 1 cm.

Complications
- Haematoma
- Visceral puncture.

Transversus abdominis plane (TAP) block

Indications

- No visceral analgesia, simple analgesics must be given preoperatively.
- The standard approach does not generally spread more cephalad than T10.
- Unilateral indications:
  - Open appendicectomy
  - Stoma closure
  - Open cholecystectomy (subcostal TAP)
  - Inguinal herniotomy
  - Iliac crest graft
  - Laparoscopic nephrectomy.
- Bilateral indications:
  - Laparoscopic appendicectomy
  - Laparotomies with infraumbilical incisions crossing the midline.

Contraindications

- General.

Anatomy

- The anterior branches of the spinal nerves form a plexus between the two innermost lateral muscles: the transversus abdominis muscle and the IOM.

US technique

- Patient is supine.
- Linear US probe is placed transversely over the midaxillary line halfway between the subcostal margin and the iliac crest.
- Count the lateral muscle layers from inside to out; this prevents potential confusion in obese patients, where there may be fascial planes within the adipose tissue.
- The needle approach is IP from anterior to posterior. The needle tip must be placed within the TAP at a point where the TA is inserting posteriorly.
- It may be difficult to place the tip between within the TAP, and it is sometimes useful to place the tip of the needle in the TA muscle and start injecting as the needle is withdrawn

Complications

- Haematoma
- Visceral puncture.

Pectus blocks

- PEC 1 block targets the pectoral nerves; it is suitable for surgery on the pectoralis major muscles.
- PEC 2 block targets the lateral and possibly the anterior spinal nerve branches and, in conjunction with PEC 1, is suitable for more extensive surgery.

Indications

- Pacemaker insertion
- Portacath (consider a superficial cervical plexus block for neck incision)
- Gynaecomastia surgery.

Contraindications

- General.

Anatomy

- Lateral (C5–7) and medial (C8–T1) pectoral nerves supply the clavicular head of the pectoralis major and the sternocostal head of the pectoralis major and pectoralis minor, respectively. They travel between the pectoralis major and minor muscles.
- T2–6 spinal nerves give off anterior and lateral branches. The branches pierce the intercostal and serratus anterior muscles. The anterior branches innervate the medial chest wall. The lateral branches emerge at the mid-axillary line, dividing into anterior and posterior cutaneous branches.

US technique

PEC 1

- Patient is supine.
- Probe is placed in a paramedian subcoracoid position. It is often useful to rotate the probe to an oblique superomedial–inferolateral axis.
- Identify the 2nd rib is directly under the axillary artery; then count down to the 3rd rib.
- Identify the pectoralis minor and pectoralis major muscles.
- The lateral pectoral nerves are adjacent to the pectoral branch of the thoracoacromial artery (found between the pectoral muscles).
- Use an IP needling technique from cephalad to caudad, placing the needle tip between the pectoral muscles.
- Inject 0.3–0.5 mL/kg of LA.

PEC 2

- Blocks T2–4 and long thoracic nerves.
- Continue needle to fascial plane between the pectoralis minor and serratus anterior.

Complications

- Haematoma
- Pneumothorax.

Penile nerve block

Indications
- Circumcision
- Distal hypospadias repair (discuss with surgeon).

Contraindications
- LA containing adrenaline (epinephrine).

Anatomy
- The ilioinguinal and genitofemoral nerves supply the penile base.
- The dorsal penile nerves (S2–4) supply the remainder of the penis.
- The dorsal nerves pass under the pubic ramus within the subpubic space.
- The subpubic space is divided into left and right compartments by the suspensory ligament. In 6% of patients, the left and right interconnect.
- The anterior border of the subpubic space is formed by Scarpa's fascia.
- The dorsal penile arteries and superficial and deep veins are in the midline. The dorsal nerves run just lateral to these vessels.
- The dorsal penile nerves run close to and either side of the suspensory ligament.
- The ventral branches of the dorsal penile nerves originate in the subpubic space.

Technique: subpubic block
- Advantage of this method is ↓ risk of neurovascular or corpus cavernosum damage.
- Patient is supine.
- A neonatal spinal needle is useful for small children.
- Do not use sharp bevelled needles or artificially blunted needles.
- Locate the symphysis pubis in the midline.
- The penis is pulled down ensuring the subpubic skin is taut.
- The needle is inserted **just** through the skin in the midline. Aim the needle posteriorly, 10° caudal and 10° lateral.
- A slight 'pop' is felt as the needle first breaches the superficial fascia, then a more definite 'pop' is felt on traversing the deep (Scarpa's) fascia at a depth of 8–30 mm.
- Depth of insertion is independent of patient weight or age.
- Withdraw the needle to just under the skin and redirect it to the contralateral side.
- 0.5% levobupivacaine 0.1 mL/kg each side, maximum 5 mL each side. The volume injected is limited to ↓ the possibility of vascular compromise.
- Additionally, always subcutaneously infiltrate LA into the ventral aspect of the penis at the penile-scrotal junction.

Complications
- Superficial haematoma
- Deep haematoma potentially causing vascular compromise and ischaemia

Paravertebral block

- Thoracic approach produces unilateral sympathetic and somatic block of spinal nerves, covering at least five dermatomes.
- Lumbar approach results in two dermatomes being covered.

Indications

- Unilateral:
  - T6–7 thoracotomy
  - T8–9 renal surgery
  - L1–2 hip surgery.
- Bilateral:
  - T3–4 sternotomy
  - Pectus surgery (catheters preferable).

Contraindications

- Same as for central blocks.

Anatomy

- The thoracic paravertebral space is a wedge-shaped area either side of the vertebral column.
- It is continues laterally with the intercostal space. The medial border is the lateral aspect of the vertebral column.
- Bordered anteriorly by the parietal pleura.
- Bordered posteriorly by the transverse processes, ribs, and costotransverse ligament.
- The space communicates caudally to T12, where the psoas is adherent. Below T12, the space is segmental.
- The spinal nerve roots emerge from the intervertebral foramen and divide into dorsal and ventral rami. In addition, sympathetic fibres of the ventral rami enter the sympathetic trunk via the preganglionic white rami communicantes and the postganglionic grey rami communicantes in this space.

Landmark technique

- Patient is in lateral position, operative side uppermost.
- 18 G (19 G for neonates) Tuohy needle.
- The needle is inserted lateral to the chosen spinous process. This lateral distance approximates to the distance between the tips of the spinous processes (1–2 cm).
- The depth in mm is estimated as 0.48 × body weight/kg + 18.7.
- The space is located with a loss-of-resistance technique through the costotransverse ligament. The end point is not as definite as with the epidural space.
- As the needle is advanced, it may contact the transverse process, in which case the needle is walked off the superior aspect into and through the costotransverse ligament.
- A single injection of 0.25% levobupivacaine 0.5 mL/kg.
- A catheter can be threaded (no more than 3 cm beyond the needle tip).
- A catheter can also be placed under direct vision during surgery.

Thoracic US technique

- Place the probe in a transverse plane over the spinous process.
  A longitudinal paramedian probe position is not feasible in infants since
  the ribs are too close together.
- Move the probe laterally and slightly angled to fit the space between the
  ribs. The transverse process and the pleura should be identified. The
  costotransverse ligament is then identified.
- IP needling is directed from lateral to medial, aiming to pierce the
  costotransverse ligament. Do not insert the needle behind the
  transverse process: this limits the risk of puncturing a dural cuff.
- A successful injection displaces the pleura anteriorly.
- Post injection, rotate the probe into a paramedian longitudinal position
  and assess caudad and cephalad spread.

Lumbar paravertebral block

- Two spinal roots can be blocked at a time by injecting above and below
  any given transverse process.
- The needle is guided onto the process and then walked off and inserted
  a further 1 cm.

Complications

- Vascular puncture
- Pneumothorax
- Horner syndrome
- Epidural or spinal injection.

Digital nerve blocks

Indications
- Finger and toe surgery, e.g. nail bed repair.

Contraindications
- LA containing adrenaline (epinephrine)

Anatomy
- The digital nerves of the fingers are derived from the radial and ulnar nerves dorsally, and the median and ulnar nerves ventrally.
- Dorsal and ventral nerves on the medial and lateral aspect innervate each finger. They are positioned at 2, 5, 7, and 10 o'clock in relation to the phalanx.

Technique: ring block
- The needle is inserted lateral to the extensor tendon. The needle is directed subcutaneously along the side of the phalanx until the volar skin surface tents. The syringe is aspirated and, as the needle is with-drawn, LA is injected.
- The needle is removed and reinserted medial to the extensor tendon and the process repeated.

Technique: metatarsal/carpal block
- When the operative site is at the base of the digit, a metacarpal or metatarsal block can be performed. The needle is inserted at 90° to the skin between the metacarpals/tarsals approximately midway along the bone.
- The needle is advanced until resistance from the palmar aponeurosis is felt. After aspiration, LA is injected as the needle is withdrawn. The process is repeated on the other side.

Dose
- 0.25% levobupivacaine 1–2 mL/side.

Complications
- Ischaemia of the digit. This is prevented by avoiding adrenaline in the LA and limiting the volume injected.

Axillary brachial plexus block

- Transarterial approach is not advised.

Indications
- Hand, wrist, or forearm surgery.

Contraindications
- General.

Anatomy
- Within the axilla, the three cords form the four main nerves: median, musculocutaneous, radial, and ulnar.
- The axillary and musculocutaneous nerves depart from the sheath around the level of the coracoid process.
- With the patient supine, the classic nerve distribution in relation to the artery has the median and musculocutaneous nerves lying superior, the ulnar nerve inferior, and the radial nerve posterior. However, US assessment in adults shows great variability in nerve distribution.

Technique
- Patient is supine with elbow flexed and arm abducted to 90°. Hand rests on or is taped to pillow.
- US probe is placed transversely; use either OOP or IP needling. Aim to surround all four nerves, starting with the deepest first.
- If no US is available, palpate the axillary artery as proximal as possible within the axilla. The needle is inserted (with a slight cephalad angulation) just above the artery and then redirected below the artery.
- The initial insertion aims to produce a fascial click on entering the sheath, and stimulates the median nerve (wrist flexion and pronation, flexion of the first fingers should be observed). Half of the total volume of LA for the block is injected.
- Redirection of the needle again elicits a fascial click and stimulates the radial nerve (wrist and finger extension should be observed) with a current of 0.3–0.5 mA. The remainder of the LA is injected.
- A total volume of 0.5 mL/kg of LA (0.25% levobupivacaine ± 1:200,000 adrenaline (epinephrine))
- When inserting a continuous nerve catheter, a more cephalad needle direction will aid threading.

Complications
- Arterial puncture with possibility of vascular occlusion
- Haematoma
- Intravascular injection
- Nerve damage.

Supraclavicular brachial plexus block

Indications
• Surgery on the elbow and upper arm.

Contraindications
• General
• Contralateral phrenic or recurrent laryngeal nerve palsy
• Relative: previous neck surgery, contralateral pneumothorax.

Anatomy
• The nerve roots of the plexus travel between the scalene muscles, forming the trunks in the lower half of the posterior triangle of the neck.
• The plexus lies slightly cephalad and posterior to the subclavian artery.
• The trunks become divisions prior to passing beneath the clavicle.

Ultrasound technique
• Patient is supine with the arm by their side, and head turned slightly contralaterally.
• A head ring is useful to stabilize the head. In small children, a small roll between the shoulders improves access to the posterior triangle.
• When performing a right-sided block, a right-handed anaesthetist should stand at the head of the bed with the US machine on the patient's left.
• A linear transducer of ≥10 MHz is placed behind and parallel to the clavicle, looking down into the chest. Unless the child's neck is too small, a large probe (50 mm) is preferable since it encourages a shallow needle trajectory.
• Firstly, the subclavian artery lying on the first rib is identified; beneath the rib, the cervical pleura and lung are visualized. The brachial plexus is located between the anterior and middle scalene muscles, superficial and posterolateral to the subclavian artery (Fig. 11.2).

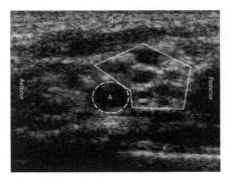

Fig. 11.2 Ultrasonographic appearance of the brachial plexus (dotted area) highlighting the proximity to the pleura (P), rib (R), and subclavian artery (A).

- IP needling is in a posterolateral-to-anteromedial direction.
- The pleura should be visible on screen at all times.
- The needle is guided into the sheath (a 'click/give' may be felt).
- Inject 0.1–0.3 mL/kg LA (e.g. 0.25% levobupivacaine ± 1:200,000 adrenaline (epinephrine)).
- For hand surgery, ensure the inferior trunk is blocked by guiding the needle tip where the brachial plexus is bordered by the first rib and subclavian artery—'pocket'.

Complications

- Pneumothorax
- Intravascular injection
- Nerve damage
- Phrenic nerve palsy
- Recurrent laryngeal nerve palsy and Horner syndrome are common side effects.

The potential complications mean that this block should only to be performed by experienced paediatric regional anaesthetists, preferably under US guidance.

Psoas block

- Aims to anaesthetize the lumbar plexus and some of the sacral plexus by injecting between the quadratus lumborum and psoas major muscles.
- Analgesia in the distributions of the obturator and femoral nerves and the lateral cutaneous nerve of thigh, with some upper branches of the sciatic plexus also affected.
- May be a good choice following previous hip surgery, since adhesions can limit the spread of LA through tissue plains required for efficacy of a 3-in-1 block or an illiacus sheath block.

Indications

- Unilateral hip, femur, thigh, or knee surgery.

Contraindications

- General as for central blocks.

Anatomy

- The lumbar nerve (and T12) roots' anterior rami enter the psoas and merge within it to form the lumbar plexus and the ilioinguinal, hypogastric, obturator, femoral, and lateral cutaneous nerves of the thigh.

Technique

- Use a PNS; do not paralyse the patient. US can be used to facilitate this block.
- Patient is positioned laterally with hips and knees flexed to 90°. Operative side is uppermost.
- Insertion point:
  - Identify point 5 cm lateral to the spinous process of L4, then 3 cm caudal from this point (cm in adults, fingerbreadths in children).
  - Alternatively, two-thirds of the distance down a line from the spinous process of L4 with the posterior superior iliac spine.
- An insulated needle is inserted perpendicular to the skin and advanced with a slight medial direction.
- The needle is advanced until it makes contact with the transverse process of L5, then 'walked off' the cranial border until either contractions of the quadriceps are visible (or a loss of resistance is felt as the needle exits the anterior edge of quadratus lumborum). Either of these end points should be reached <20 mm deeper than contact with the transverse process (Fig. 11.3).
- A nerve stimulator is attached to the needle and correct positioning is determined by contractions in the quadriceps femoris muscles at about 0.5 mA.
- This is a deep block, with the end point one and a half times the depth of the epidural space.
- LA is injected, with immediate loss of contractions.
- A catheter may be introduced into this fascial space.

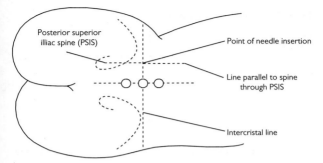

Fig. 11.3 Landmarks for psoas plexus block.

Dose
- 0.5 mL/kg of LA
- Maximum volume 30 mL.

Complications
- Epidural block from medial LA spread
- Retroperitoneal haematoma (rare)
- Dural cuff puncture and spinal anaesthesia (rare).

Femoral nerve block

Indications
- Fractured femur
- Surgery on anterior aspect of thigh or medial aspect of calf and ankle.

Contraindications
- General.

Anatomy
- The nerve is formed by L2–4 nerve roots.
- It enters the thigh beneath the inguinal ligament, lateral to the femoral artery.
- The nerve lies on the iliopsoas muscle and is deep to the fascia lata and fascia iliaca.

Technique
- Patient is supine.
- US probe just below and parallel to inguinal ligament. Check for branches of femoral artery using Doppler.
- OOP or IP needling.
- If no US is available, the needle is inserted perpendicular to the skin at a point 0.5 cm lateral to the femoral pulse and 0.5 cm inferior to the ilioinguinal ligament.
- The first 'click' felt is the fascia lata; this is followed by a second 'click' as the fascia iliaca is traversed.
- The accuracy of this technique may be improved by the use of a PNS. Contraction of the quadriceps is the desired end point.
- Volume of LA 0.1–0.3 mL/kg.
- If a 3-in-1 block is required, then use 0.5 mL/kg to allow medial and lateral spread (blocking the obturator nerves and lateral cutaneous respectively); cephalad spread towards the lumbar plexus is uncommon.
- For catheter techniques the needle should be angled 10–20° cephalad to allow threading of the catheter. Insert the catheter 1–3 cm beyond the needle tip.

Complications
- Arterial puncture
- Haematoma
- Intravascular injection
- Nerve damage.

Fascia iliaca compartment block

- Blocks the femoral, obturator, and lateral cutaneous nerve of the thigh with a single injection.
- The success rate is higher than that for a 3-in-1 block. The injection site is distant from nerves or vessels and a PNS is not required.

Indications

- Fractured femur
- Surgery on anterior and lateral aspects of thigh.

Contraindications

- General.

Anatomy

- The lumbar plexus forms the femoral, lateral cutaneous, and obturator nerves.
- The nerves pass through the iliac fossa in the potential space between the iliacus muscle and the fascia iliaca.
- The nerves become superficial at the inguinal ligament and pass beneath this in to the upper thigh. Here they are covered only by skin, subcutaneous fat, fascia lata, and the underlying fascia iliaca (which extends slightly beyond the iliac fossa beneath the inguinal ligament).
- LA injection deep to the fascia iliaca at this point may result in cephalad spread in the potential space between fascia iliaca and iliacus—blocking the three nerves in the iliac fossa.

Technique

- Patient is supine.
- Use a Huber tipped needle for catheter placement, since this provides the correct angle of insertion.
- If using a nerve catheter, angle the needle slightly cephalad and thread the catheter 2–3 cm beyond the needle tip after the second click.

US technique

- US probe in longitudinal paramedian plane just medial to ASIS.
- IP needling is from caudad to cephalad. LA is placed beneath the fascia iliaca.
- The LA can be seen to lift the fascia iliaca off the muscle. The needle is inserted into the LA space.
- This LA hydro-dissection process is repeated. Beware that the needle is directed cephalad towards the peritoneum.

Landmark technique

- Locate the ASIS and pubic tubercle. Divide the distance between these two points into thirds. Make a puncture in the skin 0.5 cm inferior to the junction of the medial two-thirds and lateral third of the line between the ASIS and pubic tubercle.
- The needle is inserted perpendicular to the skin. The initial 'click' is due to the fascia lata; a second 'click' is felt on passing through the fascia iliaca.

Dose

- Volume of LA 0.5–1.0 mL/kg. 0.25% levobupivacaine ± adrenaline (epinephrine) 1:200,000. Maximum 30 mL.

Complications

- Haematoma.

Ankle block

Indications
- Foot or toe surgery.

Contraindications
- General.

Anatomy
- The tibial nerve travels posterior to the medial malleolus, behind the posterior tibial artery. It supplies the medial heel, medial two-thirds of the sole, and the plantar aspect of the medial three and a half toes.
- The sural nerve travels midway between the lateral malleolus and the calcaneum, supplying the lateral aspect of the foot and little toe.
- The superficial peroneal nerve travels superficially over the lateral half of the ankle and the dorsal aspect of the foot. It supplies the dorsal aspect of the foot and toes, excluding the first web.
- The deep peroneal nerve is lateral to the anterior tibial artery and extensor hallucis longus tendon at the level of the malleoli. It supplies the first web space.
- The saphenous nerve passes anterior to the medial malleolus. It supplies the medial aspect of the ankle, rarely extending to the foot. Not necessary to block for most foot surgery.

US technique
- Select a small-footprint high-frequency probe. OOP or IP needling, depending on access.
- The tibial nerve is easily identified posterior to the posterior tibial artery and its accompanying veins.
- The deep peroneal nerve is identified by following the dorsalis pedis artery from mid fore foot to the level of the ankle joint where it sits on the navicular bone. The nerve is seen as a small ellipse crossing anterior to the artery from lateral to medial.
- The superficial peroneal nerve is identified more easily at the mid calf level. It is found subcutaneously in the groove between the lateral and anterior compartments.
- It is often difficult to identify the saphenous nerve: perform either a perivascular injection around the saphenous vein or a subsartorial block.
- It is may be difficult to locate the sural nerve; therefore, inject perivascularly around the short saphenous vein.

Landmark technique
- The posterior tibial nerve is blocked by inserting the needle posterior to the posterior tibial artery perpendicular to the skin.
- The sural nerve is blocked by inserting the needle at a point midway between the lateral malleolus and the calcaneum perpendicular to the skin.
- The deep peroneal nerve is blocked by inserting the needle lateral to the anterior tibial artery (at the intermalleolar level) perpendicular to the skin.

- The superficial peroneal is blocked by superficial infiltration between the two malleoli.
- The saphenous nerve is blocked by infiltration anterior to the medial malleolus in the region of the long saphenous vein.
- Blocks of the posterior tibial, sural, deep peroneal, and saphenous nerves at the ankle require about 2 mL of LA each. The wider infiltration to block the superficial peroneal may require 6–8 mL, depending on the size of the child. 0.25% or 0.5% levobupivacaine is usually used.
- Do not exceed maximum recommended LA dose.

Complications
- Haematoma
- Nerve damage.

Sciatic nerve block

- Cerebral palsy patients may prove difficult, since fixed flexion contractures may limit the use of PNS, and US anatomy may be difficult to interpret by the novice.

Indications

- Surgery on the posterior aspect of the thigh and the lateral aspect of lower leg.
- It is less suited to ankle and foot surgery, since a patchy block is possible (inner nerves not blocked owing to greater diffusion distance for LA).
- The saphenous nerve can supply sensation distal to the medial malleolus, up to the medial aspect of the great toe. Therefore, foot surgery may also require a saphenous or femoral nerve block.

Contraindications

- General
- Relative: risk of compartment syndrome.

Anatomy

- The sciatic nerve is actually two nerves within a common fascial sheath: the tibial and common peroneal nerves, originating from the lumbar and sacral plexuses (L4, L5, and S1, S2, and S3 roots).
- On leaving the pelvis via the greater sciatic foramen, the sciatic nerve passes midway between the greater trochanter and ischial tuberosity.
- The nerve travels deep to the gluteus maximus muscle.
- The posterior cutaneous nerve of the thigh lies superficial and medial to the sciatic nerve.
- The sciatic nerve divides into its two components approximately two-thirds of the way down the thigh. The level of division is variable.

US technique

- Patient is in recovery position with operative leg uppermost.
- Linear probe in transverse plane; nerve can be blocked at any point.
- A curvilinear probe may be required for obese adolescents.
- To locate the nerve, follow the fascial planes to a point just medial and level with the posterior border of the femur.
- To aid nerve identification, try scanning from lateral to medial with the probe in a longitudinal plane, seeking a narrow band of hyperechogenicity.
- OOP or IP needling. In obese patients, the former may be necessary.
- To block the posterior cutaneous nerve of the thigh, a subgluteal crease level or above is required.

Landmark technique
- Patient is supine with leg flexed at the hip.
- Locate the ischial tuberosity and greater trochanter. At the midway point insert the needle perpendicular to the skin.
- A PNS needle is used and is inserted until plantar or dorsiflexion of the foot is elicited.

Dose
- 0.25 or 0.5% levobupivacaine (± adrenaline (epinephrine) 1:200,000) depending on circumstances. Volume 0.1–0.3 mL/kg.

Complications
- Nerve damage.

Popliteal nerve block

Indications
- Any operation below the knee when combined with a saphenous or femoral nerve block, e.g. club foot surgery.
- Otherwise suitable for surgery on the lateral aspect of the leg, ankle, and whole of foot.
- As most surgery is under GA, tourniquet pain can be ignored.

Contraindications
- General
- Relative: risk of compartment syndrome.

Anatomy
- The popliteal fossa is bound superiorly by the semitendinosus and semimembranosus tendons medially and the tendon of biceps femoris laterally. The inferior border is demarcated by the medial and lateral heads of gastrocnemius.
- The fossa is divided in two by the popliteal crease or intercondylar line.
- The popliteal artery is palpated at the apex of the fossa.
- The sciatic nerve is found superficial and lateral to the artery.
- The division into tibial and common peroneal nerves is variable, and can occur as proximal as the piriformis muscle.
- US is the only reliable means of locating the division of the sciatic nerve.
- A US study in children located the nerve division 32–76 mm proximal to the knee joint. The nerves were 7–18 mm deep to the skin.

US technique
- Patient is prone or in recovery position (operative side uppermost).
- Linear probe in transverse plane.
- OOP or IP (lateral to medial).
- With children with femoral external rotation, it is possible to perform the block supine using an IP technique (medial to lateral).
- To aid definition of the nerves employ the 'See-saw' sign, dorsiflexing and plantarflexing the foot.
- Aim to place the needle tip at the division of the nerve, since this increases the available nerve surface area.
- An OOP needling technique works well for PNB catheter placement. Aim to place the catheter at the division just deep to the pre-popliteal fascia. Thread the catheter proximally up the length of the nerve.
- Threading usually meets some resistance.
- Catheter tip may be visualized; if not, try agitating the catheter or injecting saline.

Landmark technique

- Patient is prone or in recovery position (operative side uppermost).
- Insert the needle on a line between the midpoint of the popliteal crease and the apex of the popliteal fossa is identified.
- The popliteal artery is palpable. The needle is inserted perpendicular to the skin just lateral to the arterial pulsation.
- Plantar flexion and inversion indicates tibial nerve stimulation, dorsiflexion and eversion indicates common peroneal nerve.

Dose

- 0.3–0.5 mL/kg of 0.25% or 0.5% levobupivacaine.

Complications

- Nerve damage
- Vascular damage.

Caudal epidural block

- Easier in children than in adults, since:
  - The sacrum feels flatter and the angle of injection is easier, probably because the gluteal muscles are less bulky and the natal cleft lower.
  - The sacral hiatus is relatively large, since there is less ossification around the sacrococcygeal membrane (SCM).

Indications

- Infraumbilical surgery in infants:
  - Circumcision
  - Hypospadias repair
  - Inguinal herniotomy
  - Orchidopexy
  - Anorectal surgery
  - Lower limb surgery.

Contraindications

- General.
- Local skin changes, e.g. pigmentation, dimples, or hairy patches, are rarely associated with spinal dysraphism; US should be performed to exclude this.
- Mongolian blue spots are not a contraindication.

Anatomy

- See Figs. 11.4 and 11.5.
- The neonatal sacrum is composed of five cartilaginous sacral vertebrae that gradually ossify and fuse to form the adult sacrum.
- The sacral hiatus results from the failure of fusion of the posterior arches of the fifth, sometimes fourth, and occasionally third sacral vertebrae. This deficiency in the neural arch is covered by a ligament called the SCM.
- Anatomy changes with age:
  - Hiatus width toddler > neonate.
  - Antero-posterior diameter ↑ with age
- In neonates and infants, the pelvis is proportionally smaller than in adults and the sacrum is higher in relation to the iliac crests.
- As the pelvis grows, the position of the sacrum relative to the pelvis descends to the adult position by 4 years of age.
- The termination of the dural sac ascends from S3/4 at birth to S2 by 3 years of age.
- The posterior laminae begin to fuse around 7 years of age. The posterior wall is largely ligamentous until puberty.
- Ossification results in reduction in size of the hiatus. Bony fusion is complete by the late 20s.
- Sacral anomalies are found in 3–5% of individuals and can result in a reduced distance from the sacral hiatus to the dural sac.

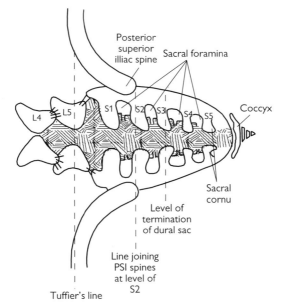

Fig. 11.4 Sacral anatomy in the neonate.

Technique

- Patient is in the lateral position with hips flexed to 90°.
- Styletted needles are used to avoid transporting into the epidural space skin plugs that may contain bacteria or dermal cells (potential for epidermoid tumour development).
- Cannulas are a popular alternative, since it is thought the blunt cannula tip reduces the chances of venous perforation, dural puncture, or damage to neural tissue.
- Finer needles cause less trauma, but may lead to false-negative aspiration tests.
- Select a 24 G cannula for a neonate or a 22 G for an infant.
- The hiatus can be considered a triangle whose base lies between the sacral cornua (inferiorly) and whose apex is formed by the fusion of sacral bones of the fourth vertebra (superiorly).
- Insertion point is the most cephalad point of the hiatus.
- The needle is gently inserted 90° to the skin. A pop may be felt as the SCM is penetrated. Usually, however, resistance is felt as the cannula touches the posterior surface of the sacral vertebral column.
- At this point, the needle angle should be flattened to approximately 20° to the skin.

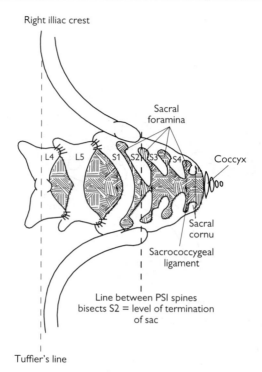

Right iliac crest

Sacral
foramina

L4   L5   S1 S2 S3   S4   Coccyx

Sacral
cornu

Sacrococcygeal
ligament

Line between PSI spines
bisects S2 = level of termination
of sac

Tuffier's line

Fig. 11.5 Sacral anatomy at 8 years old.

- Advance the needle 2–3 mm into the epidural space
- The needle is withdrawn and the cannula advanced. The cannula is left open to air for a few seconds to detect blood or CSF; this is then followed by an aspiration test.
- Much has been written about the relative merits of various tests to confirm a safe cannula position. None are 100% sensitive or specific and so LA should always be injected slowly and incrementally with ECG monitoring.
- US of the caudal space is simple, and effectively confirms epidural injection in children <2 years of age. Use a large linear probe (50 mm) and use a transverse and longitudinal midline position to observe the saline test injection (as little as 0.25 mL is readily visible). Once epidural position is confirmed, the LA is injected; the US is used to monitor the height of the spread real time.

Dose
- Usually 0.25% levobupivacaine is used, though 0.125% is often used <6 months of age.
- 0.5% may be used to provide a longer-lasting dense sacral nerve root block, e.g. hypospadias repair.
- Armitage formula for LA volume required to obtain a given block height:
  - 0.5 mL/kg sacral nerve roots
  - 1.0 mL/kg lower thoracic and upper lumbar nerve roots
  - 1.25 mL/kg mid-thoracic (T6) nerve roots.
- However, although 0.5 mL/kg consistently produce a sacral block, 1.25 mL/kg of LA may result in erratic and occasionally alarming cephalad spread! For this reason, it is more common to block thoracic dermatomes using a caudal catheter technique (➲ p. 226) or an intervertebral epidural (➲ p. 224).
- The Armitage guide is simplified to:
  - 0.3–0.5 mL/kg for sacral nerve roots
  - > 6 months 1 mL/kg of 0.25% bupivacaine will block upper lumbar nerve roots, i.e. the groin in children <20 kg (>20 kg, the technique becomes inconsistent at blocking these nerve roots).

Use of adjuncts to prolong LA effect
- Opioids, whilst effective, are not suitable owing to:
  - The risk (particularly in infants) of respiratory depression, though small, may present up to 12 h after administration.
  - Nausea, itch, and urinary retention.
- Clonidine (1–2 mcg/kg) has some effect in prolonging analgesia, but this may result from its systemic sedative and analgesic effects.
- Ketamine (0.5 mg/kg) significantly prolongs the duration of blockade. However, evidence of its neuroapoptotic effects have ↓ its use, especially in <1-year-olds. Where it is still used, a preservative-free preparation is advised.

Complications
- Failure—especially in children < 10kg, where difficulty in identifying the caudal hiatus occurs in about 10%
- Urinary retention (usually resolves spontaneously)
- Motor block
- Dural puncture
- Intravascular injection
- Rectal perforation.

Epidural block

- Less popular with the advent of US-guided peripheral nerve catheters.
- Despite enthusiasm, there is limited objective evidence that postoperative epidural analgesia is more effective than IV opioid analgesia after major surgery.
- Paediatric epidural catheters often have one end hole only and no side holes.

Indications

- Usually as an adjunct to GA, and for postoperative analgesia for thoracic, abdominal, or lower body procedures.
- Of most benefit after major surgery associated with protracted and severe postoperative pain.

Contraindications

- General.
- A ventriculo-peritoneal shunt is not a contraindication consider prophylactic antibiotics.

Anatomy

- The depth of the epidural space is extremely variable.
- Depth = 1 mm/kg for identification of the lumbar epidural space in children >1 year old (a rough guide).
- In young children, the spinal cord terminates at a lower vertebral level than in older children.

Technique

- Almost identical to the technique used in adults, apart from the fact that the child is usually anaesthetized.
- Approach may be caudal, sacral intervertebral, lumbar, or thoracic.
- Loss of resistance to saline is preferred to loss of resistance to air, which has resulted in air embolism and central neurological complications.
- The 'microdrip' method uses loss of resistance to an open saline drip, and allows both of the operator's hands to guide the Tuohy needle.
- In the lumbar region, the best angle for needle insertion is 74° cephalad. The very steep angles used for adult thoracic epidurals are unnecessary in younger children.
- The paramedian approach is possible. Here the needle is inserted slightly lateral to the midline, advanced to a lamina and then 'walked off' the superior edge of the lamina until the ligamentum flavum is reached.
- Checking of the catheter tip position may be by radiography, by US (in infants), or by Tsui's methods of ECG morphology or electrical stimulation (⊃ p. 226).
- Sacral intervertebral epidural block is possible because bony fusion of the sacrum is incomplete.
  - Easiest at S2/3 level just below the line joining the posterior superior iliac spines.
  - Angulation of the needle is unnecessary.
  - The distance to the epidural space is less because there is no lordosis.

Dose

- There is no perfect formula for LA dose.
- A reasonable initial bolus dose for a lumbar epidural is 0.7 mL/kg of 0.25% levobupivacaine.
- For postoperative infusions, most centres use 0.1% or 0.125% as a standard concentration ± fentanyl or clonidine.

Complications

- Fewer cardiovascular effects, owing to immaturity of the sympathetic system and lower vascular tone in small children.
- If hypotension does occur in the absence of bleeding, then suspect a subarachnoid or subdural catheter site.
- Hypotension more common >8 years of age.
- Bloody tap, especially if there is IVC obstruction or excessive spinal flexion at the time of insertion.
- Leak around catheters. Neonatal epidural catheter sites leak. This frequently leads to the dressing lifting off, with potential loss of the catheter. This can be minimized by tunnelling the catheter and using tissue glue to occlude the puncture sites.

Caudal catheter technique

- In neonates, it is possible to produce thoracic epidural blockade without having to perform an intervertebral approach.
- Fat in the epidural space of neonates and infants is loculated, with distinct spaces between individual lobules.
- A catheter introduced through the caudal hiatus reaches the desired thoracic position in 85% of premature neonates and 95% of term infants.
- It is less reliable with increasing age and the catheter often coils in the lumbar region. This is due to the development of the lumbar lordosis and the increasing density of epidural fat when lobules become more densely packed and are connected by fibrous strands.
- The epidural catheter is introduced via an IV cannula through the sacral hiatus and threaded cranially.
- The catheter is threaded up the epidural space to a distance estimated to correspond to the appropriate nerve roots for blockade. Often a greater length is required, since the catheter does not take a direct route.
- The catheter tip position is confirmed by:
  - X-ray
  - A styletted epidural catheter with an ECG adapter cathode at the hub allows electrical motor root stimulation from the catheter tip using a peripheral nerve stimulator. Observation of the truncal motor response (in an unparalysed patient) during catheter advancement indicates the level of the catheter tip.
  - US allows the catheter to be visualized as it is threaded up the epidural space.
  - Use a large-footprint probe: 50 mm.
  - A median and paramedian longitudinal probe position is required. If the tip is difficult to identify, try gently agitating it or inject 0.25 mL saline
- There is a greater risk of colonization compared with a thoraco-lumbar approach (with Gram-negative organisms), but actual infections are rare with short term use (< 72 h).

Subarachnoid (spinal) block

- Less common than epidural blockade, but is technically easy and carries a low risk of systemic toxicity from the small doses of LA used.

Indications

- Two groups are commonly considered for subarachnoid block:
  - Ex-premature neonates, who may prove difficult to extubate even after limited surgery, e.g. inguinal hernia repair. There is evidence that these patients experience a lower rate of postoperative apnoea after spinal blockade compared with GA. Apnoea may still occur after a spinal, so postoperative monitoring is the same as for GA.
  - Older children with muscular or neuromuscular disease who are at ↑ risk of the complications of GA. Performing a spinal block in these children is essentially the same as in adults: with a small amount of sedation, sensible 12-year-olds will cooperate sufficiently to allow successful spinal anaesthesia.
- Spinals do not provide postoperative analgesia.

Contraindications

- Procedures > 1 h (unless an epidural block is performed simultaneously).

Anatomy

- The spinal cord of the term neonate generally ends at the level of the L3 (possibly L4) vertebra.
- The volume of CSF in infants is 4 mL/kg (2 mL/kg in adults) with 50% being in the spinal canal compared with 25% in adults. These factors produce proportionately greater dilution of LA solution in the CSF in children than in adults and contribute to the shorter duration of subarachnoid anaesthesia in children.
- The depth of the subarachnoid space in the lumbar region is approximately 10 mm at birth and 16 mm at 3 years.

Technique

- Similar to adult subarachnoid block.
- Surgeon should be scrubbed and ready.
- Performed with the infant held in the sitting or the lateral position. This is largely a matter of personal preference. Care is taken to avoid flexing the neck and obstructing the airway.
- IV access is mandatory.
- A midline approach at L4/L5 or L5/S1 below the termination of the cord is easiest.
- Short pencil-point needle. Excessively fine needles are unhelpful, since speed of recognition of CSF flow is important in these patients, who will invariably attempt to move.
- The speed of onset in neonates is impressively fast. Similarly, the block wears off quickly, often regressing rapidly after 30–60 min. This is presumably partly due to the relatively greater CSF volume in neonates (➲ Chapter 1).

- It is common to perform a caudal block as well as a spinal to prolong the duration of analgesia.
- Assessing the block is difficult. The response to cold spray can be useful, as may observation of paradoxical respiratory muscle movement and loss of response to a low amperage tetanic stimulus.
- Spread of the block is less predictable than in adults, and high blocks are relatively common.
- The feet must not be raised above the head, e.g. when placing a diathermy pad, or a high block may be produced.
- Sedation is avoided because, like GA, it carries the risk of postoperative apnoeas.

Dosage

- Heavy bupivacaine is recommended in a dose of 0.3–1 mg/kg = 0.07–0.2 mL/kg of 0.5% solution.
- Lidocaine is relatively contraindicated since it produces a very short duration of anaesthesia and is associated with transient neurological symptoms.
- Spinal opiates may produce respiratory depression up to 18 h post administration and their use in children is rare.

Complications

- Relatively high failure rate of 10–20%.
- Although hypotension is rare, bradycardia occasionally occurs.
- Post-dural-puncture headache (PDPH) is rare in neonates, but persistent CSF leak has been described. Headache will not be reported, but irritability or other behavioural changes should raise suspicion.
- In older children, the incidence of PDPH is relatively high and probably under-recognized.
- Symptoms are more variable in children, who may experience dizziness, nausea or hearing loss more than headache.
- Bed rest probably only serves to delay the onset of any symptoms.
- The patient should be kept hydrated and given simple analgesics. Caffeine may be of benefit.
- Most PDPH resolve within 6 days with conservative management.
- Prophylactic epidural blood patch is not recommended unless conservative management fails (0.3 mL/kg of blood is taken with full asepsis). Blood patch is associated with side effects—back stiffness, paraesthesias, and subdural haematoma.

Further reading

℗http://www.euroespa.com/science-education/specialized-sections/espa-pain-committee/
us-regional-anaesthesia/
℗http://www.neuraxiom.com/

Section 4

Pain management

Pain and sedation

Acute Pain Service, Alder Hey Children's NHS Foundation Trust

Overview

- Babies and children feel pain in the same way adults do.
- Children have a right to effective pain management (Children's National Service Framework, DH2004).
- Nevertheless, they often do not receive analgesia in hospital and even less so at home.
- Pain management in children presents additional challenges:
  - The influence of age and immaturity.
  - Dose calculations based on both age and weight.
  - Dose formulations available and the palatability of medicines.
  - Restrictions on the marketing authorization/product licence of the medicine.
- A pragmatic approach to postoperative pain management includes:
  - Preventing predictable pain.
  - Recognizing pain.
  - Safely minimizing moderate to severe pain in all children.
  - Rapidly controlling and continuing to control pain after discharge from hospital.

Pain assessment

- Young children and those with developmental delay cannot communicate easily. Healthcare professionals need to use observational measures, behavioural measures, and parent report to identify pain.
- Pain assessment should exclude other reasons for distress and monitor efficacy of analgesia.
- Children can cry because they:
  - Are frightened.
  - Are hungry.
  - Are missing parents/family/friends/pets.
  - Want attention.
  - Have pain.
- Reassure the child you are there to help: this makes a huge difference and supports communication.
- The life experiences of children may be limited and this may impact on their ability to verbalize a painful experience.
- Ask the child:
  - Are you sore?
  - Where are you sore? Is it what you expect, e.g. abdominal pain following laparotomy; if not, investigate further.
  - What is the pain like, e.g. sharp? Remember the words they use may be different, e.g. 'headache in my tummy'.
  - How sore are you? (➔ 'Pain assessment tools' later in this section).
  - How frequently does the pain occur? If it 'comes and goes', this may indicate cramp or bladder spasm pain.
  - Most importantly—is this level of pain (whatever the score) 'okay' or does the child think they need more help. Everyone is individual and tolerance to pain is varied.
- Talk to the parents/carers—they know their child best. Ask if the child is:
  - Behaving as 'usual'.
  - Joining in conversations.
  - Playing with family/friends.
  - Doing things they enjoy.
  - Sleeping well.
  - Eating and drinking as their condition permits.
  - Mobilizing as their condition allows.
- Watch the child when they are moving, breathing, or being picked up and cuddled by their parent. Infants in pain may desaturate on being handled.
- Assess functionality as a measure of effective analgesia by, e.g., asking the child to breathe deeply after a thoracotomy or wriggle their toes after lower limb surgery.
- Never assume a child is pain-free because they are 'playing'—children are very good at distracting themselves.
- Children with complex and additional needs often report pain in a way not easily understood, e.g. self-harming, unusual movements (changing the position of a limb, licking lips, etc.). It is vitally important to discuss the child's individual pain behaviours with parents and carers. A special assessment tool is available—the Paediatric Pain Profile.

Pain assessment tools
- These tools provide an objective measure for a subjective experience. Self-report tools are the gold standard.
- An effective pain assessment tool is:
  - Quick and easy to use.
  - Valid and reliable.
  - Age and developmentally appropriate.
- The child should choose the tool they feel happiest using.
- No tool provides all the answers—use clinical acumen to ascertain a fuller picture.

C.R.I.E.S.
- Babies from 32 weeks' gestation.
- Behavioural/physiological parameters giving a score of 0–10:
  - Crying
  - O_2 required to maintain saturations >95%
  - Increased vital signs
  - Expression (grimace/grunt)
  - Sleeplessness.

F.L.A.C.C.
- 2 months–7 years.
- Behavioural/observational parameters giving a score of 0–10.
  - Facial expression
  - Legs—activity/position
  - Activity—general position/posture
  - Cry—none to constant
  - Consolable.

Faces
- From 3 years.
- Self-report using a series of faces identifying pain scores from 0 to 10.
- The tool must be explained properly.
- The child must have the capability of numerical reasoning.
- Useful when a patient needs some guidance rather than using a 'pain ruler' or visual analogue scale (VAS).
- Be aware younger children often make a rating primarily by matching their experience with the expression on one of the faces rather than selecting a point along an underlying continuum, e.g. a crying face because they are crying rather than in pain.

VAS
- From 4 years.
- Self-report.
- A line is divided into single or double gradations, and the child indicates where along the line their pain lies.
- Using the term 'worst pain possible' can be misleading; using 'the worst pain they have had' can be more useful.
- Remember children may think you will stop their painkillers if their pain score is low or will give them 'needles' or 'horrible medicine' if their pain score is high.

Paediatric Pain Profile
- For children with complex needs who are unable to communicate.
- Behavioural tool.
- Document held by parents/carers.
- Contains information regarding the child's behaviour related to:
  - The types of pain they experience
  - The types of behaviour they display depending on the origin of pain, e.g. moaning with abdominal pain, rigid leg and arms flaying with hip pain
  - Pain score on 'good days' and 'bad days'
  - Professionals already involved in their pain and general healthcare management
  - Read more at ℬ https://ppprofile.org.uk/

Acute pain management

- All ages of children experience pain in hospital; analgesics and non-pharmacological means of relieving pain are generally underused.
- Palatability of oral preparations is a factor in compliance.
- There is a reticence about using rectal analgesia in school-aged children, usually on the part of the nurse or parent, rather than the child.
- Consider PR route if child is NBM, nauseous, or refusing PO medication.
- A strict 6-hourly administration schedule does not usually fit with a child's normal sleep/wake cycle. Optimize analgesia during the day, but leave scope for as-required rescue analgesia overnight, e.g. paracetamol (QDS) at 07.00, 13.00, and 19.00. 4th dose PRN if wakes overnight in pain. Ibuprofen (TDS) at 07.00, 13.00, and 19.00

Paracetamol

- PO paracetamol is licensed for mild to moderate pain from 2 months of age (Box 12.1).
- Weight-based and age-banded doses are available.
- Age-banded doses (printed on the side of the bottle) may be conservative and may not provide adequate analgesia.
- There is a small possibility of toxicity in 'at risk' children given 90 mg/kg daily for >2 consecutive days.
- Maximum daily PO/PR dose is 75 mg/kg (maximum 4 g).
- Maximum daily IV dose is 60 mg/kg (maximum 4 g).
- Caution with obese children and those >12 years old who weigh <50 kg.

Box 12.1 Top tip

Standardize PO dose to 15 mg/kg (maximum 1 g) (in line with IV dosing). In challenging pain, optimize PO dose to 20 mg/kg (maximum 1 g) and review need for higher dosing every 24 h.

NSAIDs

- Ibuprofen is the first-line NSAID for acute pain because:
  - It is licensed from 3 months of age (>5 kg) for mild to moderate pain.
  - It is available as a palatable PO suspension (100 mg/5 mL).
  - Both weight-based and age-banded doses are available.
  - Weight-based dose of ibuprofen is 30 mg/kg daily (maximum 2.4 g) in three or four divided doses
- Diclofenac is the second choice owing to lack of a child-friendly formulation.
  - Suppositories are available in 12.5 mg and 25 mg doses, licensed from 6 years of age.
  - Doses of 150 mg/day are associated with a small increased risk of thrombotic events in adults.

Oral opioids

- Morphine is the preferred opioid for moderate to severe pain.
- PO morphine is licensed from 1 year of age.

- Below this age, the strength of the licensed liquid preparation (10 mg/5mL) means that accurate measurement of small doses is difficult, potentially leading to 10-fold errors.
- Specially manufactured solutions are available for smaller doses, e.g. 100 mcg/mL, 500 mcg/mL.
- In June 2013, the MHRA recommended restrictions on the use of codeine in children:
  - Only to be used for acute moderate pain in children >12 years if it cannot be relieved by paracetamol or ibuprofen alone.
  - Contraindicated in all children <18 years undergoing tonsillectomy or adenoidectomy for OSA.
- Tramadol is licensed from 12 years of age, and is not available in a licensed child-friendly formulation in the UK. Note that ondansetron may ↓ tramadol efficacy.
- Dihydrocodeine has poor analgesic activity in children.

PCA/NCA analgesia

- For the management of severe pain.
- Suitable for all age groups from 37 weeks gestation.
- Delivers a continuous infusion and boluses to meet individual need.
- Careful explanation is essential if it is to be useful to the individual.
- Nursing staff caring for children with PCA/NCA must receive additional training.
- Generally children >8 years old can use PCA; however, always consider:
  - Development, some younger children can use PCA well, whilst some older children find it difficult. Always assess the individual.
  - Patient's condition, e.g. PCA is impractical for a child who has both hands bandaged, or who is simply too unwell to manage their own pain relief.
  - Language barrier—may impede the ability to explain the concept of PCA.
- For optimal analgesia, prescribe regular paracetamol and NSAID (unless contraindicated).
- Parents should not use bolus button for PCA/NCA analgesia, since they do not have the ability to monitor and assess their child for adverse effects.
- Morphine toxicity in babies may present as myoclonic jerks, this may be misdiagnosed as pain and lead to inappropriate boluses of morphine.
- If boluses are ineffective, this may indicate pain is not the issue.
- Also prescribe:
  - Naloxone for respiratory arrest/depression
  - Ondansetron for PONV
  - Dexamethasone for PONV
  - Chlorphenamine for pruritus.
- Follow hospital guidelines.

Opioids and programmes

- Morphine is the first drug of choice (Table 12.1).
- Reasons to choose or change to fentanyl:
  - Poor analgesia (Table 12.2).

- Adverse effects, e.g. pruritus and vomiting.
- Renal failure: morphine metabolites are eliminated via the kidneys. Reduced kidney function can cause morphine metabolites to accumulate, and therefore fentanyl becomes the first-choice opioid.

Systemic adjuvants
- Used to complement and enhance acute pain management.
- They can complement a multimodal analgesia regime, can be opioid-sparing, or can help in reducing other issues commonly seen postoperatively, e.g. muscle spasms post multilevel orthopaedic surgery, or may help ↓ incidence of transition to chronic pain.

Gabapentin
- An antiepileptic well established in chronic and neuropathic pain management.
- Use as a part of a multimodal analgesia regime for complex and painful surgeries, e.g. spinal fusion, pectus repair, and patients with complex pain history.
- In acute pain setting it may ↓ postoperative opioid consumption.
- Dosage and duration should be locally agreed; author's recommendation is 10 mg/kg (maximum 300 mg) per dose.
  - Day 1: one dose preoperatively
  - Day 2: twice daily
  - Day 3, 4, and 5: three times a day
  - Stop on day 5 or on discharge, whichever is earlier.

Table 12.1 Morphine PCA/NCA programmes

Age	Concentration mcg/kg/mL	Infusion (mL/h)	Bolus (mL)	Lockout (min)
0–14 days OR <3 kg	10	0	0.5	30
2–12 weeks AND >3 kg	10	0.5	0.5	15
From 13 weeks	20	1	1	15
From 8 years	20	0.2	1	5

Table 12.2 Fentanyl PCA/NCA programmes

Age	Concentration (mcg/kg/mL)	Infusion (mL/h)	Bolus (mL)	Lockout (min)
From 13 weeks	1	1	1	30
From 8 years	1	0.5	0.5	10

- Dosages may need to be adjusted in patients with complex needs. 2.5 mg/kg (maximum 100 mg/kg) per dose, as per regime above.
- Commonest side effects are sedation, drowsiness, nausea and vomiting, and lethargy; dose may have to be adjusted or omitted depending on severity.

Ketamine

- Effective analgesic even at low doses.
- NMDA receptor antagonist.
- Was used with LA in caudal block, but it has been implicated in neuroapoptosis. Avoid in children <1 year of age for epidural blocks; some institutions avoid altogether.
- Commonly used IV bolus 0.1–0.3 mg/kg as part of multimodal analgesic regime for painful and major surgeries. Side effects are rare at these small doses.
- Infusions are reserved as second-line analgesic treatment, 0.05–0.2 mg/kg/h (ketamine 5 mg/kg (maximum 250 mg) made up to 50 mL with 0.9% sodium chloride).
- It can also be added to morphine PCA (1:1 concentration).
- Commonest side effects with infusions are hallucination (prescribe PRN diazepam), nystagmus, and mood swings.

Magnesium

- Mechanism of action is not fully understood; acts on NMDA receptor, as a cell membrane stabilizer and physiological antagonist to Ca^{2+}.
- Evidence is equivocal.
- Used in major general surgical, orthopaedic, and spinal fusion surgeries.
- May prevent muscle spasms post lower limb reconstruction.
- Dosage 30–100 mg/kg (maximum 4 g) given as slow IV infusion over 10–20 min.

Clonidine

- α_2-receptor agonist. Commonly used as an antihypertensive, but also has analgesic and sedative/anxiolytic properties.
- It can be administered as a single bolus IV 1–2 mcg/kg. This can prolong the duration of any LA technique administered.
- Also used as an adjuvant to paravertebral and central blocks to prolong their duration of action.
- When added to epidural solution, it can help in reducing intensity and severity of muscle spasms after multilevel orthopaedic surgery.
- Also can be given PO in the perioperative period or occasionally as an IV infusion.
- Commonest side effects are sedation, hypotension, nausea and bradycardia.

Diazepam

- Benzodiazepine used to alleviate muscle spasms in immediate postoperative period after multilevel orthopaedic surgery.
- Dosage 0.1 mg/kg 6-hourly as and when required.

Epidural analgesia

- Used as an adjunct to GA, providing pain management intra- and postoperatively.

- Paediatric epidural management should be heavily protocol-driven.
- Epidural solutions include:
  - levobupivacaine 0.125%
  - levobupivacaine 0.125% with clonidine 1 mcg/mL
  - levobupivacaine 0.1% with fentanyl 2 mcg/mL
- Epidural infusion rates are 0.1–0.3 mL/kg/h (maximum rate 15 mL/h).
- Children <13 weeks of age receive plain levobupivacaine 0.125%; owing to toxicity concerns, they are limited to a maximum of 48 h duration.
- Epidurals in children >13 weeks typically run for 3–4 days, depending on the extent of surgery and patient need. However, owing to infection concerns, the maximum duration is 7 days.
- Qualified nurses with additional training, skills, and experience should care for epidural infusions.
- Patients require regular monitoring and observation recording:
  - Hourly observation of:
    —HR
    —RR
    —BP
    —SpO$_2$
    —Pain score/assessment
    —LA toxicity
    —Sedation score
    —Infusion rate.
  - 4-hourly observation of:
    —Temperature
    —Motor block (Bromage score)
    —Nausea and vomiting
    —Pruritus.
  - 6-hourly observation of:
    —Epidural insertion site (redness/leaking/tenderness)
    —Dressing integrity (still covering epidural site)
    —Patency of IV access
    —Pressure area care.

Management of side effects
- Generally avoided by use of low-dose clonidine (1 mcg/mL) instead of an opiate additive.
- Nausea and vomiting: administer ondansetron ± dexamethasone, consider changing to opiate-free epidural solution.
- Pruritus: administer chlorphenamine and consider changing to plain or clonidine solution.
- Respiratory depression/sedation: consider naloxone—stat dose 4 mcg/kg, maximum 200 mcg (this dose reverses opioid side effects whilst maintaining analgesia). Consider changing to clonidine solution.
- Urinary retention: urethral catheterization.
- LA toxicity (➔ Chapter 11): signs include tinnitus, tingling around mouth, visual disturbances, light-headedness, and muscle twitching. Stop epidural immediately. Note that muscle twitching is the only sign a baby can show—stop infusion immediately if it occurs.

- Hypotension: usually hypovolaemia, but can occur with clonidine epidurals. Give fluid challenge and consider changing from clonidine solution.
- Pressure sore: pressure area care is vital owing to ↓ sensation and movement. Nursing care should be meticulous and it may be advisable to use a pressure-relieving mattress.

Problem-solving
- If you are asked to see a distressed child:
  - Assess pain: Where is the site of pain? Is it surgical pain? Is surgical review required? Is it cannula pain? Sore throat? NG tube? Urinary retention?
  - Leg pain: think compartment syndrome, refer for urgent senior surgical review.
  - Check block level. Is epidural on maximum rate? Is a bolus required?
  - If child <13 weeks of age and epidural is ineffective, the epidural must be removed prior to starting an NCA.
  - In child >13 weeks of age, a PCA/NCA can supplement incomplete epidural analgesia. Change the epidural solution to levobupivacaine ± clonidine.
- Epidural occlusion:
  - Is the catheter clamped?
  - Is it positional, i.e. it occurred 1–2 h after moving the patient? If so, change patient position to relieve obstruction
  - Is the catheter kinked? Can this be resolved by withdrawing the catheter 1–2 cm?
- Epidural leaking: an excessively leaking epidural may need removing if it is causing the sterile dressing to lift off. Can be avoided by tunnelling and gluing in situ at insertion.
- Any major change in motor block should be assessed to detect complications, e.g. spinal compression.

Continuous local anaesthetic nerve blocks
- For specific techniques, ➲ Chapter 11.
- Continuous PNB infusion is used to provide postoperative analgesia where prolonged analgesia is required, e.g. major lower limb surgery.
- Continuous LA solution is used: levobupivacaine 0.125%.
- Infusion rate 0.1–0.3 mL/kg/h (maximum 15 mL/h). However, if two PNB catheters are used (e.g. femoral and sciatic, bilateral PVB or TAP catheters), the infusion rate is reduced to 0.1–0.2 mL/kg/h (maximum 10 mL/h) per block.
- Currently no adjutants are added to LA solutions.
- Problem solving and monitoring for signs of LA toxicity and pressure sores are as for epidural care.

Management of transition to oral analgesia
- Prescribe regular simple analgesics and ensure they are administered prior to stopping the epidural.
- Stop the epidural at 07.00–08.00; leave it in place for 6 h to check the patient is comfortable prior to removal. If the patient is uncomfortable, restart and try again the following morning.

- Once the epidural has stopped, if the patient has had excellent analgesia, this might be their first experience of postoperative pain.
- On discharge, epidural advice should be given to patient, including signs of epidural abscess. Any signs of infection, e.g. pyrexia, back tenderness, or site redness/swelling/discharge, should be reviewed and brought to the attention of the on-call consultant anaesthetist to assess and rule out epidural abscess.

Transcutaneous electrical nerve stimulation (TENS)

- Safe and effective in young children who are able to understand its concept and control the settings (Box 12.2).
- Indicated for both acute and chronic pain.
- The type of stimulation delivered is thought to work in two ways:
  - On a high pulse rate of 90–130 Hz, A-beta sensory fibres are stimulated, activating the pain gate mechanism, reducing transmission of noxious stimulus from C fibres
  - A much lower rate of 2–5 Hz stimulates A-delta fibres, activating the release of endogenous opiates to ↓ activation of noxious sensory pathways.
- Most effective when worn for >30 min, and preferably all day.
- Electrode placement:
  - The TENS machine should be turned off before applying/removing the pads.
  - Pads can either be applied at the site of pain or either side of the spine at the appropriate dermatome.
  - Pads should be applied to clean/dry undamaged skin. Do not place them over the front/side of the neck, close to eyes, or internally.
- Suggested areas for pad placement:
  - Lower abdominal pain: T12
  - Back pain: at same level of pain either side of spine
  - Hip pain: L1
  - Knee pain or sciatica: L4
  - Pads can also be worn directly on the site of pain, although wearing them on the back seems to be better tolerated.
- Machine settings:
  - Modern TENS machines have various dials and switches to control current intensity, pulse rate/frequency, pulse width, and a selection of modes
  - A pulse width setting of 200 microseconds is standard and effective
  - Mode functions include burst, continuous, and modulation
  - It is unlikely that there is a single frequency or setting that works best for every patient; therefore, the patient should explore all settings.

Box 12.2 Top tip

Practice using the TENS machine with the patient by placing the pads on top of their forearm (or any site which is not painful) so they can explore the different settings prior to applying them to the site of their pain.

- Contraindications:
  - Pacemaker
  - Current or recent bleeding/haemorrhage
  - Caution in epilepsy
  - Do not use near water, e.g. the bath
  - Sleeping
  - Driving
  - During pregnancy, electrodes should not be used over the trunk, abdomen, or pelvis.

Procedural pain

- Clinical guidelines provide clear, effective pharmacological and non-pharmacological approaches to individual procedures, e.g. LP.
- They commonly combine all or some of the following: LA, sedatives (e.g. midazolam), analgesics (e.g. morphine or ketamine), and distraction techniques.
- Prepare all equipment prior to approaching the patient.
- Plan your approach, including best position and use of distraction.
- Involve the parent in terms of how they can assist their child.
- Be aware of the importance of your non-verbal cues and behaviours. A nervous patient will be assessing you as soon as you approach. Be calm, confident and engage them in small talk and/or humour to ↓ their perception of the threat.
- In the preschool child, focus on the parent first, since young children decide whether to trust you based on their parents' response.
- Always apply topical LA prior to any procedure involving needles unless contraindicated or patient preference.
- Topical LA can be used from birth.
- Mark the site where the topical LA is to be applied, especially where the preferred site is not obvious.
- Allow time for the topical LA to work.
- To reassure the child, demonstrate the LA effect by stroking a pen over the treated area and another patch of skin; ask if it 'feels different?' Avoid using the word 'numb', since this may heighten anxiety.
- In babies, oral sucrose/expressed breast milk (± sucking on a dummy) or breast feeding ↓ the behavioural response to painful procedures. Onset of action is approximately 2 min; dose can be repeated.
- Where there is no time to wait for topical LA, ethyl chloride spray provides rapid onset but short-acting (up to 10 s) anaesthesia. Only use in children who are old enough to be warned about the sensation of intense cold.
- Entonox® may be a useful adjunct providing anxiolysis, analgesia and amnesia. In older children, it can also give a sense of control over events.
  - No fasting required.
  - May cause deep sedation if given with other sedatives or where there is existing CNS depression.
  - Use in a well-ventilated quiet area with access to O_2, suction, and emergency drugs.
  - Child must be able to self-administer gas; encourage deep breaths 'like blowing out birthday candles'.
  - Contraindications:
    —Abnormal airway, e.g. tracheomalacia
    —Pneumothorax
    —Cough/cold or chest infection
    —Central or OSA
    —Intracranial air
    —Severe pulmonary hypertension
    —Previous allergy/adverse reaction to sedative/anaesthetic drugs

　—Child too distressed despite adequate preparation
　—Any child unable to understand and/or cooperate
　—Any child triggering any PEW parameter.
- Place child in a comfortable position with their head supported.
- Allow 2 min of effective inhalation prior to starting the procedure; anxious children will require time and encouragement to take effective breaths.
- Peak effect lasts 2–3 min.
- Side effects: euphoria, dizziness, dry mouth, tingling fingers, and nausea and vomiting (subsides 2–8 min after inhalation ceases)
- Regular Entonox® users must be monitored for onset of neurological symptoms (numbness, weakness, tingling).
- Parental involvement in the preparation of the child and during the procedure has a sedative-sparing effect.

Chronic pain

- Any continuous or recurrent pain lasting >12 weeks, or a pain that persists beyond the normal expected time for tissue healing.
- Prevalence is 15–35% of persistent or recurrent pain in <18-year-olds.
- Majority are managed in primary care with simple analgesic advice, and have little impact on daily life.
- For a minority, there are major adverse consequences for the child and family, with long-term detrimental effects on the child's education and social development.
- Incidence ↑ through childhood, peaking in early teens around 14 years.
- Higher incidence in girls compared with boys (60:40).

Causes

- Pain may have both nociceptive and/or neuropathic components.
- Chronic pain in young people can be categorized into:
  - Medically unexplained
  - Medically explained but ongoing pain not controlled by conventional analgesics, and having a detrimental effect on daily activities
  - Chronic post-surgical pain
  - Complex regional pain syndrome (CRPS).

Locations

- Common locations of chronic pain are:
  - Back pain
  - Widespread musculoskeletal pains
  - Abdominal pain
  - Headaches.

Assessment of chronic pain in children and adolescents

- Not just a numerical scale or based on physiological parameters.
- Assessment needs to encompass all aspects of the biopsychosocial model.
- Pain history: location, intensity, quality, duration, frequency, temporal variation, alleviating/aggravating factors, and accompanying symptoms.
- Impact on child's life: sleep disturbance, school attendance and achievement, participation in physical activities, and socialization with peers.
- Psychological factors: anxiety, mood, pre-existing temperament, coping style, child's beliefs, family beliefs, perceived causes, and prognosis.
- Environmental factors: family and parental behaviours surrounding pain, secondary gains, bullying, bereavement, and family breakdown.
- Child factors: age, gender, cognitive ability/developmental stage, general health, and culture.

Management

- Take into account the needs of both the child and family using a biopsychosocial model.
- The primary aims of treatment are:
  - Improve pain.
  - Improve function.
  - Promote self-management.
- Multidisciplinary team management is essential and includes pain physician, specialist nurse, clinical psychologist, physiotherapist, and occupational therapist.
- All factors in the biopsychosocial model must be addressed in the management plan.

Physical therapies

- Established in the management of chronic musculoskeletal pains and CRPS. They also have a role in improving general physical condition, since many patients develop a spiral of worsening pain, avoidance behaviours, and deconditioning, which are barriers to pain improvement.
- Techniques used include: physiotherapy, graded exercise program, hydrotherapy, desensitization exercises, TENS, and acupuncture.

Psychological interventions

- These include cognitive behavioural therapy, commitment and acceptance therapies, mindfulness, relaxation, hypnotherapy, biofeedback, guided imagery, and group therapy programmes.

Medical management

- Evidence for pharmacological strategies is limited.
- Where medication is used, it should be as part of a multimodal approach, aimed towards increasing participation in other therapies, e.g. psychology and physical therapies.
- Choice of medication is often based on presumed mechanisms of pain, aiming to ↓ intensity/frequency of pain and neurosensitization.
- Common medications include:
  - Anticonvulsants, e.g. gabapentin
  - Tricyclic Antidepressants, e.g. amitriptyline
  - NSAIDs
  - Lidocaine 5% patches
- Nerve blocks ± catheter. Very occasionally useful as part of a rehabilitation package to facilitate initial engagement with physical therapy when other strategies have failed.

Safeguarding

Anyone involved in the management of chronic pain needs to have an understanding of safeguarding issues and know how to initiate an appropriate referral within their institution. Staff involved in providing healthcare should receive regular training to acquire appropriate competencies relevant to their role.

Section 5

Medical and surgical specialities

Neonatal anaesthesia

Phil Arnold

Overview

- A neonate is a newborn baby, though the definition is often extended to any child up to 44 weeks postconceptional age.
- Whilst paediatricians often point out that children should not be considered small adults, it is even more true to say that a neonate should not be considered a small child. They present with different pathologies, are physiologically distinct, and will respond to and handle medications in a different way (➔ Chapters 1 and 2). Despite this, an anaesthetic for a neonate should look familiar to a practising anaesthetist.
- Almost any anaesthetic procedure that can be performed on an adult can be performed on a newborn, and basic standards of care will be identical.
- Risk of perioperative mortality is substantially higher in neonates than older children and they present for different surgical procedures. For specific operations, ➔ Chapter 18.

General principles

- Anaesthetists must have specific experience and training.
- Surgery should be conducted in specialist hospitals.
- Take care in preoperative assessment, though information may be limited in a child only a few hours old. Review neonatal unit records. Focus on problems related to prematurity and the presence of congenital abnormalities (especially of the airway, heart, or lungs). Parental anxiety is likely to be high.
- Choice of anaesthetic technique depends on the specific surgery and the child's condition, as well as personal and institutional preferences.
- The doses of all drugs will require modification according to body size. Those of many drugs will require further modification to account for different sensitivities to the drug or PK. IV or inhalational anaesthetic doses should be reduced.
- Take extra care to maintain normothermia; monitor core temperature. Forced air warmers have greatly simplified this for the majority of patients. Increasing the ambient temperature and humidity, using overhead radiant heaters, and covering the child with warm insulation help maintain normothermia.
- Incubators provide a thermoneutral environment for transfer and nursing post-operatively. Avoid hyperthermia.
- Use two pulse oximeters, since it is common to lose one intraoperatively.
- In babies with a PDA, one probe is placed on the right hand (pre-ductal) and the other is placed on a lower limb (post-ductal). This will help detect reversion to fetal circulation with right-to-left shunting in preterm babies (secondary to hypoxia and high airway pressure).
- Most regional anaesthesia techniques can be performed. The balance of risks and benefits will be different in neonates than in older children. Infraumbilical operations may be performed with spinal or caudal anaesthesia alone. If successful, a regional technique without GA is associated with less risk of apnoea following hernia repair.
- Combinations of GA and LA can avoid the need for systemic opiates. If systemic opiates are required, reduce the dose.
- Neonates may take a longer to wake up at the end of the procedure. Generally only patience is required.
- GA or sedation can be avoided for non-painful procedures, e.g. MRI ('feed and wrap' to promote sleep).

Airway considerations

- A neonate's airway is different to that of older children, but should not be considered 'difficult'. Mask ventilation is straightforward, though care should be taken to avoid compression of soft tissues. The large occiput will tend to flex the neck, and this should be avoided, as should excessive extension. Inflation of the stomach can compromise ventilation and is avoidable by good airway management. Supraglottic airways can be used, but are often unstable.
- During intubation, the larynx is high and anterior and it is easy to inadvertently place the laryngoscope blade too far in. If recognizable structures are not visible, the blade should be withdrawn until they are. Straight blades are often used and the blade tip placed either anterior

or posterior to the epiglottis. Gentle pressure on the anterior neck will often improve the view.

- Position the ETT tip 3–4 cm past the glottis. A 3.5 mm ID uncuffed tube is suitable for most term newborns (4.0 and 3.0 tubes may be required). An overly large ETT can cause damage: the ETT should pass easily through the glottis, with a small audible leak on positive pressure ventilation. If there is excessive leakage, change to a larger size or consider a cuffed ETT; a 3.0 cuffed ETT is the smallest size available and is suitable for a term newborn (there should be no resistance to insertion).
- Where possible, turn the head to one side, since this prevents the weight of the drapes pushing the ETT further into the trachea.
- Make a verbal and written note of the ETT length at the mouth or nose. The ETT is held by the anaesthetist or assistant until securely fixed. Nasal intubation is more secure for long procedures when the patients head will be moved often, or when postoperative IPPV is required.

Vascular access

- The veins are small, but are generally superficial. With care, they are easy to cannulate. However, cannulas do not always last long and reusing veins is often impossible. IV access may become challenging in babies who have been in hospital a long time. Early use of 'long lines' may avoid this problem.
- Percutaneous central lines can be placed in similar sites as used in adults. It is the author's opinion that US should be used for all central lines.
- Arterial cannulation can be challenging. Peripheral arterial lines often do not last long, especially if 24 G cannulas are used. A 22 G cannula is preferable in a term neonate, even for radial cannulation. Femoral and axillary arteries are alternative sites, and US can be used to facilitate cannulation. If there is evidence of distal ischemia, the line should be removed and the limb observed closely.
- Umbilical arterial catheters can be of value, but usually need to be removed during abdominal surgery.

Fluids

- Take care with fluid administration: pumps are more precise, and volumes of drugs and flushes should be measured. Isotonic solutions are suitable.
- All neonates are at risk of intraoperative hypoglycaemia, and starvation times should be minimized. Risk is ↑ if IV glucose is being given preoperatively, and in infants of low birth weight. Monitoring of glucose and continuing administration of glucose is required for all but very short procedures.
- Bolus administration to restore intravascular volume should always be an isotonic fluid or colloid and should not contain glucose. A variety of fluids and blood products may be required.
- Postoperatively, efforts should be made to re-establish enteral feeding. If this is not possible, use of TPN should be considered early. Electrolytes should be monitored at least daily when parenteral fluids are given for several days. The traditional formula of giving 150 mL/kg/day of fluid is not appropriate for postoperative crystalloid infusion. 4 mL/kg may also be excessive, and it is important that fluid prescriptions be regularly reviewed. Isotonic fluids with 5–10% glucose should be used initially, unless there is a particular risk of Na^+ overload.

Premature and ex-premature infants

- Prematurity can be defined as being born <37 weeks postconceptual age.
- Very premature is 28–32 weeks and extreme prematurity <28 weeks.
- Chance of survival increases with increasing gestational age. Survival is rare at <24 weeks and does not occur prior to 23 weeks. Low birth weight (for dates) is common and further reduces survival.
- In the NCEPOD report into children's surgery, 33% of deaths were in neonates undergoing surgery for NEC (➲ Chapter 18). The considerations above apply to a greater extent to premature than to term neonates. Special considerations include:
  - With increasing prematurity all organ systems will be increasingly undeveloped.
  - Skin is very thin in extremely premature infants. Care is required in securing equipment and positioning.
  - Fluid administration is complex, and many preterm infants will come to theatre with pre-existing electrolyte and fluid imbalance. A simple approach is to continue the preoperative fluid replacement, and give additional boluses of a colloid or isotonic fluid as required.
  - Premature infants are at risk of retrolental fibroplasia, which will be aggravated by hyperoxia; maintain SpO_2 between 90% and 95%. Avoid high inspired O_2 concentrations other than for short periods.
  - Monitoring can be challenging. Non-invasive devices can be unreliable. Invasive monitoring can be difficult to achieve, can also be unreliable, and can be associated with morbidity. Transparent drapes allow direct observation of the patient. Looking after an extremely sick infant with limited monitoring is a worrying experience.
  - The high RR and low V_T may be beyond the ability of even modern anaesthetic machines. Manual ventilation may be required, but should be avoided whenever possible for long periods.
  - In the postoperative period, the patient is at risk of apnoea. Even following short surgery, the patient should be observed in hospital at least overnight using an apnoea alarm and O_2 saturation.
  - Risk of apnoea is increased with increasing prematurity, O_2 dependency, anaemia, hypothermia, hypoglycaemia, and use of opiate analgesia.
  - The risk of apnoea persists in premature infants, even after their expected delivery date. The balance of risks, in particular with regard to day case surgery, is controversial. The author's practice is to admit overnight ex-premature babies up to 55 weeks postconceptual age.
  - Chronic lung disease, feeding problems, and delayed neurodevelopment are common persistent complications of prematurity.

The transitional circulation

- At birth, the cardiovascular system undergoes dramatic changes. However, these are not complete at birth, but mature further over the first weeks of life (➲ Chapter 1). This process may be affected by disease processes.

- In response to severe stress, e.g. birth asphyxia, severe illness, or lung injury, the PVR will be elevated further. This can result in shunting of poorly oxygenated blood from the pulmonary to the systemic circulation. This will result in a lower SpO_2 in the lower limb (relative to the upper limb). If more than transient, this is termed pulmonary hypertension of the newborn (PPHN, formerly persistent fetal circulation) and is a life-threatening situation.
- A similar picture of pulmonary hypertension can be associated with severe lung abnormalities, e.g. lung hypoplasia associated with diaphragmatic hernia or severe lung disease in prematurity.
- Treatment:
  - Optimize oxygenation and ventilation.
  - Support the cardiovascular system with inotropes and fluid.
  - Alkalization using $NaHCO_3$.
  - Inhaled NO.
- Higher arterial CO_2 will further elevate the PAP; however, in the context of severe respiratory failure, attempts to increase ventilation will cause further lung damage, and permissive hypercapnia is associated with improved survival. ECMO may be required for children with pulmonary hypertension and severe respiratory failure.
- Right-to-left shunting via the PDA can also occur in the context of CHD, e.g. coarctation of the aorta.
- Surgical manipulation in the heart and great vessels (with an open PDA) can also cause right-to-left shunting. This usually responds to stopping the manipulation.

Anaesthesia and the developing brain

- Animal experiments demonstrate neurological injury (primarily cell apoptosis) and deficits in development and learning in association with GA exposure in healthy neonatal animals.
- Early experiments were exclusively on rodents; however, better-controlled studies have now been conducted on larger newborn animals, including primates and piglets.
- Effect is less in primates than other animals, and is less apparent at dates further from the point of exposure
- Observational human studies are inconclusive.
- The putative mechanism of injury is suppression of neurotrophic synaptic signalling, which is required to prevent apoptosis in the distal neurone.
- The relevance of these findings to human health is currently unknown; prospective studies are currently underway that may clarify this issue.
- Most GA and sedatives have been implicated; excluding α_2- antagonists and xenon, which may be protective.
- LA appear to be safe; however, intrathecal ketamine is associated with neurological injury in animals.
- Neurological injury may also be associated with inflammation associated with pain and surgery. In this context, GA may be protective.
- Factors such as underlying illness, drug withdrawal, periods of hypoxaemia or cardiovascular instability, hospitalization, separation from family, and altered nutrition may all impact on neurological outcome to a greater degree than any direct effect of GA.
- This has led to a wider discussion of how anaesthetic care can be modified to prevent injury to the developing brain. There is, however, a general lack of evidence for specific interventions proposed; such as enhanced monitoring of cerebral circulation or more aggressive maintenance of BP.
- The degree of uncertainty makes it difficult to know what to tell parents. The majority of UK paediatric anaesthetists would not mention this issue, unless asked by the parents. Specific questions should be answered honestly and openly, taking into account the discussion above. A minority of parents may be considering taking decisions on the basis of incomplete information, with the potential to be detrimental to their child's health. Position statements produced by professional societies, e.g. the Association of Paediatric Anaesthetists, are helpful.
- If there is a good reason to operate, then concerns over neurotoxicity should not influence this decision. Alternatively, if surgery can be delayed until the child is older, without compromising the outcome, then there are good reasons to do so other than the concerns over neurotoxicity.

Further reading

Disma N, Davidson A, de Graaff J, et al; Gas Study Consortium. The GAS study: the postoperative apnea outcome in a RCT comparing spinal and general anaesthesia for infant hernia repair: ESAPC1-4. *Eur J Anaesthesiol* 2014;31:2.

Hansen TG, Lönnqvist PA. The rise and fall of anaesthesia-related neurotoxicity and the immature developing human brain. *Acta Anaesthesiol Scand* 2016;60:280–3.

Morton NS. Anaesthesia and the developing nervous system: advice for clinicians and families. *BJA Educ* 2014;15:118–22.

Sanders RD, Hassell J, Davidson AJ, et al. Impact of anaesthetics and surgery on neurodevelopment: an update. *Br J Anaesth* 2013;110(Suppl 1):i53–72.

Day-case surgery

Steve Roberts

Overview

- Children benefit hugely when managed through a day-case pathway, particularly the avoidance of a daunting overnight admission.
- Current recommendations are that 75% of elective paediatric surgery be performed as day cases.
- Ideally, minor semi-urgent surgery, e.g. plastics trauma, should be performed as a day case. This requires access to dedicated theatre time.
- Success requires careful patient selection, an experienced multidisciplinary team, child-friendly facilities, and effective protocols for analgesia, discharge, and postoperative follow-up.
- Increasingly, more complex procedures and patients are managed as day cases.

Facilities and staffing

- The child should be admitted to a designated day-case ward.
- If there is no inpatient paediatric cover, a geographically close neighbouring children's service must provide practical support and take formal responsibility for the arrangement. A clear assistance and transfer protocol must be agreed.
- If inpatient paediatrics is unavailable, then the consultant anaesthetist and surgeon must be experienced in the condition and must remain available until the patient is discharged.
- One team member must be APLS-trained, the rest must have basic PLS.
- At all times, one basic PLS provider must be present on the unit.
- The environment should comply with child safety standards and be child-friendly.
- Children should not be admitted or treated alongside adults.
- Recovery should be physically separate from adult recovery.
- An environment for children with special needs must be provided; a quiet room and a sensory room are essential.
- Thought should be given to a quiet route into the hospital for children who are hypersensitive to bright colours and noise.
- Children should not be mixed with acutely ill inpatients.

Selection and exclusion criteria

- Should be clear and relevant to the expertise of the unit. The four key areas are:
  - The patient
  - Social circumstances
  - The procedure
  - Anaesthetic considerations.

The patient

- As the majority of patients are ASA 1 and 2, nurse-led preoperative assessment is appropriate (➔ Chapter 3).
- Preop is also an opportunity to highlight significant patient preparation issues, e.g. autism; the anaesthetist can assess further either by phone or in clinic.
- ASA 1 and 2 term infants >44–50 weeks (units vary) postconceptual age and preterm infants >52-60 weeks (units vary) post-conceptual age can be treated on a day-case basis for minor procedures.
- Children <1 year of age listed for cosmetic surgery, e.g. excision of accessory digit: parents should be offered LA or defer procedure until the child is >1 year old, when GA complications are less frequent.
- Stable ASA 2 conditions, e.g. asthma, epilepsy, or cerebral palsy, are suitable.
- Experienced units accept ASA 3 patients.
- Asymptomatic, uncomplicated cardiac lesions, e.g. small VSD, or well children with surgically corrected cardiac lesions may be suitable.
- Stable IDDM is suitable (➔ Chapter 26).
- Inborn errors of metabolism are unsuitable.
- Sickle cell disease is unsuitable.
- Morbid obesity is a relative contraindication, depending on the proposed procedure; e.g. tonsillectomy for mild OSA would be inappropriate.

Social circumstances

- This is clinician- and operation-dependent, making hard and fast rules difficult.
- It is generally recommended that families live <1 h drive away. However, in our institution (Alder Hey), it is not unusual to have a simple day case, e.g. GA MRI, take a short flight to get home.
- Telephone and transport to return are necessary.

The procedure

- Should be superficial and of short duration, with postoperative pain managed by PO analgesics.
- Modern GA techniques mean longer procedures are feasible, e.g. mastoidectomy.
- Should not be associated with significant risk of postoperative haemorrhage or cardiovascular instability.
- The day-case procedure 'basket' is expanding, e.g. some institutions perform tonsillectomy in mild–moderate OSA patients.

- Adenotonsillectomy for non-OSA indications is acceptable in children >3 years old. Require a period of 3 h recovery to observe for haemorrhage.
- Urgent cases, e.g. minor trauma, must have a designated list to access, have a specific pathway, and be able to reasonably wait 1–2 days before admission.
- Longer and more painful procedures, e.g. tonsillectomy, squint, orchidopexy, and metal work removal, are listed early on the list.

Anaesthetic considerations

- MH or difficult airway are not a contraindication.
- Prolonged GA is associated with delayed recovery and complications, e.g. PONV. Consider use of TIVA or desflurane, and prophylactic antiemetics.

Patient pathway

- The most important function is an integrated admission plan delivering efficient preoperative assessment and preparation.
- Ideally delivered in the actual DSU, allowing difficult patients to familiarize themselves with the staff and ward. This facilitates patient experience and theatre utilization.
- Popular methods include structured questionnaires and a nurse-led pre-admission clinic. Assessment is performed in person or via the telephone, with major issues escalated to the anaesthetist.
- Clear verbal and written fasting instructions are essential. Liberal regimes for oral fluids ↓ preoperative distress in patients and parents and improve perioperative behaviour.
- Specific written advice on GA and the listed procedure should be provided in clinic or via online resources.
- Age-appropriate patient information should be available.
- A reminder phone call/text 72 h prior to admission confirming attendance, reiterating fasting guidelines, and enquiring about present health, e.g. URTIs, is essential.
- In our unit, a 'batched' admission process is used whereby each theatre session has two admission times, e.g. 07.30 and 09.30 for morning sessions. This improves patient flow and experience, decreasing fasting times, preoperative waiting, and frequency of premedication.
- Ideally, there should be a dedicated paediatric operating list; if not, then patients should be placed first on an adult list.

Anaesthetic considerations

- Sedative premedication is not contraindicated.
- Good analgesia is essential.
- If not contraindicated, administer preoperative paracetamol and NSAID (ibuprofen is more palatable) to all patients having a painful procedure; if refused, administer IV and PR, respectively intraoperatively.
- LA techniques for all appropriate cases.
- Consider the use of small doses of clonidine (2mcg/kg) and ketamine (0.2–0.3 mg/kg) where LA is impossible.
- Use antiemetics for high-risk PONV cases, e.g. orchidopexy.
- Dexamethasone has additional advantage of improving postoperative analgesia, especially where swelling contributes to pain, e.g. dental extractions.
- Avoid opiates.
- Discharge with paracetamol and NSAID; plus oral morphine for painful procedures, e.g. tonsillectomy.

Discharge criteria

- Airway reflexes intact and no respiratory distress or stridor.
- Stable vital signs and conscious level appropriate for individual child.
- No bleeding or surgical complications.
- No or minimal pain and no PONV.
- Ambulation appropriate for child.
- Able to drink (not essential).

- Pass urine—only following specific procedures, e.g. cystoscopy.
- Written and verbal instructions given with hospital contact details.
- Essential documentation completed to ensure aftercare by school nurse, community nurse, or GP.
- Escort home by responsible adult in private car or taxi.

Audit and quality control
- The commonest problems requiring admission are surgical observation, pain, and PONV.
- Regular audit should address cancellation, unplanned admissions, postoperative morbidity, and parent and child satisfaction.

Cardiothoracic surgery

Phil Arnold

Congenital heart disease (CHD)

Overview
- Incidence 0.5–1% of live births.
- There is a wide range of severity. Small septal defects, mild pulmonary stenosis, or small patent ductus arteriosus (PDA) may remain asymptomatic for life. Other lesions, e.g. hypoplastic left-heart syndrome (HLHS), will require complex interventions during neonatal life, have high procedural mortalities, and are associated with continuing functional limitation and shortened life expectancies.
- Treatment is increasingly successful; therefore, more patients with complex disease are surviving into later childhood and adult life.
- CHD patients are at risk of infective endocarditis. Current UK guidelines are not to give additional antibiotics during procedures that carry a risk of endocarditis.
- In the UK, around 10,000 procedures (including 6,000 surgical interventions) are performed yearly (7,500 in patients <16 years of age).
- These patients require GA for investigation of CHD and for the treatment of other associated or incidental illnesses.
- CHD is a predictor of adverse events during GA. In data from the Pediatric Perioperative Cardiac Arrest Registry, 34% of patients who experienced a perioperative cardiac arrests had CHD. In a single-centre study, 80% of 'anaesthetic-related' deaths were in children with cardiovascular disease.

Classification
- It is helpful to classify patients into groups. From the perspective of the anaesthetist, it is useful to approach this from a physiological perspective:
  - Left-to-right shunts, in which blood is diverted owing to the pressure gradient primarily from the systemic to the pulmonary circulation.
  - Right-to-left shunts, in which blood is diverted owing to the pressure gradient primarily from the pulmonary to the systemic circulation.
  - Lesions in which there is relatively free mixing between pulmonary and systemic circulations.
  - Obstructive lesions.
  - Valvular regurgitation.

Left-to-right shunts
- Ventricular septal defects (VSD), atrial septal defects (ASD), and PDA.
- Size and position of the defect will affect the volume of blood shunted between circulations and therefore the clinical impact. The volume shunted may be several times the systemic blood flow.
- Pulmonary blood flow is ↑, leading to volume overload of the right heart and ↑ pulmonary artery pressure (PAP).
- In the case of a VSD, the left heart will also be disadvantaged, since a large part of its ejection will be through the VSD.
- If the additional flow exceeds the heart's capacity, then heart failure develops.
- Infants with heart failure present with poor weight gain, poor feeding, and tachypnoea. Medical management includes nutritional supplements, diuretics, and ACE inhibitors. Closure of the shunt (by surgery or trans-catheter procedures) usually provides lifelong treatment.

- Raised PAP will cause damage to the pulmonary vasculature. This leads to raised pulmonary vascular resistance (PVR). At first, this is 'reversible' and will drop in response to high O_2 concentration, drug treatment, or reducing the flow by closure of the shunt. With time, the raised PVR becomes irreversible.
- Once the raised PVR become irreversible, closure of the shunt will result in failure of the right ventricle (RV) due to pressure overload. If the increased PVR is such that the RV pressure exceeds the left-ventricular (LV) pressure, the direction of flow reverses and the patient becomes cyanosed—Eisenmenger syndrome. These patients are at a very high risk from GA.

Right-to-left shunts

- The most common lesion is tetralogy of Fallot (i.e. VSD, pulmonary stenosis, overriding aorta, and RV hypertrophy).
- Pulmonary stenosis obstructs the RV outflow, leading to elevated RV pressure; if this exceeds the left-sided pressure, then blood shunts from right to left.
- Right-to-left shunt causes desaturation and often visible cyanosis.
- Features such as heart failure or failure to thrive do not occur unless hypoxaemia is severe and prolonged. Pulmonary hypertension does not occur.
- The degree of cyanosis and the presentation will depend on the degree of RV outflow tract obstruction (RVOTO). Severe obstruction will lead to cyanosis at birth and the blood flow to the pulmonary circulation will be largely via a PDA. Around 20% of patients have no physical outflow to the RV (pulmonary atresia). Children with less severe obstruction will not be visibly cyanosed in the first months of life.
- RVOTO is complex. As well as pulmonary stenosis, there is usually subvalvular obstruction due to hypoplasia of the outflow tract and hypertrophic muscle growth into the outflow tract. There may be supravalvular obstruction due to stenosis of the main or branch pulmonary arteries, or hypoplasia of the pulmonary vessels. There may also be other sources of blood to the lungs: major aortopulmonary collateral arteries (MAPCAs).
- 'Tet spells' are acute periods of ↑ cyanosis. They occur due to ↑ subvalvular obstruction caused by muscle spasm around the outflow. Incidence and severity increases with age. They can be life-threatening. 'Spells' may be provoked by GA. Beta-blockers are often used to ↓ the frequency of spells. The management of severe spells is discussed later.
- Surgical correction includes VSD closure and augmentation of the RV outflow tract. This may involve extensive resection of RV muscle and insertion of a patch along the outflow tract.
- Most patients do well following a Fallot's repair. Late morbidity includes ventricular arrhythmia. This is often associated with pulmonary regurgitation, dilation of the RV, and residual RVOTO.
- In very small infants exhibiting severe hypoxia (or with duct-dependent circulations), palliative procedures may be preferred to a surgical repair. This may include BT shunts (discussed later) or endovascular stenting of the ductus or outflow tract.

Lesions with mixing between left and right circulations

- In complex lesions, there may be considerable mixing between blood from the systemic and pulmonary circulations. Blood, in effect, shunts both left to right and right to left.
- These may include situations in which there is effectively only a single ventricle, and situations in which two ventricles are functioning as a single pump.
- The circulation can be described as a 'parallel' circulation. The flow to each circulation largely depends on the respective resistances of these circulations.
- When the flow to the two circulations is approximately equal, the circulation is balanced. The patient will remain cyanosed (usually with a SpO_2 of around 80%) and the single ventricle will be producing twice as much flow as the systemic circulation (it is 'volume-loaded').
- If the pulmonary flow is much less than the systemic flow, the child will become increasingly hypoxaemic.
- If the pulmonary flow is much greater than the systemic flow, the child is likely to have symptoms of heart failure. They may also be at risk of coronary insufficiency (due to steal from the coronaries to the pulmonary circulation) and damage to the pulmonary vasculature (due to high PAP).
- Either the systemic or pulmonary circulation may be dependent on flow through the PDA. Infusions of prostaglandin may be required to maintain patency of the ductus, usually as a bridge to an intervention.
- Examples of single ventricle conditions include: HLHS, tricuspid atresia, and unbalanced atrioventricular septal defect (AVSD).

Surgical palliation

- This is any surgical or endovascular procedure designed to modify the circulation but not restore normal continuity of the circulation.
- Used as an interim measure prior to a surgical repair (or longer-lasting palliation) or as 'destination' therapy for circulations that cannot be repaired.
- A large part of mortality in CHD surgery is related to palliative procedures performed in small infants.

Modified Blalock–Taussig shunt (BT shunt)

- A synthetic tube is placed between the subclavian artery and the pulmonary artery (PA) on that side (usually the right).
- It is used to ↑ pulmonary blood flow or as a replacement for the PDA (which may be allowed to close or be ligated).
- May be used with severe tetralogy of Fallot (or variants) or in patients with single ventricles and 'duct-dependent' pulmonary blood flow.
- The BT shunt is 'restrictive', i.e. it is of a small calibre and aims to limit excessive flow to the lungs.
- May be performed as an emergency lifesaving procedure or relatively electively.
- Creates (or sustains) a 'parallel' circulation as described previously.
- Most shunts are 'too big' when placed, with a tendency to excessive flow. This can cause heart failure with possibility of 'steal' from the coronary and other circulations.

- As the child grows, the shunt becomes relatively smaller. Heart failure will become less of an issue; however, SpO_2 will fall.
- Shunt thrombosis is immediately life-threatening. Patients are usually on an antiplatelet drug, e.g. aspirin.

Pulmonary artery band:
- Used to limit pulmonary blood flow.
- A band is placed around the main PA to produce obstruction to the RV outflow. This increases the pressure proximal to the band, reducing right-to-left shunt, and reduces the pressure distal to the band, providing protection to the pulmonary vasculature.
- Historically, PA bands have been used to treat simple VSDs. Today, most patients will have the VSD repaired. Patients undergoing PA bands will either have severe comorbidities (commonly respiratory disease) or have more complex lesions (often with a single ventricle) that preclude repair.
- As the child gets larger, the PA band will become increasingly restrictive. Pulmonary blood flow will fall resulting in reduced SpO_2.

Norwood procedure
- Used for treatment of HLHS.
- Aim is to construct a systemic outflow path committed to the (single) RV and to stabilize pulmonary blood flow independent of the PDA.
- Classically consists of division of the MPA, MPA stump is used to construct the proximal aorta (such that RV output is directed systemically), a patch to augment the aortic arch, PDA ligation, atrial septectomy, and a modified BT shunt.
- Rather than a BT shunt, a small (restrictive) conduit is often placed from the RV to the PA (Sanno modification).
- This complex surgery is conducted in the first weeks of life; the postoperative period is prolonged and often unstable in the early stages.
- As with the shunts discussed elsewhere, this still represents a 'parallel' circulation with inherent instability in the relationship between pulmonary and systemic flow.

Cavopulmonary connections
- In the first month of life, the pulmonary vasculature is immature. PVR remains both high and labile. A high 'driving' pressure is required to produce a reliable pulmonary blood flow. As the child matures, in the absence of pulmonary hypertension or intrinsic anomalies of the pulmonary vasculature, the PVR will fall and become more stable. At this point, a lower pressure is required to provide adequate flow. This can be achieved by diverting blood from the vena cavae to the pulmonary vasculature.
- This is usually conducted in two stages. First, the SVC is connected to the pulmonary arteries (a superior cavopulmonary connection or Glenn shunt). Later, the IVC is also diverted to the pulmonary arteries: the Fontan operation.

- Following a superior cavopulmonary connection, the IVC blood still returns to the heart and mixes with more oxygenated blood from the pulmonary veins. The child is still cyanosed, with SpO_2 75–85%.
- Following a Fontan operation, most of the venous return will go via the lungs. SpO_2 will be higher: high 80s to low 90s. Some blood will bypass the lungs owing to collaterals or surgically created fenestrations. There is likely to be increased VQ mismatch.
- As most of the blood flow is now diverted through the pulmonary vasculature, any impediment to this flow will ↑ systemic venous pressure and ↓ CO. As there is no subpulmonary ventricle, pulmonary blood flow and therefore CO are limited.
- Poor function of the single ventricle, non-sinus rhythm, ↑ PVR or atrioventricular valve regurgitation will ↑ the risk of failure of the Fontan.
- A failing Fontan circulation is marked by signs of reduced CO (tiredness, reduced exercise tolerance, and end-organ dysfunction), and high venous pressures (ascites, malabsorption due to gut wall oedema, and hepatic dysfunction). SpO_2 will fall.
- Fontan failure can occur gradually or more acutely following surgery. Fontan failure during childhood is largely avoidable by careful selection of patients. With increasing age, SVR will ↑, leading to back pressure on the abnormal heart and elevation of the end-diastolic pressure. This reduces forward flow in the Fontan. This is the likely situation in adults with Fontan failure.

Non-cardiac surgery and congenital heart disease

- Many children, in particular those who have undergone repair of 'simple' CHD, will not have a significantly increased risk from GA and will not require modification of the anaesthetic plan.
- Others, in particular those with pulmonary hypertension or ventricular dysfunction, will have significant risk even during 'minor' procedures (Table 15.1).

Table 15.1 Risk stratification of cardiac pathology

Low risk*	Medium risk	High risk	Highest risk
'Innocent' murmur	Uncorrected moderate to large VSD	Infants with shunted circulations	Severe pulmonary hypertension
Corrected ASD, VSD	History of SVTs	Aortic stenosis	Severe ventricular dysfunction
Simple ASD		Uncorrected tetralogy of Fallot	Persistent arrhythmia
Mild pulmonary stenosis		Following Fontan with symptomatic limitations	
Small VSD			

*Unlikely to require modification of anaesthetic plan.

Assessment

- Even for 'minor' surgery, it is important for the anaesthetist to be aware of the underlying cardiac diagnosis and previous treatment. If this is unavailable, discuss with the responsible cardiology team.
- Clinical assessment is informative. If the child is well, with no or minimal restriction to their lifestyle, it is likely they will tolerate GA well.
- Poor weight gain in infancy can be a sensitive indicator of systemic disease.
- Baseline SpO_2 should be noted.
- Cardiovascular medications should generally be continued perioperatively.
- Manage anticoagulation and antiplatelet therapy in consultation with cardiologist.
- Comorbidities are common.

Anaesthesia and pulmonary hypertension

- These patients require careful management and have a high risk of intraoperative complications.
- Risk is related to the severity of pulmonary hypertension, ventricular function, and mechanism of the pulmonary hypertension. It is highest for patients with primary pulmonary hypertension.
- There is a difference between a patient with a large left-to-right shunt, high pulmonary flow, and high PAP and a patient with no shunt (normal PA flow) and high PAP. In the former, the predominant clinical problem will be congestive heart failure. The latter group is at risk from severe decompensation, due to acute right heart failure and 'pulmonary hypertensive crisis' (an acute rise in PVR, often in response to noxious stimuli).
- A variety of anaesthetic approaches have been taken with this group of patients.
- 'Careful' GA, which should be adequate but not excessive, skilled airway management, and a sense of alertness to adverse events, are more important than the choice of any particular drug. Adequate oxygenation should be maintained.
- When faced with deterioration, initial assessment should follow the principle of 'ABC'. Deteriorations should not be presumed to have a cardiovascular cause.
- A pulmonary hypertensive crisis will be associated with desaturation, arterial hypotension, ST changes on ECG, and arrhythmia.
- Management should include 100% O_2, use of vasopressors to maintain diastolic BP, use of fluid and inotropes, and specific measures to ↓ PVR (hyperventilation and inhaled NO). Adequate GA and muscle relaxation are maintained.

Anaesthesia and ventricular dysfunction

- Severe ventricular dysfunction may be seen as a complication of CHD or as a consequence of cardiomyopathy or myocarditis.
- As with pulmonary hypertension, a variety of anaesthetic techniques have been described and it is difficult to recommend any particular approach.
- A careful and observant approach is required.

- Coronary perfusion (diastolic BP) should be actively maintained.
- A disproportionate number of adverse events will occur during 'minor' procedures, e.g. imaging, vascular access, or PEG.

Anaesthesia and shunted circulations

- SpO_2 will reflect, among other things, pulmonary blood flow.
- Reduced BP will result in reduced pulmonary blood flow and reduced SpO_2.
- High inspired O_2 concentrations and low arterial CO_2 will ↓ PVR and ↑ shunt flow.
- Factors that ↑ pulmonary flow can lead to worsening of heart failure, systemic low perfusion, and coronary ischemia. Patients with relatively large shunts, with poor ventricular function, who are systemically unwell or are in the period immediately after shunt placement are most at risk.
- Patients with low SpO_2 preoperatively may have small shunts. They are at risk of developing critical hypoxaemia if BP drops further. Measures to restore BP or even maintain supranormal BP can improve SpO_2. Urgent involvement of cardiology to plan ongoing care is required.

Anaesthesia and Fontan circulation

- Careful preoperative assessment is essential.
- Patients who are doing well in normal life are likely to tolerate GA for minor surgery well.
- An exaggerated reduction in BP is common during GA. This is usually well tolerated and unlikely to require any therapy beyond judicious administration of IV fluids.
- Positive pressure ventilation will cause a further ↓ in CO and BP. This is often tolerated for short periods; even so, inflation pressures, inspiratory time, and duration of ventilation should be minimized. Avoid very high inflation pressures or high PEEP.
- Major surgery is associated with significant morbidity.
- Laparoscopic surgery is possible, but carries a risk of haemodynamic compromise. Direct arterial pressure measurement is preferred, IV fluid should be given, intra-abdominal pressure should be limited to 10 cmH_2O, and extreme positioning should be limited.
- MDT discussion, involving anaesthesia, cardiology, and the operating surgeon, is useful prior to major surgery. Risk–benefit should be carefully considered.

Anaesthesia and tetralogy of Fallot

- Uncorrected tetralogy of Fallot patients have a significant risk of hypercyanotic Tet spells perioperatively. Monitor SpO_2 throughout.
- To ↓ risk of Tet spells:
  - Continue perioperative medication.
  - Maintain an adequate level of GA and analgesia.
  - Maintain normovolaemia.
  - Avoid hypothermia.
- Tet spells require an 'ABC' approach. Cardiovascular causes should only be pursued after exclusion of inadequate airway or ventilation.
- Tet spell management: high inspired O_2 concentration; sedation/analgesia; administration of a systemic vasoconstrictor, e.g. phenylephrine 2–4 mcg/kg; fluid bolus and correction of acidosis.

Anaesthesia for cardiac surgery

- A highly specialist area within which many management controversies exist. There are, however, common elements to how a case is approached.

Preoperative assessment

- Well-functioning cardiac units will have MDT meetings attended by surgeons, cardiologists, and other members of the cardiac team. The precise diagnosis is defined and a definite surgical plan made. Anaesthetists should be actively involved in this disuccsion.
- Care should be taken with patient assessment, pay particular attention to the child's functional status, and to comorbidities. Surgery should generally be postponed in the presence of respiratory tract infections.
- Children are often very anxious. Consider anxiolytic premedication for children >1 year old.
- Parental anxiety is common and requires a sensitive approach.
- Routine investigations are often performed and, when available, should be reviewed. The value of many of these investigations is uncertain. Adequate blood should be prepared according to institutional policies.
- Vital medication, e.g. prostaglandin, should be continued.
- Starvation times should be kept to a minimum.

Induction and preparation

- Both inhalational and IV induction are acceptable.
- Preparation should include:
  - Secure airway and means to ventilate
  - Ability to rapidly transfuse fluid and blood
  - Direct arterial BP monitoring
  - Means to take ABG samples
  - Means to administer bolus doses of medication into a central vein
  - Means to deliver infusions of vasoactive drugs into a central vein
  - Means to maintain GA throughout, including during cardiac bypass
- How this is achieved can vary; arterial and central lines can be placed at several sites. Generally the position of lines is not critical, though some operations will require care in choosing an appropriate site. Access to the patient is restricted during surgery, and planning must be made to ensure access to lines.
- The anaesthetist must not be distracted by performing practical tasks as to not be observing the patient's condition.

Pre-bypass phase

- Most heart surgery is conducted via a median sternotomy and involves the use of cardiac bypass. The exceptions are repair of coarctation of the aorta and PDA ligation, which are conducted via a left thoracotomy without bypass. BT shunts and PA bands may be conducted via sternotomy or thoracotomy.
- Median sternotomy can cause a marked stress reaction and adequate analgesia is required.
- Following sternotomy, the thymus (if present) is removed and the pericardium opened.

- Bypass will require cannulation of the venous and arterial side: most commonly the ascending aorta and the venae cavae.
- Cardiovascular instability during cannulation is common, especially in sicker and smaller patients.
- Irritation of the heart can cause arrhythmia.
- Redo-surgery is common and requires special precautions on the part of the anaesthetist and surgeon.
- Heparin 300-400 units/kg is given prior to cannulation. Activated clotting time (ACT) is a simple and crude bedside test that confirms administration of heparin. An ACT >300 is required for cannulation, whilst an ACT >400 is required for cardiac bypass.

Bypass phase
- The principles are similar in children and adults. Specialist techniques are required during certain surgeries, e.g. surgery on the aortic arch.
- Bypass is a complex technique and represents a significant physiological insult. Failure to achieve 'good bypass' can lead to serious injury to the child.
- 'Good bypass' is indicated by an empty heart, an appropriate perfusion pressure and evidence of adequate perfusion. 'Bad bypass' usually indicates a technical problem with bypass—most often misplacement of the bypass cannula.
- Continuous monitoring of arterial BP, aortic line pressure, mixed venous saturation, and direct observation of the heart are mandatory. More advanced techniques are often used, e.g. monitoring of cerebral perfusion with near-infrared oximetry.
- The components of the bypass circuit for use with children are smaller than in adults but larger relative to the size of the patient. In the case of small infants much larger. This will dilute blood components. It is often necessary to add red cells to the circuit in infants to avoid anaemia.
- Efforts should be made to limit the size of the circuit and to avoid administration of excessive fluid during bypass.
- The BP and flow aimed for should be appropriate to the size of the child.
- Techniques to ↑ the haemoglobin concentration at the end of bypass include cell salvage and ultrafiltration.
- Adequate GA must be maintained. Inhalational agents can be given via the oxygenator, IV agents can be given intermittently or (by preference) infused continuously. Propofol should not be administered directly into the circuit.

Separation from bypass
- Prior to separation, ensure there is:
  - Adequate ventilation
  - Acceptable heart rhythm
  - Adequate cardiac function
  - Virtually normal temperature
  - Acceptable electrolytes.
- Cardiac function is judged by direct observation of the heart, ECHO and haemodynamic parameters. Partial occlusion of the bypass venous line will allow filling of the heart. Dilation of the heart and a failure to produce pulsatile flow is an indication of poor function or residual pathology.

- Once the heart is adequately filled, the venous line is completely occluded. Blood can be transfused via the aortic cannula to achieve adequate filling.
- Problems include residual pathology, myocardial dysfunction, arrhythmia, and respiratory insufficiency.
- Following separation from bypass, there should be attempts to assess the repair with the aim of excluding residual surgically correctable pathology prior to the patient leaving the operating room. Whilst true of all patients, it is particularly important if the patient is unstable.
- This may include:
  - Direct measurement of pressures within the heart and implied pressure measurements using indwelling lines. The degree of residual stenosis can be assessed by measurement of pressures above and below the stenosis. A high RV pressure (in the absence of outflow obstruction) may indicate a residual VSD.
  - Measurement of saturations in different parts of the vascular system can indicate the presence and degree of residual shunts. An ↑ in saturation from the RA to the PA indicates a residual VSD. An estimate of the size of the shunt can be made using a modification of the 'shunt equation'. The pulmonary venous saturation is usually assumed to be 100%. The ratio of pulmonary to systemic flow is given by

$$\frac{Qp}{Qs} = \frac{SaO_2 - SsvcO_2}{SpvO_2 - SpaO_2}$$

  where SaO_2 = arterial oxygen saturation

  $SsvcO_2$ = superior caval saturation

  $SpaO_2$ = pulmonary arterial saturation

  - ECHO provides imaging of the heart and of residual defects. It is performed either by placing a probe directly on the heart (epicardial) or into the oesophagus (TOE). Interpretation for CHD requires considerable experience. An anaesthetist can be the primary provider of TOE; however, a team approach is required in decision-making.
  - Making critical decisions on the basis of these findings requires experience and a considerable knowledge of outcomes for different lesions. A decision to return to bypass to close a VSD will depend also on how easily the VSD can be closed. A Qp:Qs of >1.5 is an indication for further efforts to close the defect or placement of PA band. Decisions around further relief of valvular stenosis or regurgitation can be complex.
- On rare occasions, further imaging may be required to assess the quality of the surgical repair. This may include cardiac catheter, CT or MRI. Wider availability of 'hybrid' operating rooms (which include facilities to perform angiography) may ↑ the use of these modalities. If ECMO is required postoperatively, ensure correctable pathology is excluded.

Myocardial dysfunction

- Some degree of dysfunction always occurs, though not always severe enough to cause a clinical problem or require treatment.
- Longer periods of cardiac ischemia (cross-clamping), more complex repairs with greater surgical manipulation, and poor preoperative condition of the child are likely to be associated with worse dysfunction.
- Filling of the heart should be optimized. The central venous pressure (CVP) is often used as an index of filling; however, the relationship is complex. A higher CVP is often required following surgery on the RV to produce adequate filling. Left-atrial pressure can also be measured directly. Very high filling pressures are likely to reflect residual pathology or myocardial dysfunction. Response to fluid administration, observation of the heart, and ECHO can add to the assessment of filling.
- Check: electrolytes (especially ionized Ca^{2+}), haemoglobin, and heart rhythm.
- Monitoring lines can mislead; assess the clinical situation as a whole.
- Vasoactive drugs are often required after complex surgery. Choice is often guided by institutional preference, but should also be mindful of individual patient factors (especially the underlying pathology).
- The author's preference is to initiate milrinone in patients at risk of dysfunction, prior to separation from bypass. Dopamine is then titrated to maintain an adequate BP. Following very complex surgery, adrenaline (epinephrine) and noradrenaline (norepinephrine) (in combination with milrinone) are used in preference to dopamine. Rarely, vasopressin is added for refractory hypotension.
- In patients at risk of myocardial dysfunction, vasoactive drug infusions should be connected to the patient prior to separation from bypass, though not necessarily started.
- Severe haemodynamic compromise may require recommencement of bypass. If refractory, it may require longer-term mechanical support of the circulation using extracorporeal membrane oxygenation (ECMO).
- If the degree of haemodynamic compromise appears out of proportion to the surgery or is severe, an effort should be made to exclude residual surgically correctable pathology.

Haemorrhage

- A common problem due to the extent of vascular surgery and derangement of coagulation (secondary to cardiac bypass and anticoagulation).
- Risk factors for severe bleeding include small patient size, neonates, long cardiac bypass, extensive surgery, and use of deep hypothermia.
- Heparin should be reversed by protamine in all patients. There are various regimes. The author's practice is to administer 4–6 mg/kg of protamine.
- The need for treatment of coagulation in the operating theatre depends primarily on clinical assessment.
- Coagulation tests can guide management. ACT is widely used but crude. Thromboelastography is more sophisticated and able to differentiate effects of residual heparin, excessive fibrinolysis, and deficiencies of platelets, fibrinogen, and other clotting factors.

- In the presence of clinical suspicion of coagulopathy, following adequate reversal of heparin, the most common defects are of platelets and fibrinogen. Platelet concentrates must be available (10–20 mL/kg). Fibrinogen can be corrected by infusion of cryoprecipitate (5–10 mL/kg) or fibrinogen concentrates (70–90 mg/kg). Fresh frozen plasma has little role in initial management of coagulopathic bleeding.
- Recombinant factor seven (rVIIa), prothrombin complex concentrates, and warm fresh whole blood have all been used in treatment of severe bleeding. Risks and benefits are unclear.

Arrhythmias
- Bradycardia is most likely due to heart block, which can result from damage to the conducting system (AV node or bundle of His). Placement of epicardial pacing wires allows temporary pacing. Ventricular pacing (VVI) will restore ventricular rate; however, sequential pacing of atrium and ventricle (DDD) will often produce improved haemodynamic results.
- Tachyarrhythmias may be supraventricular or ventricular. With an open chest, cardioversion is straightforward. SVTs may also be terminated by applying cold saline to the epicardium, adenosine, or by 'overdrive' pacing. Arrhythmias will often result from surgical stimulation of the heart; however, other underlying causes e.g. electrolyte disturbance, should be excluded. Ventricular arrhythmia may indicate coronary insufficiency.
- Recurrent arrhythmia is likely to require antiarrhythmic drugs. Amiodarone 5 mg/kg is often used (correct Ca^{2+} to ↓ risk of hypotension). Junctional ectopic tachycardia (may complicate neonatal and RV surgery) is often refractory to treatment, and may require therapeutic cooling to 35°C to control the ventricular rate.

Transfer to intensive care
- The patient should be stable prior to transfer.
- As far as possible, care should continue to the same standard as during surgery.
- Sufficient personnel and equipment should be available to treat adverse events during the transfer and handover.
- Handover to ICU staff should be comprehensive. Standardized handover forms facilitate this.

Fast tracking
- Traditionally patients have been ventilated for prolonged periods postoperatively. It is increasingly recognized that this is unnecessary even following relatively complex surgery.
- Patients should remain intubated if unstable or bleeding or if the surgical result is uncertain.
- Many patients benefit from early extubation, but this requires a high standard of perioperative care. In particular, it demands good analgesia without excessive sedation. This can be difficult, but can be facilitated by regional anaesthesia.
- Regional techniques include thoracic epidurals, intrathecal catheters, surgical parasternal blocks, caudal opiates, and local infiltration. Both the

effectiveness and safety of some of these techniques is questionable.
The author's practice is to place bilateral single-shot US-guided PVBs;
this provides reliable wake-up, good early analgesia, and haemodynamic
stability. Opiates are still required; however, the total dose needed is
substantially reduced.
- With careful planning, patients can bypass ICU. They still require HDU
care immediately after surgery and availability of medical input. The
objective is faster progress through all levels of care, including discharge
from hospital.

Extracorporeal membrane oxygenation and ventricular assist devices (VADs)

- Mechanical devices are used to support the function of the heart and
lungs (ECMO) or the heart in isolation (VADs).
- An ECMO circuit is similar to a modified bypass circuit. Blood is taken
out of the circulation, passed through an oxygenator and pumped back
into the circulation. ECMO can be veno-arterial (VA) or veno-venous
(VV). VA ECMO will involve cannulation of the atrium or a large vein(s)
and the aorta or other large artery (commonly the internal jugular
vein and carotid arteries). The function of both the heart and lungs
are supported. VV ECMO involves only cannulation of a large vein. It
provides gas exchange but does not directly support the circulation.
- Compared to a bypass circuit, ECMO is simplified and modified for
longer use.
- A variety of VADs are available. A single device will support a single
ventricle. To provide bi-ventricular support, 2 devices are required.
These devices do not contain an oxygenator and cannot provide gas
exchange. Compared to ECMO, VADS are commonly used when longer
periods of support are required. They may be used to bridge the patient
until the heart recovers or until the patient receives a transplant. Very
long periods of support (>1year) are infrequent but possible.
- Thrombosis and bleeding are common complications. Anticoagulation
is required. During ECMO, this is usually a continuous heparin infusion.
During longer periods of ventricular assist, more complex regimes are
required.
- Patients may require surgical interventions whilst on such support. This
will be a major undertaking requiring careful planning.

Anaesthesia in the cardiac catheter laboratory

- CHD patients often present to the catheter laboratory for assessment
or treatment. The principles of GA are similar to those discussed
above and it is the author's practice to provide GA with endotracheal
intubation for almost all procedures. Procedures fall into three
groups: diagnostic cardiac catheters, interventional cardiac catheters,
and electrophysiological studies.
- Improvements in the quality of echocardiography and other imaging
modalities, e.g. MRI and CT, means that the need for diagnostic cardiac
catheters has diminished. Common exceptions are in the assessment
of pulmonary hypertension, studies conducted prior to the Fontan
operation, and sick postoperative patients (in whom there is diagnostic
uncertainty).

- The primary objective of a diagnostic catheter is haemodynamic data. GA will alter haemodynamics. An effort to minimize these changes is important.
- High inspired O_2 concentrations should be avoided initially when measuring PAP or shunt size.
- Catheter interventions include balloon dilatation of vascular or valvular stenosis, placement of endovascular stents, closure of defects, e.g. ASD, or creation of septal defects, e.g. balloon atrial septostomy.
- Many patients will be relatively well and procedures will be uneventful. Some patients may be extremely unwell with complex disease and undergoing more involved procedures, e.g. a neonate with single-ventricle anatomy undergoing stenting of a PDA. These patients can be a considerable challenge to cardiologist and anaesthetist. Occasionally, patients will require surgical 'rescue', owing to failure of treatment or misplacement of a vascular device.
- Electrophysiological studies are intended to study the conducting system to guide arrhythmia management. Radiofrequency or cryoablation allows modification of conduction. The usual patient is an adolescent with a well-tolerated supraventricular tachycardia. GA may alter the ability to induce (and therefore treat) the arrhythmia. Avoid high doses of volatile agents.

Thoracic surgery

Overview

- Surgery on either hemithorax will usually involve a thoracotomy or a thoracoscopy. Indications include:
  - Vascular surgery within the chest (PDA ligation, coarctation repair, PA band and BT shunt).
  - Treatment of congenital abnormalities of the lung include lobar emphysema (where a portion of lung shows emphysematous changes), congenital cystic adenomatoid malformation (CCAM, where a part of the lung, often an entire lobe, is replaced by a large cystic abnormality), and sequestrations (segments of abnormal lung not connected to the airway receiving a blood supply from systemic arteries).
  - Surgery on other structures within the chest, e.g. repair of trachea-oesophageal fistula and oesophageal atresia (➔ Chapter 18) or anterior release in scoliosis repair (➔ Chapter 22)
  - Infections may require chest tube placement, decortication, and rarely lung resection
  - Tumours are rare. Most common tumours will be haematological malignancies in the mediastinum, which rarely require resection (➔ Chapter 20). Rarely, lung metastases require resection (usually osteosarcoma).

Preoperative assessment

- As for other surgery.
- Indication for surgery.
- Presence of respiratory compromise.
- Presence of infection within the chest. In particular, potential for spreading of infection within the tracheobronchial tree.
- Presence of active sepsis.
- Discuss with the surgeon: blood loss and the need for one-lung ventilation (OLV).
- Postoperative care should be planned and discussed with the patient (if appropriate) and family. This should include analgesic techniques and anticipated need for PICU or respiratory support.

General conduct of anaesthesia

- Induction IV or inhalational.
- Positive-pressure ventilation and reliable wide-bore IV access for all cases.
- Consider invasive monitoring and the potential for more rapid transfusion.
- Patient is in lateral position with operative side uppermost.
- Surgery is usually possible with both lungs ventilated or with OLV.
- The respiratory physiology of small children may make hypoxaemia more likely: closing volume > FRC, perfusion is preferential to the non-operated side, hypoxic pulmonary vasoconstriction is poorly developed, chest wall compliance is higher, and O_2 consumption is higher than in adults relative to body size.

- Severe hypoxaemia or cardiovascular compromise is most likely to be due to poorly placed surgical retractors—compressing the airway or vascular structures. It responds to repositioning of the retractors. Increased FiO_2, periodic re-inflation of the lung, insufflation of O_2 to the collapsed lung, and manipulation of ventilation may be required. Long periods of hand ventilation should be avoided, though this may be necessary to ensure oxygenation.
- Intraoperatively, there should be the facility to provide endobronchial suction and a bronchoscope to confirm airway device position.
- Concerns during thoracoscopy are similar, though there is less pain. Avoid excessive inflation pressures that may cause respiratory and cardiovascular compromise.

OLV techniques

- Selective endobronchial intubation. The ETT tip is advanced into the main-stem bronchus corresponding to the non-operated lung. In small children, both main-stem bronchi are short (in particular the right), making optimal positioning difficult and precarious. Further problems are variations in airway anatomy (including 'pig bronchus', where the right upper lobe bronchus arises directly from the trachea). This technique is not generally favoured by the author, but can be useful when very urgent lung isolation is required, e.g. a catastrophic air leak or airway haemorrhage.
- The smallest double-lumen ETT available is 26 Fr. This is unsuitable for children <10 years old.
- Bronchial blockers are the author's preferred technique. Potentially, any catheter with a distal balloon can be used; however, specially designed blockers are available in age-appropriate sizes (smallest 5 Fr). Blockers should always be placed under vision using a bronchoscope. When a smaller ETT is used, the technique of placement is modified, since it is no longer possible to place the blocker and a bronchoscope through the ETT. A variety of techniques are described. The author's experience is that a blocker placed outside of the ETT can be manipulated into either bronchus relatively easily (though bending the end to make a slight 'hockey stick' can ease placement).
- ETT with integrated bronchial blockers are available, e.g. the smallest Univent tube has an uncuffed 3.5 mm internal diameter tube; however, the external diameter of larger sizes prohibits use in small children.
- Whenever lung isolation is intended, a fibreoptic bronchoscopy is conducted to define the airway anatomy and confirm device placement. These devices can move during surgery and bronchoscopy may be required to reconfirm position (in particular after repositioning the patient).
- The main indication for OLV is to improve surgical access. Other indications are to protect a relatively disease free lung from soiling from an infected lung, in the management of air leak, and to prevent 'ball-valve' inflation of bullae.

Analgesia

- Thoracotomy is very painful. Inadequate analgesia can result in retention of secretions and respiratory insufficiency.
- Techniques include use of potent opiates or regional techniques. Other analgesic modalities should also be employed, including regular paracetamol and NSAIDs. Other adjuncts to analgesia may be used as appropriate.
- Regional techniques include thoracic epidural, lumber epidural, PVB, intercostal block, intrapleural block and wound infiltration.
- A PVB ± catheter can be placed at the start of the procedure; ensure the catheter avoids the surgical field. Alternatively, the surgeon can place a catheter intraoperatively.

Management of pleural drains

- Use of pleural drains is common and usually uneventful; however, mishaps in management may be disastrous.
- A one-way seal is usually provided by use of an underwater seal. If the drain bottle falls over, this can compromise the function of the seal.
- Gentle suction of 5 mmHg is often placed on drains to aid drainage of blood and fluid. Suction should be adapted to this purpose ('high-volume low-pressure') to prevent excessively high suction, since this is dangerous.
- Nursing must be by experienced staff.
- Intercostal drains are painful. Provide adequate analgesia.

Surgery on mediastinal structures

- Midline sternotomy or limited sternotomy may be used to access other structures in the mediastinum:
  - Thymectomy may be performed for myasthenia gravis (➋ Chapter 26).
  - Major airway surgery includes tracheal reconstruction and tracheoplasty. This is highly complex surgery, usually involving cardiac bypass.
  - Aortopexy is a procedure in which the aorta is attached to the back of the sternum to ↓ external compression of the trachea or bronchi. It is performed via a limited upper sternotomy or thoracotomy.
  - Resection of mediastinal tumours is uncommon. This can be extremely major surgery and may involve cardiac bypass if the tumour is invading the heart or major vascular structures.

Chest wall surgery

- The commonest major procedures are for correction of pectus deformity.
- The indication is almost entirely cosmetic. These deformities do not produce any respiratory or cardiac compromise (though they may be a consequence of cardiac surgery or respiratory disease when younger). Most patients are otherwise-fit teenagers.
- The Ravitch procedure is performed for pectus carinatum. It involves a submammary incision, resection of costal cartilages and an osteotomy of the sternum. The lower sternum is flail at the end of the procedure.

- The Nuss procedure is performed for treatment of pectus excavatum. It involves placing a metal bar behind the sternum. The bar is shaped such that when rotated it reduces the deformity. In doing so, the integrity of the thoracic ring is altered, probably displacing the costosternal joints. The procedure may be performed using a thoracoscope or without. Pleural drains may or may not be required. The bar is usually removed after 2 years.
- Both these procedures are always extremely painful postoperatively. Extensive efforts are required to manage this pain. A significant proportion of patients will still require analgesics several months after surgery.
- Thoracic epidurals are often used. However, at our institution, standard practice is to use a combination of bilateral PVB catheters and a fentanyl PCA. Use of this technique has markedly reduced inpatient stay (from 6 to 3 nights) and improved analgesia.
- A number of analgesic adjuncts are also used, including NSAIDs, paracetamol, gabapentin during the admission, and Mg^{2+} intraoperatively. Early mobilization and chest physiotherapy are encouraged.

Further reading

Ramamoorthy C, Haberkern CM, Bhananker SM, et al. Anesthesia-related cardiac arrest in children with heart disease: data from the Pediatric Perioperative Cardiac Arrest (POCA) registry. *Anesth Analg* 2010;110:1376–82.

van der Griend BF[1], Lister NA, McKenzie IM, et al. Postoperative mortality in children after 101,885 anesthetics at a tertiary pediatric hospital. *Anesth Analg* 2011;112:1440–7.

Hammer GB, Fitzmaurice BG, Brodsky JB. Methods for single-lung ventilation in pediatric patients. *Anesth Analg* 1999;89:1426–9.

Dental and oral surgery

Ed Carver

Elective surgery

- Comprises:
  - Extractions of decayed teeth
  - Restorative work
  - Surgical exposure of impacted or unerupted teeth
  - Removal of supernumerary teeth
  - Extraction of healthy permanent teeth to facilitate orthodontic treatment.
- 28% of 5-year-olds have signs of dental disease with three or four teeth affected.
- In the UK, GA for dental surgery in children is provided in hospitals or in clinics equipped and staffed to the same standard as a hospital. It is mandatory that facilities and staff be able to support a collapsed patient pending recovery or transfer to an HDU or ICU (potentially on a separate site).
- Simple extractions of deciduous teeth may only take few minutes. Complex extractions, restorations, or oral surgery may take 1–2 h.
- The majority of simple extractions are performed under LA.
- GA is used in children:
  - Too young or anxious to cooperate with LA only
  - With developmental delay or behavioural problems
  - With complex medical conditions where LA alone will not be tolerated
  - For complex or prolonged procedures
  - LA allergy.

Preoperative assessment

- Usually between 3 and 8 years old.
- Anxiety about the procedure and previous unpleasant experience under LA is common.
- A small number need sedative premedication.
- These lists often contain patients with comorbidities, e.g. developmental delay or cardiac or neuromuscular disease. Make a thorough assessment.
- Document any loose teeth.
- Enquire regarding any history of abnormal bleeding in patient or family.

Anaesthetic technique

- Airway management depends on the procedure, patient, and preferences of anaesthetist and dental surgeon.
- Extraction of one or two deciduous teeth, e.g. incisors, can be effected by preoxygenation, quick removal of teeth, and reapplication of face mask without the need for other airway adjuncts.
- A nasal mask (McKesson or Goldman) can be used for simple extractions in short procedures. The mask is held at the same time as applying jaw thrust to maintain the airway. Often used with a pack at the back of the mouth placed by the dentist; however, this does not guarantee protection from blood or debris entering the pharynx. Beware of airway obstruction due to dental pack or pressure from

operator. An NPA may provide superior airway control, but can provoke bleeding. Airway seal is poor with a nasal mask and $ETCO_2$ trace may be poor. The anaesthetist must remain vigilant to signs of airway compromise by observing breathing and listening for breath sounds. The patient will often entrain room air through the mouth and therefore the level of inhaled volatile agent may need to be kept relatively high.

- LMA (usually flexible) provides 'hands-free' airway maintenance and some protection from debris, but it can restrict surgical access. It is easily displaced in small children during insertion of packs, when bite blocks are placed/repositioned, and from pressure by the dentist during extraction. An LMA is usually suitable for extractions but less so for longer oral surgery procedures.
- Do not secure the LMA, since the dentist needs to move it around to gain access.
- ETT: south-facing preformed RAE or north-facing nasal ETT. Used when there are multiple extractions or restorations in a small child, a risk of reflux, or a requirement for IPPV. Provides a more secure protected airway, and greater access for surgical manoeuvres. Preferred for oral surgery. It may be helpful to size ETT orally first before attempting nasal route.
- Use nasal decongestant, e.g. Otrivine or another vasoconstrictor to ↓ risk of bleeding. Use soft ETT or soften in warm sterile water and lubricate outside of ETT to ease passage. Advancing a nasal ETT over a suction catheter may help to ↓ nasal trauma during insertion and avoid plugging the ETT with secretions.
- Throat packs are used with LMAs and ETTs to protect against aspiration of blood or debris.
- Usually SV is appropriate, but consider IPPV in compromised children.
- Maintenance is usually with volatile. Alternatively, for longer cases, TIVA with propofol ± remifentanil 0.05–0.2 mcg/kg/min.
- The dental surgeon usually inserts a bite block, taking care not to displace the LMA/ETT.
- Analgesia:
  - Paracetamol 15 mg/kg PO preoperatively or IV if patient refuses.
  - NSAID: ibuprofen 10 mg/kg PO preoperatively. If patient refuses, then obtain verbal consent for PR diclofenac sodium 1 mg/kg (or, if available, IV diclofenac 0.3–1 mg/kg).
  - LA infiltration or nerve block: lidocaine 2% with 1:80,000 adrenaline (epinephrine), maximum dose 7 mg/kg (each cartridge contains 2.2 mL = 44 mg lidocaine; maximum = 1 cartridge/7 kg body weight). Prilocaine 3% with felypressin 0.03 IU/mL (felypressin is a synthetic hormone with properties similar to vasopressin; it does not cause local or distal ischaemia at injection site) is useful if adrenaline is contraindicated (maximum 6 mg/kg). Articaine 4% with adrenaline 1:100,000 is also available for infiltration only, maximum 7 mg/kg.
  - Opioids, e.g. fentanyl 1 mcg/kg or morphine 50 mcg/kg IV, are restricted to major procedures.
- Antiemetic, especially for longer cases or if opioids administered: ondansetron 0.1–0.15 mg/kg IV (maximum 4 mg).

- Except for simple extractions, give dexamethasone 0.1 mg/kg to ↓ swelling and pain.
- All extracted teeth and any loose teeth should be accounted for.
- Remove throat pack and document as per hospital procedure.
- Patients are recovered in the left lateral head down position, especially if bleeding from extractions.
- Always remove LMA/ETT awake.

Postoperative care

- Rescue analgesia: morphine 0.1–0.2 mg/kg PO.
- Encourage oral fluids.
- Most simple extractions can be discharged within 1 h.
- Patients who needed premedication or those with comorbidity may need a longer recovery.
- Post-discharge analgesia: paracetamol and ibuprofen.
- Mouth care and diet instructions according to unit.

Emergency dental anaesthesia—dental abscess

- A dental abscess is a collection of pus originating in the centre of a tooth that may spread to bone and surrounding tissues.
- 4% of 5-year-olds and 2% of 15-year-olds have signs of dental sepsis as part of the PUFA examination – (open pulp, obvious ulceration, fistula, and abscess). Only a small number of these will need emergency treatment under GA.
- Symptoms and signs include pain, pyrexia, swelling of gums/face, redness and inflammation, anorexia, malaise, trismus.
- Treatment may require extraction of one or more teeth under GA and IV or PO antibiotics.
- Serious complications include systemic sepsis and brain abscess.

Preoperative assessment

- Examine for signs of dehydration and sepsis. Are IV fluids or antibiotics warranted?
- Pay particular attention to airway: is there any obstruction, altered speech or limitation of mouth opening? Inability to protrude the tongue is a warning sign of sublingual involvement and the potential for airway compromise. Mouth opening may be limited by pain, swelling, or muscle spasm in the awake child. Usually, but *not always*, this relaxes on induction of GA, and laryngoscopy is straightforward.
- It is usually appropriate to wait until the child is fasted.

Anaesthetic technique

- If there is any doubt about your ability to manage the patient's airway, it is wise to use an inhalational induction.
- Assess your ability to control the airway and breathing as well as ease of intubation before administering muscle relaxation.
- Advanced airway techniques may be needed for a difficult airway (→ Chapter 9).
- A south-facing RAE ETT is the best way to control the airway and protect the trachea from soiling.
- Antiemetic.
- Throat pack to protect against aspiration of blood and pus.
- Extubate awake after removal of throat pack and oropharyngeal suctioning.

Postoperative care

- Analgesia can be provided by a dental nerve block by the operator.
- Most children are managed with e.g. PO paracetamol and ibuprofen.
- Occasionally an opioid, e.g. morphine sulfate solution 0.1 mg/kg, will be needed.
- An overnight stay may be needed for further doses of IV antibiotics.
- Oral intake can usually be resumed after the procedure.

ENT surgery

Kate Thomas

General considerations

- Requires sound knowledge of anatomy, physiology, and pathology of the paediatric airway.
- Often high-turnover lists with many challenges:
  - Shared airway requires excellent communication between surgeon and anaesthetist.
  - Anaesthetist is often remote from the airway.
  - Unusual conditions or syndromes can be associated with airway and intubation difficulties.
- Many procedures are suitable as day cases, with large numbers performed in general hospitals. Complex patients or procedures are managed in specialist centres.

Myringotomy and grommets

- One of the commonest paediatric operations in the UK—usually a day case.
- Indication: recurrent otitis media and persistent middle-ear effusions.
- Usually infants and toddlers.

Surgery

- Short procedure; patient supine with head turned to the side.
- Usually bilateral.
- Myringotomy—incision in the tympanic membrane and suction of middle-ear secretions. This may be combined with placement of grommets (tympanostomy tubes).

Preoperative assessment

- High incidence of respiratory symptoms in this patient group: assess risk : benefit (→ Chapter 3). Often proceed with anaesthesia as operation is short and URTIs are common. But there is an increased incidence of laryngospasm and hypoxia.
- A minority have underlying congenital conditions notably Down syndrome (→ Chapter 16).

Anaesthesia

- Induction as preferred.
- LMA or face mask with SV.
- Ensure deep level of GA prior to incision; failure to do so can result in coughing, laryngospasm, and LMA displacement.
- Have a syringe of propofol readily available.
- Use head ring.
- Maintenance with volatile agent in O_2 and air/N_2O.
- If bilateral the head is turned mid-way; this is when the LMA can be displaced.
- Analgesia:
  - Preoperative PO paracetamol and ibuprofen usually suffices.
  - Opiates not recommended.

Postoperative management

- Postoperative pain is unpredictable, ranging from none to severe. Pain mainly results from trauma to the external auditory meatus and possibly acute pressure changes in the middle ear.
- PRN PO morphine 0.1mg/kg (100 mcg/kg).
- TTO paracetamol and ibuprofen.

Tonsillectomy

- Common operation, often performed with adenoidectomy and/or grommets; regularly performed as a day case.
- Adenoidectomy may be carried out in isolation. Anaesthetic considerations similar to those for tonsillectomy.
- Indications:
  - Recurrent tonsillitis (tend to be older patients)
  - Adenotonsillar hypertrophy with upper airway obstruction ± OSA
  - Unilateral hypertrophy of tonsil.
- Pre-existing comorbidities may predispose to upper airway obstruction:
  - Congenital or acquired craniofacial abnormalities, e.g. Pierre Robin, Treacher Collins, Down syndrome
  - Neuromuscular disease, e.g. cerebral palsy.

Sleep disordered breathing (SDB)

- Spectrum that includes snoring, upper airway resistance syndrome, and OSA.
  - Incidence 10%.
- History of mouth breathing, snoring, restlessness, poor-quality sleep, apnoeas.
- Daytime somnolence, irritability, poor concentration at school, and rarely enuresis.
- Hyperactivity and or failure to thrive in cases of moderate to severe OSA.

OSA

- 2% incidence.
- Majority have mild OSA.
- Moderate or severe OSA includes at least two of:
  - Hourly apnoeas 10–20 or more
  - Minimum saturations <90%
  - Transcutaneous CO_2 measurements elevated 10–15 mmHg or more.

Surgery

- Supine with neck in extension.
- The surgical mouth gag can cause obstruction, kinking, or displacement of ETT. Watch capnography trace as the gag is inserted; a temporary change is common, but if sustained there is a problem with the tube position or patency.
- Traditionally performed by dissection and diathermy.
- Coblation uses high-frequency energy to create a plasma field to dissect or vaporize the tonsil. It is less painful in the initial recovery period.
- Tonsillotomy may be indicated for OSA. It removes just enough tonsil tissue to improve breathing; it may be less painful and have lower risk of bleeding.

Preoperative assessment

- Suitable for day surgery if:
  - >3 years old
  - Day-case criteria met (➲ Chapter 14)
  - Mild OSA.

- Admission overnight if:
  - <3 years old
  - Moderate or severe OSA
  - Craniofacial abnormalities
  - Failure to thrive or significant obesity
  - Hypotonia
  - Chronic medical problems.
- Seek history of SDB.
- SDB patients may have had overnight SpO_2 or polysomnography (shows apnoea frequency and duration, plus associated fall in SpO_2).
- Severe prolonged OSA can result in right-heart strain, pulmonary hypertension, and cor pulmonale. Seek cardiology advice, ECG, and ECHO.
- In OSA patients, the application of Ametop® (tetracaine) or EMLA™ (lidocaine/prilocaine) (even if an inhalational induction is planned) may enable early insertion of IV cannula during induction without stimulating the child and enable a dose of propofol to be given to aid depth of GA.
- Upper airway respiratory symptoms are common. This is not necessarily a contraindication to proceeding if the child is apyrexial, well, and the chest is clear (➲ Chapter 3).
- An URTI predisposes to anaesthetic complications and tonsillar bleeding.
- Children with adenoidal hypertrophy may have a constant nasal congestion and discharge; ask the parents what's normal for their child.
- Exclude cervical spine instability (as per Grommets).
- Prewarn parents and children that it is impossible to prevent all pain postoperatively. Subjectively older children with a history of recurrent tonsillitis have more discomfort.
- Encourage the use of regular analgesia postoperatively.

Anaesthesia

- Sedative premedication is used with caution in OSA. If deemed necessary, e.g. severe behavioural issues, ensure the presence of a skilled anaesthetist with means of maintaining the airway on the ward whilst the premedication takes effect.
- Induction as preferred.
- Children with OSA may have a prolonged inhalational induction; patience and expert airway skills are required. Consider asking for a second pair of hands to gain IV access promptly.
- In SDB patients (especially if there are associated craniofacial abnormalities), upper airway obstruction may occur during induction. Management:
  - Ensure the mouth is open (not closed by application of fingers to the mandible).
  - Apply a jaw thrust.
  - Apply CPAP.
  - Insert oral airway when GA depth is adequate.
  - Consider an NPA; with care if adenoidal hypertrophy, since significant bleeding may occur. Use topical decongestant drops, e.g. xylometazoline, before insertion

- Intubation facilitated by:
  - Deep inhalational anaesthesia
  - Propofol bolus
  - Topical LA to the larynx (NBM for 1 h after application)
  - Short-acting muscle relaxant.
- Preformed 'south-facing' RAE ETT (cuffed or uncuffed) secured in the midline; be aware that in syndromic children these ETTs can be too long—always auscultate the chest.
- Whilst in anaesthetic room, if using an uncuffed ETT, assess the leak with the child's neck in extension, i.e. mimicking surgical position; a small leak can become too large.
- LMA can be used in children >3 years of age. A standard LMA usually suffices, but flexible, reinforced, or armoured may be better. Advantages are protection of lower airway from soiling and an improved list turnover. Disadvantages include difficulty positioning the mouth gag (risk of obstruction and laryngospasm), decreased surgical access, and extra surgical care and respect for shared airway required.
- In the UK, all surgical and anaesthetic airway equipment used in adenoidectomy or tonsillectomy is single-use owing to concerns regarding prion disease transmission.
- Patient position is supine with neck extended by a shoulder roll, recheck that there is no cervical instability, e.g. Down and Morquio syndromes.
- Maintenance as preferred: generally volatile agent in O_2 and air/N_2O.
- SV or IPPV.
- 20 mL/kg of IV fluid.
- Analgesia:
  - Preoperative PO paracetamol and ibuprofen.
  - IV morphine sulfate 50 mcg/kg.
  - An alternative opiate-free protocol includes clonidine 2 mcg/kg and ketamine 0.3 mg/kg.
  - Dexamethasone (also antiemetic). Note: avoid in unilateral tonsillar hypertrophy).
  - Topical or LA infiltration.
- OSA patients have increased sensitivity to opiates; therefore ↓ dose, especially if morphine. In severe OSA patients, avoid opiates and clonidine.
- IV ondansetron.
- Prior to extubation, the surgeon or anaesthetist must suction the airway under direct laryngoscopy to ensure the tonsillar bed is dry, and a head lift to check for blood clots in posterior nasopharyngeal space is also performed.
- Ensure muscle relaxants are reversed. In severe OSA where rocuronium is used, sugammadex provides excellent reversal.
- Extubate 'deep' or 'awake' depending on preference. Extubate OSA patients awake.
- Moderate to severe OSA patients may take a while for SV to recommence at the end of surgery; they may have apnoeas and obstruct their airway after extubation. Prolonged recovery often needed.
- Recover in head-down lateral position unless extubated awake, when this may not be needed.

- If airway issues develop post extubation, the patient may need to be placed supine (after excluding blood in airway) to facilitate assessment of airway and situation as a whole. For obese and large children, extubating in upright position may work better.

Postoperative care

Healthy or mild OSA patients

- Mild OSA patients will be admitted to a general ward bed, with the ability to monitor the patient as required.
- Regular PO paracetamol and ibuprofen.
- PRN PO morphine; in some institutions this is also prescribed as a TTO.
- Encourage PO intake (if topical LA used on larynx, ensure 1 h since application).
- In older children, chewing gum aids analgesia.
- Pain can last for up to 2 weeks; parents need clear instructions regarding regular analgesia. A comfortable child will eat and drink, which promotes healing of tonsillar bed and reduces risk of secondary bleeding.

Moderate–severe OSA patients

- Patients without a recognized syndrome affecting the airway but with moderate or severe OSA will be admitted to a high-acuity monitored bed on the ward.
- Admit to HDU if:
  - Syndrome affecting the airway (e.g. Down, Treacher Collins, or Pierre Robin)
  - NPA required.
  - <1 year old
  - Obesity or malnourishment (BMI > or < 2 standard deviations from mean).
- If unable to extubate, or severe OSA with multiple comorbidities, admit to PICU.
- Regular PO paracetamol and ibuprofen.
- PRN PO morphine omitted or prescribed at a reduced dose.

Tonsillar bleed

- Up to 3% incidence. Most are managed conservatively.
- Either primary (within 24 h) or secondary (within 28 days).
- Main issues:
  - Possible hypovolaemic shock
  - Pulmonary aspiration at induction of swallowed blood or food
  - Potential difficult intubation—bleeding and airway oedema
  - Second GA in potentially short time period.
- Assess, resuscitate, plan for theatre imminently.
- Send FBC, clotting, and blood crossmatch.
- Check previous GA chart.
- Make preparations:
  - Obtain senior help.
  - Have two suction devices ready.
  - Laryngoscope—correct size of blade and ready for use
  - ETT size as used before, plus 1/2 a size smaller in case of laryngeal oedema. Have two of each size, since the first may become blocked with clot.

- Fluid bolus and vasoconstrictor drawn up and ready.
- NGT to empty the stomach of blood at the end of surgery.
- Surgical team scrubbed and ready.
- Have patient head-up in comfortable position. Induction as preferred, but generally an IV RSI is recommended.
- Rarely, a large clot obstructs the trachea: management includes suctioning with a tracheal suction catheter, suction applied to the ETT, FOB or rigid bronchoscopy suction and lavage, and thrombolytics.
- Give further dose of dexamethasone, and paracetamol if possible. Opiates not required.

Middle-ear surgery

- Both mastoidectomy and tympanoplasty are suitable for day-case surgery; some patients may need overnight stay if PONV persists.
- High risk of PONV: a multimodal approach is required.

Surgery

- Mastoidectomy is performed to remove infected air cells within the mastoid bone, usually caused by cholesteatoma. Cholesteatoma arises from migration of squamous epithelium into the middle ear and accumulated desquamated epithelium that accumulates in the middle ear as a result of chronic middle-ear infection. It erodes middle-ear structures and remains a source of ongoing infection.
- Now relatively unusual because of the widespread use of antibiotics.
- Several surgical procedures may be performed:
  - Simple (or partial) mastoidectomy. The operation is performed through the ear or through an incision behind the ear. The surgeon opens the mastoid bone and removes the infected air cells. The eardrum is incised to drain the middle ear.
  - Radical mastoidectomy. The eardrum and most middle-ear structures are removed, but the innermost small bone (the stapes) is left behind so that a hearing aid can be used later to offset the hearing loss.
  - Modified radical mastoidectomy. The eardrum and the middle ear structures are saved, which allows for better hearing than is possible after a radical operation. The wound is stitched around a drain, which is removed 1–2 days later.
- Tympanoplasty is performed to repair a persistent perforation in the tympanic membrane. A graft of temporalis fascia is usually taken and used to repair the defect. This can be performed as an endoscopic procedure.

Preoperative assessment

- Usually older ASA 1 children.
- Often have had many GAs and may be anxious.

Anaesthesia

- Induction as preferred.
- ETT or LMA (possibly flexible) with SV or IPPV; ask surgeon about operation duration, since this may help determine airway choice.
- Maintenance:
  - TIVA with propofol and remifentanil is recommended (high risk of PONV).
  - Alternatively volatile anaesthesia in O_2/air combined with remifentanil infusion.
- Remifentanil avoids the need for muscle relaxant. If a facial nerve monitor is used, then neuromuscular blockers are avoided or only used at induction.
- Avoid N_2O during tympanoplasty because of potential pressure changes in the middle ear during and after surgery and owing to high incidence of PONV.

- 15°–20° head-up position.
- Avoid hypertension. Mild hypotension may be requested; this is delivered using a remifentanil infusion or by increasing depth of GA.
- Maintenance fluids.
- IV ondansetron and dexamethasone.
- Check with surgeon regarding antibiotics.
- Monitor temperature: may need active warming.
- Analgesia:
  - Preoperative PO paracetamol and ibuprofen.
  - LA infiltration (contains adrenaline (epinephrine))
  - Greater auricular nerve block if post-auricular incision used.
  - Avoid opioids.

Postoperative care
- Regular PO paracetamol and ibuprofen.
- PRN PO morphine sulfate.
- PRN antiemetic.
- IV fluids if delay in drinking.

Bone-anchored hearing aids (BAHA)

- Indications: conductive deafness and children who cannot wear behind-the-ear hearing aids.
- Three main groups:
  - Congenital malformation of middle/external ear, including microtia (varying severity of ear severity from an ear that is virtually absent to an ear that is perfectly formed but smaller than its fellow and aural atresia (failure of development of the external auditory canal, which is present in 80% of patients with microtia). Congenital malformations include:
    —Auditory canal atresia as seen in Treacher Collins syndrome
    —Microtia, e.g. Treacher Collins and Goldenhar syndromes and in hemifacial macrosomia
    —Narrow ear canal, such as in Down syndrome.
  - Chronically draining ear that prohibits use of air-conducting hearing aid
  - Bilateral conductive hearing loss due to ossicular disease that is not surgically correctable or aided by air-conducting devices.
- Most are suitable for day case surgery.

Surgery

- Surgically implanted abutment conducts sound through skull into inner ear, bypassing external auditory canal and middle ear.
- Usually performed at 4–5 years of age.
- Children too small for BAHA wear a headband that holds a sound processor against the skull until they are large enough.
- Two-stage surgery performed 3–4 months apart:
  - Stage 1: small post-auricular incision, hole drilled into bone, and two titanium fixtures inserted; implant is inserted into skull. Postoperative head bandage to ↓ risk of bleeding.
  - Stage 2: wound reopened and an abutment (to which the hearing aid will attach) attached to the titanium fixtures.
- Surgery takes 40–50 min.

Preoperative assessment

- Airway assessment, since some of the syndromes that have outer-ear abnormalities will also have airway issues, such as Treacher Collins, Goldenhar, and CHARGE. Assessment of cervical spine is necessary in at risk patients such as Down syndrome. Exclude URTI.
- Ascertain severity of deafness and how the child communicates.

Anaesthetic technique

- Preoperative oral ibuprofen and paracetamol usually sufficient.
- Induction as preferred.
- LMA with SV is generally suitable.
- Positioning: head turned to contralateral side to operation; use suction pillow or head ring.
- LA + adrenaline (to ↓ bleeding).

Postoperative care

- PO paracetamol and ibuprofen
- Rescue dose of PO morphine may be needed.
- Generally quick and uneventful recovery.

Cochlear implant surgery

- Indication: sensorineural deafness due to lack of development or damage to either the auditory nerve or to the sensory hair cells in the inner ear.
- Important to identify possible cause of deafness.
- Maximal benefit in speech and language development if implanted at 9–12 months old.
- Bilateral simultaneous implantation is standard.
- Surgery takes 3–5 h, depending on anatomy.

Aetiology of sensorineural deafness

- Congenital:
  - Non-syndromic sensorineural deafness is commonest genetic cause.
  - Syndromic genetic sensorineural deafness, e.g. Waardenburg, Jervell and Lange-Nielsen, Pendred, and Usher syndromes.
  - Intrauterine infections, e.g. toxoplasmosis, rubella, CMV, or syphilis.
- Acquired:
  - Those at higher risks are: neonates/infants needing prolonged IPPV (including oscillation) or ECMO, e.g. CDH
  - Kernicterus
  - Certain medications, e.g. gentamicin
  - Bacterial meningitis
  - Skull fracture or severe concussion.

How does the an implant work

- A microphone and sound processor are worn externally behind the ear; this communicates with a cochlear implant that is inserted in the mastoid bone.
- The implant translates the data into electrical pulses that are delivered to an array of electrodes that are surgically placed within the cochlea.
- The electrodes stimulate the auditory nerve, providing a sensation of hearing, though hearing is not restored.

Preoperative assessment

- Most will have had previous GA for ABR or CT/MRI scans.
- Common comorbidities include ex-prematurity and cerebral palsy.
- Thorough assessment for URTI.
- ECG to exclude pronged QT, especially those with family history of deafness and sudden cardiac death. Most children have an ECG as part of the initial investigation of the aetiology of hearing impairment.
- Important to ascertain cause of deafness and if syndromic cause look at specific issues; e.g. Jervell and Lange-Nielsen syndrome patients have bilateral profound sensorineural deafness with associated prolonged QT.
- Other syndromes to be aware of include:
  - Waardenburg syndrome: sensorineural deafness, pale eyes/brilliantly blue eyes, white forelock of hair, wide-set eyes
  - Pendred syndrome: bilateral sensorineural hearing deafness and goitre with euthyroid or mild hypothyroidism
  - Usher syndrome: sensorineural hearing loss and retinitis pigmentosa.

- Assess how the child communicates and for older children remind them they will not be able to hear anything in the operated ear when they wake; the tight head bandage must be explained too.

Anaesthetic technique

- Induction as preferred.
- RAE or armoured ETT. Flexible LMA may be suitable for older children for unilateral surgery.
- Maintenance with volatile and remifentanil, or TIVA. O_2 and air; avoid N_2O (can be used at induction).
- Avoid muscle relaxants if possible, since facial nerve monitoring is used (a single dose may be used to aid intubation). Use short-acting opiate, remifentanil, and/or topical LA to cords to aid intubation if needed.
- Prophylactic penicillin-based antibiotic (if not allergic).
- Patient positioned with head turned to contralateral side to operation: suction pillow or head ring with shoulder roll.
- Attention to pressure points, including non-operated ear. Eyes need to be protected.
- Temperature management; oropharyngeal temperature probe necessary, active warming usually not needed.
- LA + adrenaline infiltrated prior to incision to ↓ bleeding.
- Analgesia: paracetamol and NSAID (if bilateral surgery, administer PR at completion of first side when surgeon re-drapes, or IV). Use of long-acting opiates intraoperatively not normally needed.
- Dexamethasone and ondansetron (avoid if prolonged QT).
- Greater auricular nerve block or wound infiltration at end of surgery, before head bandage applied.

Postoperative care

- On emergence, patient may be unsettled owing to prolonged fasting, tight head bandage, or pain.
- Parental presence in recovery and a drink usually settles the child.
- Vertigo and PONV, especially in older children. Regular antiemetics and delayed ambulation help.
- For older children, the change in communication may be upsetting, so try visual aids.
- Possible day case depending on comorbidities and distance to hospital from home.
- Surgical risks include CSF leak and bleeding (including subdural haematoma).

GA for children with cochlear implants having incidental surgery/procedures

- MRI risks include potential device repositioning, causing injury or pain, damage to device, and also image artefact.
- Presence should be picked up by MRI safety questionnaire. 3T scanners are riskier than lower-tesla scanners. Never let a patient with a cochlear implant into the MRI without first checking with the cochlear implant team and/or manufacturer.

- You must always check with the MRI staff before taking a child into the scanner. Manufacturers will advise on up-to-date safety information.
- MRI-compatible cochlear implants are available.
- If the implant is incompatible, options include surgical removal of the external magnet (reinsertion after scan) or a different type of imaging, e.g. CT.

Diathermy
- Discuss at team brief.
- Bipolar diathermy can be used if >2 cm away from implant.
- Monopolar diathermy contraindicated in the head and neck region.
- If accidently used, contact cochlear implant team to arrange for the device to be tested.

Bronchoscopy

- Normally undertaken in specialist paediatric centres; however, an acute airway emergency may present at a general hospital.
- Performed by ENT surgeons (normally rigid bronchoscopy, although flexible nasal endoscopy used on ward/clinic) or respiratory physicians (flexible bronchoscopy). (→ Chapter 20).
- Pay attention to patient at all times, titrating the anaesthetic to the child's response (Table 17.1).
- Most patients have some degree of respiratory compromise.
- Signs and symptoms include stridor, wheeze, hoarseness, recurrent infection, cyanosis, persistent cough, and signs of respiratory distress.
- Day case, depending on patient and condition.
- Many children need overnight admission for observation and steroids.
- Commonest indication for rigid bronchoscopy is stridor (laryngomalacia, tracheomalacia, subglottic stenosis) and FB removal.

Rigid bronchoscope

- The Storz ventilating bronchoscope is the commonest rigid bronchoscope used.
- Consists of a metal tube with a removable optical telescope.
- Holes in the wall allow ventilation of the contralateral lung when the distal end of the bronchoscope is positioned in a bronchus (Fig. 17.1).
- The side arm has a 15 mm attachment for an anaesthetic T-piece circuit (Fig. 17.12).
- Ventilation occurs between the bronchoscope lumen and the outer surface of the telescope.
- The telescope occupies most of the internal diameter of smaller bronchoscopes and impedes ventilation in infants.
- With the telescope in place, a closed system exists and allows controlled ventilation, but the cross-sectional area of the lumen through which the infant can breathe is reduced.
- Using too large a bronchoscope leads to compression of tracheal mucosa and postoperative oedema with the risk of stridor.

Table 17.1 Indications

Diagnostic	Therapeutic
Recurrent pneumonia	FB removal
Tracheo-oesophageal fistula	Mucus plugs, e.g. cystic fibrosis
Airway obstruction	Lobar collapse
Laryngomalacia	Refractory atelectasis
Haemoptysis	Balloon dilation
To obtain biopsy or brushings	Stent insertion
Failure to wean from ventilator	Laser treatment

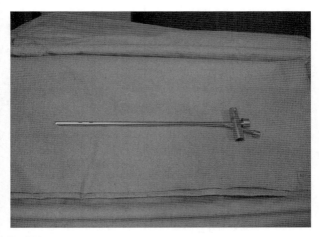

Fig. 17.1 Storz rigid ventilating bronchoscope. Note distal side holes for ventilation of contralateral lung.

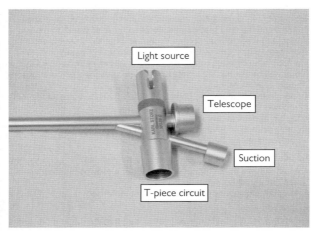

Fig. 17.2 Storz bronchoscope: close up of proximal end.

- Venturi bronchoscopes are commonly used in adults, but in paediatrics are limited to patients weighing >40 kg because of the risk of barotrauma. Ventilation occurs via jet insufflation with O_2 and entrained air using a Sanders injector. Anaesthesia is maintained with IV agents. CO_2 retention is a greater problem with this method.

Flexible bronchoscope

- Greater field of vision, and the smaller diameter allows access to the distal airways.
- The smallest diameter used has an ED 1.8 mm distally and 2.2 mm proximally.

Preoperative assessment

- Ascertain indication for bronchoscopy
- Careful history and examination focusing on airway and respiratory system: e.g. how do symptoms change with position, crying, and feeding?
- If stridor present, is it inspiratory (likely laryngomalacia), expiratory (likely tracheomalacia), or biphasic (obstruction at glottis or subglottic area, subglottic stenosis)?
- Review flexible nasal endoscopy findings from clinic.
- Review previous GA charts for ventilatable on face mask, laryngoscopy grade, airway obstruction, ETT size, and difficulties encountered.
- Airway FBs are potentially life-threatening. In children with less severe obstruction, there may be oedema and airway hyperactivity, especially with peanuts. There may be a history of choking episode that has either brought them to hospital, potentially in an acute state, or has settled down, and the child has become unwell a couple of weeks to months later with wheeze and infection. A chronic case may show atelectasis or consolidation on CXR. Acute airway obstruction due to an FB will present with choking, cough, stridor, and respiratory distress. A CXR may well be normal, but air-trapping can be seen if the object is creating a ball-valve effect.
- Specific investigations may be indicated, e.g. CXR for suspected FB, CT for lower airway obstruction.
- Explain to parents that breath-holding and coughing may occur during the procedure and that symptoms, e.g. stridor, may be worse postoperatively.

Anaesthesia

- Avoid sedative premedication if evidence of airway obstruction or respiratory compromise.
- Anticholinergic agents are no longer commonly used.

Rigid bronchoscopy

- SV is needed for diagnostic examinations so that the surgeon can assess dynamic and functional status of the upper airway.
- Inhalational induction is frequently used to maintain SV in children with possible airway obstruction. Induction may be slower if marked airway obstruction is present.

- Inhalational induction with sevoflurane in 100% O_2.
- Gentle application of CPAP helps overcome upper airway obstruction.
- Once deeply anaesthetised, topical lidocaine (up to 4 mg/kg) is sprayed on the epiglottis and larynx, and between the vocal cords using a mucosal atomizer device (do not advance through the cords, since it could seed laryngeal papilloma).
- Topical LA is key to success, preventing coughing, breath-holding, and laryngospasm during the examination.
- An NPA is frequently used to provide a good airway and deliver anaesthetic.
  - First instil xylometazoline drops
  - Select ETT 1/2 size smaller than that indicated for intubation.
  - Use direct laryngoscopy to position NPA tip in oropharyngeal space, avoiding the laryngeal inlet.
  - Loosely tie/tape in place; ensure that this is easy to remove if necessary to remove or advance the NPA.
  - A correctly placed NPA provides a good airway when the mouth is closed and the contralateral nostril occluded; the bag on the T-piece will move appropriately and normal capnography is observed
- Alternatively, an RAE ETT can be placed orally with the tip in the oropharyngeal space,
- Patient is supine with a shoulder roll to extend the neck and push the trachea anteriorly. A suction pillow provides good stability.
- Anaesthesia is maintained with sevoflurane in 100% O_2 given from a T-piece circuit attached to the side port of the bronchoscope (lower concentrations of O_2 can be used in a stable child) or the NPA.
- Alternatively, TIVA can be used. Propofol with or without remifentanil suppresses airway reflexes and provides rapid emergence, and there is less pollution of the operating theatre atmosphere.
- The capnography trace is unreliable (often non-existent) during the procedure because of leakage. The reservoir bag of the T-piece may also not move; closely observe the child's respiratory pattern; this may include a hand placed on the chest wall. Transcutaneous CO_2 monitoring may be useful.
- When the telescope is introduced, the cross-sectional area of the bronchoscope is reduced and the work of breathing may be significantly increased, especially in infants where narrow bronchoscopes are used. Adequate gas exchange may require intermittent removal of the telescope from the bronchoscope to allow uninterrupted ventilation.
- If assisted ventilation is used, a long time constant may be needed to avoid air-trapping.
- If coughing or lightening-up from anaesthesia occurs, give 1–2 mg/kg propofol.
- FB may be dislodged with IPPV; therefore, SV is generally preferred.
- Dexamethasone (100–250 mcg/kg IV) may be given to ↓ postoperative airway oedema.
- Surgeons often assess vocal cord function as the child emerges from anaesthesia.

Fibreoptic bronchoscopy
- Usually elective cases, and many of them, e.g. CF patients, will attend regularly.
- Sedative premedication if needed
- Induction as preferred.
- Topical lidocaine is applied as for rigid bronchoscopy.
- The method of airway management depends on the indication. If laryngomalacia is queried, then a facemask (fitted with an angle piece modified for passage of a bronchoscope) with SV allows examination of the larynx during normal breathing. Under these circumstances, an LMA may distort the larynx and impede vocal cord movement. Examination of the trachea is performed through an LMA. Examination of the bronchial tree and/or broncho-alveolar lavage is usually feasible with an LMA, though an ETT may be required.
- An appropriately sized LMA (with no bars, e.g. P3) allows the passage of a larger fibrescope than with an ETT.
- SV and CPAP are used to aid management of airway obstruction. The endoscopist may want to examine the airway with and without CPAP to identify tracheomalacia.

Postoperative care
- SpO_2 monitoring for at least 2 h to detect hypoxia secondary to hypoventilation.
- NBM for 1 h after topical anaesthesia to the larynx.
- PRN PO paracetamol and possibly an NSAID will provide adequate analgesia.
- IV fluids and antibiotics may be indicated, depending on the situation.
- If stridulous, administer a further dose of steroid, and nebulized adrenaline 1:1,000 0.5 mL/kg (maximum dose 5 mL).

Microlaryngeal surgery

- Indications: congenital or acquired anatomical laryngeal lesions, e.g. laryngomalacia, subglottic stenosis, and laryngeal web.

Laryngomalacia

- Neonate presenting with soft inspiratory stridor. Worse when feeding and lying flat.
- Bronchoscopic findings: short aryepiglottic folds, redundant arytenoid tissue, and long curled epiglottis, resulting in inward collapse during inspiration.
- Once diagnosed, only a minority need an aryepiglottoplasty. This involves division of the aryepiglottic folds, resection of excess arytenoid tissue, and suspension of the prolapsing epiglottis if needed.
- GA as for bronchoscopy; surgery performed with NPA or ETT (surgical preference).

Subglottic haemangioma

- Biphasic stridor develops at 2–6 months old.
- Laser surgery or direct excision for small lesions, tracheostomy for large lesions.
- Recent advances mean propranolol is used to shrink the haemangioma; often first-line treatment (provided airway not at risk).

Subglottic stenosis

- Commonly seen in premature babies who have been intubated.
- Present with inspiratory or biphasic stridor.
- Degree of stenosis directs management:
  - Mild is managed conservatively (monitor as child grows) or by balloon dilation.
  - More severe stenosis may need an anterior cricoid split or tracheostomy if severe. Anterior cricoid split involves division of first and second tracheal rings. Postoperatively, remain intubated on PICU (tip of ETT positioned distal to split). If reintubation needed, perform orally.
  - Severe stenosis necessitates a tracheostomy, followed by airway reconstruction surgery when older. This reconstruction involves anterior ± posterior costal cartilage graft(s) to trachea. A stent may be used to secure the graft. Prolonged PICU stay; treat as precious airway—if reintubation needed, perform orally.

Surgery

- Performed using a suspension laryngoscope and operating microscope.
- Often involves laser surgery to the airway and the relevant precautions that go with this.
- Camera and video display allow the anaesthetist to observe the airway and surgical field.

Preoperative assessment

- Patients often present for repeated procedures and may have significant airway obstruction.
- Many patients present with significant obstructive symptoms, especially from recurrent papillomatosis, and may develop total airway obstruction after induction of anaesthesia.
- Many patients have a tracheostomy: enquire after size, duration, and when last exchanged.

Anaesthesia

- Sedative premedication can be used if no significant airway compromise.
- Similar anaesthetic principles apply as for bronchoscopy.
- An inhalational induction with sevoflurane and 100% O_2 is commonly performed; if the child has a tracheostomy, it is connected to the anaesthetic circuit for induction.
- The larynx is sprayed with 2% lidocaine (up to 4 mg/kg).
- Options for maintenance include:
  - SV of volatile in 100% O_2 through an ETT (placed through the nose/mouth or via dedicated channel in the suspension laryngoscope) with the distal end in the oropharynx above the laryngeal inlet so as not to obscure the surgical field.
  - Apnoeic insufflation where the child is paralysed and volatile and 100% O_2 insufflated through an ETT placed as above. Arterial CO_2 rises during apnoea and during prolonged procedures surgery is interrupted to allow a period of IPPV.
  - ETT and IPPV. A narrow ETT is used to allow visualization of the larynx. However, the view is impaired, and hence other techniques are often preferred.
  - TIVA can be used.
  - Jet ventilation combined with TIVA in a paralysed patient. Risk of barotrauma and infrequently used in children

Postoperative care

- SpO_2 monitoring for at least 2 h to detect hypoxia secondary to hypoventilation.
- NBM for 1 h after topical anaesthesia to the larynx.
- PO paracetamol ± NSAID provide adequate analgesia.
- IV fluids and antibiotics may be indicated, depending on the situation.
- Further dose of steroid and nebulized adrenaline if patient is stridulous.

EXIT procedure

- The ex utero intrapartum treatment (EXIT) procedure is an important strategy in the management of prenatally diagnosed congenital malformations that will have an immediate and critical problem when the baby is separated from the mother at delivery, e.g. airway obstruction.
- The aim is to intervene before the umbilical cord is cut, ensuring the baby is safe as possible.
- Multidisciplinary (obstetricians, neonatologists, anaesthetists, ENT, and general surgeons) and requires careful coordination. A designated team leader is necessary to provide an overview, including time-keeping and deciding what the next step should be and when to stop.
- Three main types: EXIT to airway, EXIT to ECMO, and EXIT to resection.

EXIT to Airway

- Commonest form. Under GA, a midline caesarean section is performed. The uterus is kept relaxed to ensure good placental blood flow.
- The baby is partially delivered so the head and arms are accessible, whilst placental perfusion is maintained. Monitoring and IV access are performed at this point.
- The next step is to address the critical problem, usually an airway issue, e.g. neck or chest mass, CHAOS, or severe micrognathia. The aim is a secure airway for the baby, either via oral or nasal intubation by the anaesthetist or neonatologist or via a surgical airway by the ENT surgeon.
- Once the airway is secured, the remainder of the baby is delivered and the caesarean section is completed.

EXIT to ECMO

- Undertaken when the lungs are inadequately developed or if there is pathology preventing ventilation, e.g. CDH, bronchopulmonary sequestration, neck masses, or severe CHD. Also used to slow transition from fetal to neonatal circulation, hopefully avoiding the hypoxia associated with pulmonary hypertension.
- In essence, the baby goes from placental bypass to ECMO bypass. The intravascular cannula needed for ECMO are inserted before the umbilical cut is cut.

EXIT to resection

- Indicated when there is a large life-threatening tumour or mass, e.g. sacrococcygeal teratoma or congenital cystic malformation.
- The mass is resected whilst the baby is still attached to the placenta. Only performed when the baby cannot receive O_2 without removal of the mass.

Preoperative assessment

- Thorough assessment of all available information, including MRI or US.
- If there is airway obstruction, identify the level and extent.

- Multidisciplinary team need to plan procedures and allocate specific roles.
- Plan for airway intervention includes direct laryngoscopy, rigid or flexible bronchoscopy, or tracheostomy.
- Paediatric anaesthetic role is to aid securing the airway, help with haemodynamic stability and oxygenation of the baby, administer anaesthetic agents, and assist with resuscitation.

Anaesthetic technique

- A second experienced paediatric anaesthetist is preferable.
- Two-person airway controls may be needed, including displacement of large tumours to allow airway to be secured.
- Barotrauma is a significant risk; ensure equipment to decompress pneumothorax is available.
- Aspiration of cystic component of mass may be useful to aid securing the airway.
- IV access is secured in one of delivered hands.
- Risk of haemorrhage with immediate tumour resection: have packed cells in theatre.

Postoperative care

If the procedure is successful, transfer to NICU.

General surgery and urology

Naveen Raj

Elective

Circumcision

- Partial or complete removal of foreskin.
- Preputioplasty, i.e. a dorsal slit with transverse closure, may be performed as an alternative to treat phimosis with conservation of foreskin. Management is similar to circumcision.
- Usually a day case.
- Indications:
  - Religious/cultural: perform when >1 year of age to minimize GA risks.
  - Medical: phimosis and paraphimosis, recurrent balanitis, balanitis xerotica obliterans, and rarely recurrent UTI.

Pre-operative assessment
- Usually ASA1.
- Some institutions require both parents to be present to consent for religious/cultural circumcisions.

Anaesthesia
- Induction as preferred.
- LMA with SV.
- Maintenance as preferred.
- Analgesia:
  - Preoperative paracetamol and NSAIDs
  - Dorsal penile nerve block (use 0.5% levobupivacaine)
  - Caudal block—commoner in infants, where penile nerve block may be difficult
  - Subcutaneous ring block and topical LA cream least effective option
  - IV opioids if block not performed or failed
  - Dexamethasone.
- At the end of the procedure, the wound area is covered with chloramphenicol ointment, paraffin, or lidocaine gel.

Cystoscopy

- Involves the passage of a rigid scope for examination of the urethra and bladder.
- Indications:
  - Investigation: haematuria, UTI, voiding dysfunction or outflow obstruction.
  - Therapeutic uses include:
    —Treatment of urethral strictures
    —Removal of stents
    —STING procedure (vesicourethral reflux)
    —Botulinum toxin injection (neurogenic bladder)
    —Nephrolithiasis
    —Resection or ablation of posterior urethral valves
    —Obtaining biopsies and excision of polyps and other abnormal tissues.

Anaesthesia

- Usually short day-case procedures.
- Usually LMA and SV. ETT and IPPV considered for patient-specific issues.
- IV fluids and warming measures as indicated.
- Procedural considerations include:
  - Lithotomy position—take measures to prevent nerve injuries
  - Antibiotic prophylaxis—follow local policy.
  - Warm irrigation fluid to avoid hypothermia.
- Analgesia: preoperative paracetamol and NSAID usually sufficient.

Epigastric, ventral, and umbilical hernias

- Usually a day-case procedure.
- Rarely incarcerated.

Preoperative assessment
- Usually ASA 1.

Anaesthesia
- Induction and maintenance as preferred.
- LMA and SV unless specific contraindications.
- Analgesia:
  - Preoperative PO paracetamol and NSAID
  - Bilateral US-guided rectus sheath or TAP block
  - LA infiltration by surgeon
  - IV opioids rarely required.

Postoperative care
- Regular paracetamol and NSAIDs for up to 48 h.

Fundoplication

Overview
- Gastro-oesophageal reflux disease (GORD) is symptomatic reflux severe enough to require medical treatment or associated with complications.
- GORD results from a failure of the normal anatomical and physiological barriers.
- GORD is associated with:
  - Prematurity: abnormal relaxation of the lower oesophageal sphincter (LOS)
  - Severe impaired neurological function: disorder of motility of the distal oesophagus and abnormal relaxation of LOS
  - Congenital defects:
    —OA: reduced intraabdominal oesophageal length with loss of normal high-pressure zone
    —CDH: increased IAP
    —Abdominal wall defects: increased IAP
  - Obesity
  - Gastrostomy
  - Sandifer syndrome: spastic torticollis and dystonic body movements.
- GORD causes:
  - Recurrent vomiting with failure to thrive
  - Recurrent chest infections from aspiration
  - Epigastric, retrosternal, or back pain from oesophagitis
  - Oesophageal ulceration and stricture
  - Anaemia
  - Chronic airway issues
  - Dental erosions
  - Acute otitis media
  - Apnoea or apparent life-threatening events (ALTE).
- Diagnosis by:
  - pH study
  - Upper GI contrast studies
  - Endoscopy—more useful to assess oesophageal ulceration or stricture.
- Conservative treatment includes:
  - Feeding:
    —Reduced volume and more frequent feeds
    —Thickening of formula milk
    —NG feeds.
  - Antireflux medication: short-term course (4 weeks) to evaluate response
    —Proton pump inhibitors, e.g. omeprazole–not recommended in infants
    —H_2 receptor antagonists, e.g. ranitidine.
- Surgery indicated in 5% of children with GORD because of:
  - Failed conservative treatment
  - Worsening symptoms, e.g. recurrent pneumonia, recurrent apnoeas

- Failure to thrive
- Anatomical defects, e.g. OA

Surgery
- Usually performed in children with impaired neurological function.
- Commonest procedure is a Nissen fundoplication (open or laparoscopic):
  - Open procedure requires a subcostal incision.
  - 360° wrap of the fundus of the stomach around the lower part of the oesophagus to increase the lower oesophageal sphincter pressure, altering the angle of His, ↑ the length of intra-abdominal oesophagus, and repair any hiatus hernia present.
  - Usually combined with vagotomy, pyloroplasty, and gastrostomy in the neurologically impaired child.
- Newer techniques include endoluminal fundoplication and radiofrequency application to the oesophagogastric junction.

Preop assessment
- Routine preoperative anaesthetic assessment focusing on:
  - Problems due to neurological disability (➲ Chapter 26)
  - Recurrent chest infection: may need perioperative chest physiotherapy
  - Failure to thrive, causing anaemia, hypoalbuminemia, and fluid and electrolyte imbalance.
- Investigations:
  - CXR
  - FBC and U+E
  - Blood group not required.
- Regular medication, especially antiepileptics, antispasmodics, and antireflux medications, should be given.
- Premedication:
  - Sedatives: benefit balanced against compromising pulmonary function and oversedation in children with impaired neurological function.
  - Antisialagogues: may already be on hyoscine patches.
  - Consider antacid medication, e.g. PO ranitidine or omeprazole.

Anaesthetic technique
- Monitoring:
  - Routine non-invasive monitoring for most cases.
  - Consider central venous line if difficult venous access.
  - Arterial line rare unless significant comorbidity.
- Active measures to maintain temperature from induction:
  - Warm theatre and anaesthetic room
  - Forced air warming blanket
  - Fluid warmers
  - Minimized surgical gut exposure.
- IV induction preferred, but may be impractical.
- Modified RSI with application of cricoid pressure and intubation as soon as possible to ↓ risk of aspiration.

- Maintenance:
  - Increased sensitivity to volatile anaesthetics; desflurane preferable.
  - Remifentanil useful for volatile-sparing qualities.
  - Increased requirement for non-depolarizing agents.
  - Reduced seizure thresholds.
- Analgesia
  - IV paracetamol and NSAID.
  - Epidural (T8 level) or other regional nerve blocks with continuous infusion (PVB/high TAP) are recommended. Positioning the patient to perform the block can be challenging.
  - Where LA blocks are impossible or contraindicated, consider opiates (note increased sensitivity) combined with other adjuvants, e.g. ketamine or clonidine.
- Laparoscopic procedures, considerations are similar to other abdominal laparoscopic procedures. Pain is not a significant issue and can be controlled by regular paracetamol and NSAIDs, and LA infiltrations of port sites.

Postoperative care

- Stable, warm, and comfortable children can be extubated and discharged to ward.
- Children with preoperative pulmonary dysfunction or significant comorbidities may need HDU or PICU.
- Maintenance IV fluids until enteral intake satisfactory.
- Analgesia:
  - Commonly difficult to assess pain; use suitable pain scoring system.
  - IV paracetamol and NSAID.
  - If continuous LA technique is employed, use plain LA solution without opiates.
  - PCA may not be possible, in which case consider NCA or opiate infusion.
  - Regular antiemetic.
  - Laparoscopic patients: simple analgesics plus PO morphine PRN.
- Prescribe laxatives for constipation.
- Continue antiepileptics, antispasmodics and antireflux medications; oral antiepileptics may need to be changed to IV whilst patient is NBM.

Hydrocele repair

- Hydrocele is a fluid collection around the testes, between the parietal and visceral layers of the tunica vaginalis.
- Primarily due to persistent processus vaginalis communicating with the peritoneum. May be associated with an indirect hernia.
- Secondary non-communicating hydrocele can be due to trauma, torsion, epididymitis, or varicocele operation.
- Commoner on right side; may be bilateral.
- Unless there is testicular pathology, inguinal hernia, or significant discomfort, surgery is deferred until 2 years of age, since spontaneous resolution can occur.
- Operation: ligation of processus vaginalis via inguinal incision, leaving the sac open.
- Anaesthetic management similar to elective open inguinal hernia repair.

Hypospadias

- Abnormal position of the urethral meatus (incidence 1:300).
- Defect anywhere along ventral aspect of penis from the glans to the perineal scrotum.
- The foreskin is abnormally formed, resulting in a hood-like effect.
- Usually associated with a downward (ventral) curve of the penis called chordee.
- Associated with undescended testes (10%) and inguinal hernia (9–15%).
- Severe hypospadias with cryptorchidism ± ambiguous genitalia may be associated with congenital adrenal hyperplasia.
- Surgery performed between 6 and 18 months of age.

Surgery

- Involves creation of a neourethra with the meatus at the tip of the glans, and release of chordee if present.
- Usually performed in a single stage, but complex proximal lesions may undergo staged repair.
- Occasionally, graft tissue is taken to repair larger defects—usually from buccal mucosa (sometimes from bladder mucosa).
- Postoperatively, a free-draining urethral stent or catheter is left in situ for up to 48 h with a specific penile dressing to stop surgical oedema preventing urination.
- 2 h duration, depending on complexity.

Preoperative assessment

- Usually ASA1.
- Suitable day case.

Anaesthesia

- Induction as preferred.
- Usually LMA with SV.
- Maintenance as preferred.
- Active warming measures.
- IV fluid to maintain hydration and UO >1 mL/kg/h.
- Analgesia:
  - Preoperative PO paracetamol and NSAID, or PR at induction.
  - Caudal block ± adjuncts; consider repeating at the end of prolonged procedures.
  - Penile nerve block for minor and distal repairs.
  - IV dexamethasone prolongs analgesia.

Postoperative care

- Continue IV fluid to ensure adequate UO until oral intake is established.
- Regular paracetamol and NSAIDs for up to 48 h.

Inguinal hernia

- Common if <32 weeks gestation (13% incidence) and <1kg (30% incidence).
- M>F.
- Usually right-sided (60% incidence), although 10% are bilateral.
- Aetiology:
  - Failure of normal obliteration of the processus vaginalis (the peritoneal covering of the testes as it descends into the scrotum)
  - Normally completed by 36–40 weeks, gestation but can be patent at birth in up to 80% of children, closing by 6 months of age. Persistent processus vaginalis can still be present at 2 years of age in 40% of children.
  - Results in a hernial sac with protrusion of abdominal contents.
- Indirect inguinal hernia common and direct inguinal hernia rare.
- Presentation:
  - Incidental finding
  - Lump in groin on crying or straining, usually asymptomatic
  - Tense swelling in groin, with local and systemic inflammatory signs—indicating incarcerated hernia
  - Intestinal obstruction
  - A strangulated hernia may present with signs of peritonitis.

Surgery

- Usually repaired electively; early repair in children <1 years of age because of increased risk of incarceration and strangulation.
- Urgent surgery if incarcerated or strangulated.
- Majority of incarcerated hernias can be reduced; listed for urgent surgery to ↓ risk of re-incarceration.
- Open or laparoscopic procedure; the latter has the advantages of allowing exploration and repair of contralateral side, reduced pain, and earlier mobilization and discharge from hospital.

Anaesthesia

- Management classified into four groups:

1. Urgent repair for irreducible incarceration or strangulation
- Those with signs and symptoms of intestinal obstruction or peritonitis are managed as an acute abdomen requiring explorative emergency laparotomy.
- Need assessment and optimization of haemodynamic and fluid status preoperatively.
- Incarceration is commoner in first year of life, but incidence is lower in premature infants.

2. Children undergoing a laparoscopic repair
- As for other laparoscopic procedures.

3. Elective open repair
- Usually a day-case procedure in age-appropriate children (for day-case criteria ➜ Chapter 14).
- Or following reduction of incarcerated hernia.

Preoperative assessment
- Usually ASA1.

Anaesthesia
- Induction as preferred.
- LMA, but ETT where indicated.
- Maintenance as preferred, usually SV with volatile anaesthetic agent $\pm$ N_2O.
- Keep anaesthetic plane deep, since traction on the cord may cause laryngospasm or bradycardia if patient is 'light'.
- Antiemetic.
- IV fluids depending on age of patient.
- Analgesia:
  - Preoperative paracetamol and NSAID
  - LA techniques:
    —TAP block
    —Caudal block for infants, especially if bilateral repair
    —LA infiltration at end of procedure, pain scores higher at 2 h when compared with caudal or nerve block patients.

4. Premature infants with significant comorbidities
- Significant comorbidities (⊃ Chapter 13) and therefore at increased GA risk.
- Benefit of using awake LA technique:
  - Reduced morbidity
  - Reduced need for IPPV
  - Conflicting evidence regarding reduction in apnoea risk.
- Disadvantages of using awake LA technique:
  - Significant failure rate
  - Short duration of anaesthesia for operation
  - Challenging to anaesthetist and surgeon
  - Postoperative apnoea or bradycardia can still occur.
- Considerations of various awake LA techniques:
  - Spinal anaesthesia:
    —Dural sac terminates at a lower level compared with adults, but the intercristal line can still be used as landmark.
    —Increased meningeal permeability and a larger CSF volume compared with adults, necessitating an increased dose of LA.
    —Shorter-duration block (60–90 min) compared with adults.
    —25 G neonatal short spinal needle.
    —0.1–0.2 mL/kg of 0.25% or 0.5% levobupivacaine (minimum volume 0.5 mL, maximum volume 3 mL).
    —Do not lift legs to place diathermy plate immediately after injection.
  - Caudal anaesthesia:
    —1 mL/kg 0.25% levobupivacaine.
    —Slower onset compared with spinal.
    —Onset of motor block may take longer, and it may be necessary to strap the lower limbs down to prevent movement during the initial stages of surgery.
    —Duration 45–90 min.

- Combined spinal and caudal block:
  —0.1 mL/kg of 0.25% levobupivacaine injected into spinal space. The rest of the maximum volume of 0.25% levobupivacaine injected into caudal space. Alternatively, a caudal cannula can be sited at the time of spinal block, with a short extension attached through which LA can be injected at a later time to prolong the duration of anaesthesia.
- Spinal combined with TAP block (performed immediately after the spinal block or at the end of the procedure).
- Spinal block with LA infiltration in the proximity of the ilio-inguinal nerve is performed by surgeon during the procedure.
- Technical considerations:
  - Preoperative discussion with parents, including risk of conversion to GA.
  - Application of topical LA cream to planned site of injection—spinal or caudal.
  - Prepare for potential GA.
  - Surgeon and theatre team scrubbed and ready.
  - Block performed in theatre on operating table to minimize delays.
  - Assistant holds child still in lateral or sitting position.
  - Standard non-invasive monitoring.
  - PO sucrose to calm the child during regional block insertion
  - Often the child will fall asleep after the block owing to loss of afferent stimulus from the lower body
  - IV access before block is ideal, but may be impossible and cause significant distress. In difficult cases, it may be easier to obtain IV access in the lower limbs after performing the block. The immaturity of the sympathetic nervous system means there are no deleterious haemodynamic effects.
  - Rescue techniques for failed or inadequate block:
    —Be prepared to convert to full GA anytime during the procedure.
    —If maximum LA dose not used, consider supplementary field block or ilio-inguinal nerve block by surgeon.
    —IV ketamine 0.5–1 mg/kg or propofol 1–2 mg/kg followed by an infusion.
    —Low concentration of sevoflurane by nasal cannula or face mask.

Postoperative care

- SpO_2 and apnoea monitoring for neonates.
- Regular PO paracetamol ± NSAIDs (older children).
- PRN PO morphine.

Laparoscopy

- Advantages over open procedures include improved cosmetic results, less pain, fewer wound complications, and quicker recovery.
- An open technique is used to insert the first trocar, and subsequent trocars are placed under direct vision to avoid visceral or vascular injury.
- CO_2 insufflates the peritoneum to provide a good visual field. CO_2 is used because it does not support combustion and has minimal effects with intravascular embolization.
- The paediatric abdominal wall is very pliable, so adequate visualization of the intra-abdominal contents is possible at lower IAP than in adults.
- Procedures may be prolonged.
- Other considerations:
  - Need age-appropriate size laparoscopic equipment and surgical experience.
  - Risk of laparoscopy converting to open procedure.
  - Gas embolism.
  - Risk of subcutaneous emphysema, pneumomediastinum, or pneumothorax due to congenital or surgical defects in diaphragm and raised IAP.
- The physiological effects of pneumoperitoneum are usually benign:
  - Cephalad shift of diaphragm.
  - FRC relative to closing volume predisposes to atelectasis, ventilation–perfusion inequalities, and hypoxia.
  - Pulmonary compliance ↓ and airway resistance ↑.
  - HyperCO$_2$ commonly due to CO_2 absorption and poor ventilatory compliance.
  - The ↓ FRC exacerbated by Trendelenburg position.
  - Reverse Trendelenburg position (used for upper abdominal procedures) may improve respiratory compliance.
  - When IAP >15 mmHg, IVC compression reduces venous return and thus CO. This is potentiated by hypovolaemia and the head-up position.
  - ↑ SVR due to aortic compression and hyperCO$_2$.
  - When insufflating pressure <12 mmHg, any cardiorespiratory changes that occur are usually within acceptable values.
  - Effects on ICP are complex. ↑ ICP during laparoscopy has been reported in patients with VP shunts, despite a low IAP and a normal arterial pCO$_2$. HyperCO$_2$ ↑ cerebral blood flow and may ↑ ICP, which is exacerbated by head-down position. A ↑ in IAP also tends to ↑ ICP. When these changes are combined with a ↓ CO and a ↑ intrathoracic pressure, the possibility of a reduction in CPP exists.
  - Decreased UO due to decreased GFR and neurohumoral response.

Preoperative assessment

- The scenario may vary from an elective procedure in a healthy child to an emergency laparoscopy to evaluate an acute abdomen in a premature neonate.
- History and examination to evaluate the patient's preoperative clinical status with investigations as appropriate.

- Assess fluid status, especially for emergency laparoscopic procedures; ensure hypovolaemia corrected.
- Assessment of comorbidities, e.g. sickle cell disease if presenting with gallstones for cholecystectomy.
- Blood must be grouped and saved for major laparoscopic procedures.

Anaesthesia
- Induction as preferred; RSI where indicated.
- ETT and IPPV.
- Where possible, a cuffed ETT is preferable. For uncuffed tubes, aim for a minimal leak at 20 cmH$_2$O inspiratory pressure. Allow adequate ventilation when PIP ↑ with abdominal insufflation.
- Owing to potential for respiratory changes, exhaled V$_T$ and PIP are monitored during insufflation. Hypoxia is overcome with supplemental O$_2$ and moderate PEEP.
- ↑ risk of endobronchial intubation due to elevated diaphragm moving the carina cephalad. Suspect if there is a ↑ in airway pressure and a fall in SpO$_2$ at time of insufflation or patient positioning.
- NGT to decompress the stomach, thus improving visualization of abdominal contents and limiting risk of inadvertent damage during trocar placement. Urinary catheter often inserted for similar reasons.
- GA maintenance as preferred, but avoid N$_2$O.
- A remifentanil (0.1–0.25 mcg/kg/min) infusion blunts the haemodynamic response to a pneumoperitoneum and aids emergence.
- Have atropine ready to treat bradycardia secondary to visceral stimulation.
- Environmental lighting may be suboptimal, and space and access is at a premium.
- Following completion of procedure, the CO$_2$ is evacuated to limit problems with pain, PONV, and diaphragmatic splinting.
- Insufflation of cold gas increases risk of hypothermia; therefore actively warm.
- Risk factors for complications:
  - Lower age group and weight of child
  - Higher pressure and duration of insufflation
  - Prolonged procedure.
- Analgesia:
  - Preoperative or intraoperative paracetamol and NSAID.
  - Pre-emptive LA infiltration of trocar insertion sites
  - IV morphine 100–150 mcg/kg IV can be given towards the end of the procedure to ensure adequate analgesia in the early postoperative period.
  - Neurologically or respiratory compromised patients should have opioids titrated once adequate spontaneous respiration is established.
  - Ondansetron and dexamethasone.

Postoperative care
- Referred shoulder tip pain can occur owing to diaphragmatic irritation secondary to incomplete evacuation of intra-abdominal CO$_2$.
- Early pain may be severe, but usually ↓ dramatically over 24 h.

- Regular paracetamol ± NSAID.
- PRN PO morphine.
- PRN antiemetics.
- Minor to moderate surgery: PRN PO morphine is usually satisfactory.
- Major procedures, peritonitic abdomens, or postoperative ileus: use NCA/PCA.
- IV fluids until drinking.

Long-term central venous access devices

- Indications:
  - TPN
  - Antibiotics
  - Chemotherapy
  - Medication
  - Repeated investigations or fluids/blood transfusion
  - Critical venous access.
- Two types:
  - Subcutaneously tunnelled cuffed venous line with external access ports:
    —Broviac line or Hickman line; the former has a smaller lumen.
    —Usually one- or two-lumen.
    —Made of silicone, Teflon, or polyurethane material.
    —Distal Dacron cuff near to exit from skin site–fixes the catheter by encouraging fibrous tissue formation and may act as barrier to infection.
  - Subcutaneously tunnelled venous line with access port is implanted under the skin:
    —PORT-A-CATH or Mediport.
    —Usually one-port.
    —Made of silicone or polyurethane.
    —The injecting port sits under the skin; it has a titanium base and a self-sealing silicone membrane that is pressure-resistant and fixes the injecting needle in place.
    —Port is accessed by a special needle–Huber.
- Subcutaneous tunnelling reduces infection risk and secures line.
- Both can be used for venous access during GA with appropriate aseptic non-touch techniques, but are unsuitable in situations where rapid large-volume infusion required.

Surgery

- Commonest vein used is internal jugular.
- MRV or Doppler US preoperatively if doubts regarding vein patency, e.g. previous insertion or thrombosis.
- Vein is accessed by open surgery or increasingly by percutaneous means.
- Percutaneous: US-guided access to vein and confirmation of placement of position of wire by fluoroscopy.
- Open surgery is performed via a small transverse incision over the neck vessels at the level of the cricoid.
- Broviac:
  - Catheter is tunnelled under the skin from the pectoral region, ensuring the distal cuff is buried under the skin at the distal entry point.
  - Catheter is trimmed to length based on measuring either directly against the corresponding rib space or with the aid of fluoroscopy.
  - In open procedures, a small venotomy is performed and the catheter inserted into the vein.

- In percutaneous cases, a split sheath introducer is used to insert the catheter.
- Catheter position is confirmed by fluoroscopy and aspiration of blood.
- Catheter is fixed and incisions closed.
- PORT-A-CATH:
  - Venous access and catheter insertion is similar to Broviac insertion.
  - Then a conveniently positioned percutaneous pocket is created in the pectoral region; the port is then sited and fixed.
  - A catheter is connected to the port and then percutaneously tunnelled to be inserted into the vein. The rest of the procedure is completed as for Broviac
  - Tip is ideally positioned in the lower SVC or RA, fluoroscopically indicated as 1 vertebral position below the carina. If inserted in the lower body, it should be at the lower border of the IVC, which corresponds to just above the 5th lumbar vertebra.
  - A Huber needle is inserted through skin into the port and its position confirmed by aspiration of blood.
- Flush with heparin saline.

Preoperative assessment
- Routine assessment with focus on the condition requiring venous access.
- Sepsis is a relative contraindication, although sepsis treatment itself might be the indication for line insertion—risks and benefits need to be assessed.
- Oncology/haematology patients commonly need clotting defects corrected preoperatively.
- Platelets should be transfused as close to the time of line insertion as possible. Aim for platelets >100,000.
- Crossmatch generally unnecessary.

Anaesthesia
- Induction as preferred; often inhalational owing to IV access problems.
- Routine non-invasive monitoring.
- Difficult venous access: venous access may be impossible and a clear plan on how to conduct anaesthesia is needed. Consider IO access or peripheral venous cut down in extreme cases.
- Surgery is close to the airway—ETT preferred.
- Ensure can access venous line (plan before induction).
- IPPV commonest option, especially in smaller children. To prevent air embolism, avoid SV until the vein is closed.
- If line insertion is part of surgical management, e.g. laparotomy, then consider optimal time for insertion:
  - Before: having central venous access is advantageous and may obviate the need for insertion of either a percutaneous central line (for CVP monitoring or giving inotropes) or an arterial line (for venous blood gas sampling).
  - After: in cases of cardiorespiratory instability, e.g. raised IAP preventing adequate ventilation, the surgical procedure may need to performed before line insertion.

- Maintenance as preferred.
- Avoid dexamethasone in oncology and immunosuppressed patients or in those on fixed protocol-driven treatment measures.
- Active warming devices and IV fluids, since procedures can be prolonged.
- Analgesia:
  - IV paracetamol
  - Superficial cervical plexus block—covers neck incision
  - Pecs block—analgesia of the pectoral region
  - TAP block—in cases of femoral lines
  - LA infiltration by surgeon—before catheter tunnelled
  - Consider opioid, e.g. fentanyl, especially before tunnelling—avoid if high risk of PONV.
- Observe for:
  - Bleeding
  - Arrhythmias
  - Pneumothorax
  - Air embolism.
- CXR not required when line position confirmed by fluoroscopy.

Postoperative care

- In neutropenic patients, avoid regular paracetamol—may mask pyrexia.
- Prescribe postoperative heparin flushes.

Orchidopexy

- Cryptorchidism is a failure of testes to descend into the scrotum; normally occurs by 6 months of age.
- Unilateral or bilateral.
- Undescended testes may be high in the scrotum, in the inguinal canal, or intra-abdominal.
- An ectopic undescended testis, which is usually well developed and histologically normal, has deviated from its normal path of descent and may be present in the superficial inguinal pouch, the perineum, the femoral canal, or the root of the penis.
- Diagnosis by history and physical examination. US is of limited value.
- Surgery is ideally performed by 18 months of age to reduce risks of:
  - Subfertility
  - Testicular cancer
  - Torsion
  - Inguinal hernia.

Surgery

- Depends on position of testis:
  - Palpable testis:
    —Scrotal orchidopexy: uncommon; scrotal incision to fix very low-lying testis.
    —Inguinal orchidopexy involves mobilization of the testis and securing it in the scrotum via inguinal and scrotal incisions. If it is difficult to bring the testis down to the scrotum, then it is fixed as low as possible in the groin and a second operation is performed in 6 months' time.
  - Non-palpable testis: surgeon examines under anaesthesia after induction to aid operative decision. Testis is impalpable on examination 20% of the time.
    —Laparoscopy to determine if the testis is intra-abdominal (50–60%), atrophic, or absent (20%). If the testis is found, it is mobilized and then a laparoscopically assisted or open orchidopexy is performed.
    —Two-stage procedure may be used: an initial laparoscopy is performed to identify the position of the testis and bring it down into the inguinal canal, then, 6 months later, a further procedure is performed to position the testis in the scrotum.
    —Attempt at inguinal orchidopexy: if testis is not found during exploration, then laparoscopy is performed.
    —Fowler–Stephens procedure. If the testis is >2 cm from the internal inguinal ring, the testicular vessels may be short and not reach the scrotum. By dividing and ligating the testicular vessels, the testis can be brought down into the scrotum with the blood supply to the testis depending on flow through vessels from the vas deferens. This is commonly a laparoscopic procedure done in two stages, with ligation as the first stage, followed by orchidopexy after 6 months to allow for establishment of blood supply to the testis, but it can also be done as a single procedure and as an open technique

Preoperative assessment
- Day case, usually ASA 1.
- Increased incidence with:
  - Prematurity
  - Abdominal wall defects
  - Myelomeningocele.

Anaesthesia
- Similar to inguinal hernia repair management.
- Similar anaesthetic considerations as for any abdominal laparoscopic procedure.
- Usually LMA and SV for open procedures.
- ETT and IPPV for laparoscopic procedures or in very young children.
- Maintenance as preferred.
- IV fluids and assisted warming devices.
- High incidence of PONV: give ondansetron and dexamethasone.
- Note: The testes have a sympathetic innervation that reaches the CNS at about T10. For this reason, even with a good block for the incision, traction on the testis can produce laryngospasm or a bradycardia mediated by the vagal nerve. Incidence is reduced by maintaining adequate depth of GA.
- Analgesia:
  - Preoperative PO paracetamol and NSAIDs.
  - Regional technique depends on patient age and surgical approach.
  - TAP block for inguinal orchidopexy, and potentially for laparoscopically assisted procedures. Both require LA infiltration of scrotal incision.
  - Caudal block for infants.
  - LA infiltration by surgeon at end when blocks are not performed
  - Consider opioids for surgically difficult cases.

Postoperative care
- Increased incidence of pain and PONV in older children.
- Regular paracetamol and NSAIDs for up to a week.
- Some institutions provide PO morphine TTO.

Nephrectomy

- Performed to remove all or part of a non-functioning kidney. Underlying pathology includes a multicystic dysplastic kidney, congenital renal dysplasia, severe reflux nephropathy, severe obstructive uropathy, and Wilms tumour (nephroblastoma).
- Increasingly performed laparoscopically.
- Open procedure uses either subcostal flank or abdominal incision, with patient commonly in lateral or semilateral position with affected kidney up.

Preoperative assessment

- Usually ASA 1 with no features of chronic renal disease or fluid and electrolyte disturbances.
- Some have comorbidities that affect the anaesthetic technique. These include spina bifida, renal artery stenosis, polycystic disease, Wilms tumour, or chronic renal failure. Considerations include anaemia, hyperkalaemia, fluid overload, hypertension, intercurrent drug treatment, and venous access.
- Patients have often had symptoms and illness for months and may have undergone multiple investigations and imaging ± GA.
- Bleeding is not usually a problem. More of a risk with heminephrectomy or duplex system kidneys. It is a major consideration in removal of a Wilms tumour, which may have invaded locally or extended into the IVC—cross-match blood.

Anaesthesia

- Induction as preferred.
- ETT and IPPV.
- Two good-sized IV cannulas.
- For lateral renal incisions, older children are placed in a lateral position with the table broken, while a flank roll is used in babies to allow access to the kidney. The lateral renal incision does not split muscle and analgesic requirements are less than for more extensive procedures using a lower abdominal incision.
- GA maintenance as preferred ± remifentanil infusion (0.25–0.5 mcg/ kg/min).
- Antibiotics as per local policy.
- IV fluids maintenance and volume replacement with crystalloid, colloid, or blood.
- Dexamethasone and ondansetron.
- Analgesia:
  - Preoperative or intraoperative paracetamol and NSAIDs (if not contraindicated)
  - Open procedures: PVB ± catheter or low-thoracic epidural
  - Laparoscopic procedure: LA infiltration plus IV morphine 100 mcg/kg.

Postoperative care
- IV fluids 12–24 h.
- Start drinking earlier after laparoscopic and retroperitoneal surgery.
- Regular PO paracetamol ± NSAIDs (if renal function normal).
- For laparoscopic procedure, PRN PO morphine, possibly NCA/PCA overnight.
- For open procedure, LA infusion or NCA/PCA.

Pyeloplasty

- Ureteropelvic junction obstruction (UPJO) prevents urine flowing from kidney into ureter, resulting in hydronephrosis; this ↑ in pressure causes progressive renal dysfunction (irreversible over time).
- Incidence 1:1,500 births, 2M:1F.
- Usually the left kidney is affected. Bilateral in 30% of cases.
- Renal associations: horseshoe kidney, megaureters, and urethral valves.
- Extrarenal associations: VACTERL and DS.
- Aetiology is unclear, both intrinsic (ureteric hypoplasia, abnormalities in the ureteric wall), extrinsic (pressure from aberrant blood vessels or tumour, malformations of the kidney, previous surgery/ instrumentation), and intraluminal (urethral valves) causes.
- Presentation depends on age, with generalized symptoms and failure to thrive common in infants, and flank pain, haematuria, UTIs, and rarely abdominal mass in older children.
- Can be diagnosed by antenatal scans and usually confirmed with postnatal radiological investigations (US scans and MAG3 gamma imaging).

Surgery

- Pyeloplasty is the surgical treatment of choice, required in up to 20% of cases before renal dysfunction becomes irreversible
- Open pyeloplasty is gold standard; laparoscopic and robot-assisted techniques are becoming popular. Endoscopic procedures are possible.
- Nephrostomy where pyeloplasty is impossible (pyonephrosis)
- Indications:
  - Failure of conservative treatment (observation and antibiotics with regular radiological follow-up) with worsening renal function
  - Symptomatic hydronephrosis (pain, infection)
  - Asymptomatic with significant US findings of dilation or renal dysfunction.
- Technique involves an ipsilateral subcostal or flank incision and rarely a dorsal incision. Retroperitoneal access to the kidney, removal of the obstructed area of the ureter and re-anastomosis ± flap, and reduction of dilated pelvis.

Preoperative assessment

- Routine assessment including associated comorbidities and clinical and biochemical parameters of renal function : fluid status, BP, anaemia, and electrolytes.

Anaesthesia

- Induction and maintenance as preferred.
- ETT and IPPV.
- Positioning: depends on incision and surgical preference.
- IV fluids and active warming measures.
- Prophylactic antibiotics as per policy.

- Analgesia:
  - Avoid NSAIDs if significant renal dysfunction
  - Consider LA block: ipsilateral PVB or TAP block
  - LA infiltration
  - IV opioids if LA blocks contraindicated.

Postoperative care
- Regular IV or PO paracetamol.
- PRN PO morphine.
- PRN antiemetics.

Emergency or semi-urgent

Appendicectomy

- Peak incidence 11–13 years of age.
- Presentation depends on severity of condition:
  - A clinical diagnosis suffices in most cases, but the false-negative appendicectomy rate is 10–30%. Diagnosis can be challenging.
  - A Paediatric Appendicitis (Samuel) Score in children or Alvarado Scoring System in adults may aid diagnosis.
  - Onset of severe GI symptoms before pain may indicate a different diagnosis.
  - Younger children may present late and be severely ill with full-blown peritonitis and shock. Perforated appendix is present in 70% of <4-year-olds at time of surgery
  - Abnormal appendix position may lead to atypical presentation and delayed diagnosis.
- Investigations including FBC, U+E, CRP, and urine analysis aid in diagnostic process. US or CT scan may aid diagnosis when there is doubt or atypical presentation.
- Clinical course varies from spontaneous resolution to peritonitis and abscess formation.
- Conservative treatment with antibiotics seem to be safe and effective in patients with uncomplicated early-presentation appendicitis (no evidence of perforation). If symptoms persist, surgery is indicated
- Surgical treatment should not be delayed, since the risk of perforation increases by 5% every 12 h, 36 h after the onset of symptoms.

Surgical technique

- Historically, open appendicectomy was the gold standard. Now, where possible, laparoscopic appendicectomy is performed because of:
  - Better visualization of the peritoneal cavity and reduced surgical complications
  - Reduced postoperative pain and length of recovery.
- Open appendicectomy involves a transverse incision at the McBurney point.
- Laparoscopic procedure utilizes one to three ports. Significant risk of conversion to open.
- Appendicular abscess/mass is treated with IV antibiotics and radiological or operative drainage. Interval appendicectomy is performed at 6 weeks if there is no clinical improvement.

Preoperative assessment

- Usually ASA 1.
- Assess hydration state (NBM and potentially septic); check antibiotics and analgesia.

Anaesthesia

- RSI.
- Signs of shock may be subtle, especially in young children, who may decompensate at induction and require resuscitation.
- Insert a large-bore IV cannula early, especially in the decompensated child.
- IPPV. Maintenance as preferred, but avoid N_2O.
- Broad-spectrum antibiotics within 1 h of surgical incision.
- Warm IV fluids and warming blanket are used. If open appendicectomy is planned, a US TAP block can be performed at induction.
- For a laparoscopic procedure, the considerations are similar to those for other abdominal laparoscopic procedures.
- Antiemetics to ↓ risk of PONV.
- Analgesia:
  - IV paracetamol.
  - PR NSAID.
  - For an open procedure, perform a unilateral TAP block (before or after operation).
  - For a laparoscopic procedure, use LA infiltration to port sites.
  - IV opioids, especially if peritonitic, e.g. morphine 50–100 mcg/kg.

Postoperative care

- Long line or PICC line inserted for TPN (and antibiotics if there is significant peritonitis or perforation).
- IV fluids and antiemetics.
- Regular IV paracetamol and NSAID.
- PO morphine for mild appendicitis.
- PCA/NCA if there are signs of peritonitis.
- No consensus on duration of antibiotics; follow local policies.
- Simple cases have feeding re-established early and are discharged home within 2–3 days.
- Complex cases have delayed recovery and prolonged hospital stay.

Neonatal laparotomy

- This section describes the various neonatal diagnoses requiring laparotomy and their perioperative management. The final subsection describes the general management of any neonatal laparotomy. For a detailed discussion of neonatal anaesthesia, ⦿ Chapter 13.

Necrotizing enterocolitis

- Necrosis of the intestinal wall, potentially leading to perforation, sepsis, and DIC.
- Commonest surgical emergency of GIT in the premature infant.
- Incidence 0.5–5:1,000 live births.
- Incidence and risk of fatality inversely proportional to gestational age and birth weight.
- Mortality varies from 15% to 90% (NEC totalis, where the entire intestine is affected).
- Unknown aetiology.
- Risk factors:
  - Formula milk feeds (90% have received); the risk is ↓ with breast milk and probiotics. The timing of initiation of enteral feeds or the rate at which they are given is inconsequential.
  - PDA.
  - Gastroschisis.
- Rare in term infants, but is associated with hypoxic/ischaemic conditions, e.g. CHD, respiratory distress syndrome, and polycythaemia.
- Bell's staging system modified by Walsh and Kliegman is used for staging severity and planning treatment. It uses clinical, radiological, and laboratory parameters.
  - Stage 1: Suspected, managed conservatively.
  - Stage 2: Proven, managed conservatively.
  - Stage 3: Advanced, often require surgery.
- Signs and symptoms:
  - Abdomen:
    - —Abdominal distension
    - —Occult or frank blood PR
    - —Vomiting and/or diarrhoea
    - —Peritonitis.
  - Systemic:
    - —Lethargy
    - —Temperature instability
    - —Respiratory distress and apnoea
    - —Signs of sepsis and shock
    - —DIC.
- Investigations:
  - Plain X-ray abdomen: pneumatosis intestinalis (intramural gas due to absorption of intraluminal gas) or portal venous gas (intravascular gas absorption) with dilated loops of bowel, pneumoperitoneum, and ascites.
  - US abdomen with Doppler: detects necrotic bowel and measures mesenteric vessel blood flow.

- Laboratory investigations:
  —ABG: acidosis.
  —FBC: anaemia, neutropenia, and thrombocytopenia.
  —Neutrophil count <150,000 and platelet count <100,000 are associated with increased mortality risk.
  —Decreasing platelet count correlates well with necrotic bowel and worsening disease.
  —Coagulation defects.
  —U+E: electrolyte imbalance, ↑ CRP.
- Most cases are managed conservatively:
  - NBM and TPN
  - Continuous low-grade NG suction to decompress bowel
  - Broad-spectrum antibiotics
  - Cardiorespiratory support as required.
- 20–40% require surgery:
  - Absolute indication:
    —Pneumoperitoneum, i.e. perforation.
  - Relative indications:
    —Abdominal wall erythema
    —Intra-abdominal mass
    —Signs of obstruction
    —Signs of peritonitis
    —Sudden and marked ↓ in platelet count
    —Worsening acidosis
    —Failure of conservative management.

Surgery

- Laparotomy, with resection of ischaemic and necrotic bowel segments. End-to-end anastomosis if possible; otherwise stoma formation to allow time for healing and growth before anastomosis.
- Insertion of peritoneal drain to decompress abdomen:
  - Performed on neonatal unit.
  - Initially used only in unstable critically ill infants usually of extremely low birth weight (high mortality rate).
  - Now being considered as an alternative to laparotomy.
- Trials have failed to demonstrate advantage of any treatment with respect to mortality.
- Immediate postoperative complications include wound dehiscence, abscesses, and intestinal strictures (mainly colonic).
- Longer-term complication: short-gut syndrome (TPN dependent).

Spontaneous intestinal perforation

- Bowel perforation without evidence of NEC.
- Differential diagnosis for NEC:
  - Not related to enteral feeds.
  - No signs of significant inflammation.
- Risk factors:
  - Prematurity
  - Birth weight
  - Indometacin and dexamethasone.

- Abdominal X-ray:
  - Absence of pneumatosis intestinalis
  - Pneumoperitoneum.

Duodenal atresia
- Incidence 3:10,000.
- Embryogenic failure in recanulization of developing intestine; commonly at junction of first and second parts of duodenum.
- Can be diagnosed by antenatal US and is associated with maternal polyhydramnios.
- Characteristic signs on abdominal X-ray: 'double bubble' with absence of air in distal intestine in cases of complete obstruction.
- Up to 50% associated with congenital anomalies:
  - Trisomy 21 (30% of cases)
  - CHD
  - Intestinal atresia and malrotation
  - Trachea-oesophageal fistula
  - Anorectal anomalies
  - VACTERL.
- Surgery involves a right upper quadrant incision, resection of the atretic segment, and re-anastomosis. Can be performed laparoscopically.

Jejuno-ileal atresia
- Incidence 1:1,500–12,000.
- Commonest site for intestinal atresia.
- May be multiple sites.
- Classified into four types, which affects treatment and prognosis
- Thought to be a result of intrauterine vascular insult.
- <1% associated with chromosomal or other system anomalies.
- Higher incidence in premature and low-birth-weight babies.
- Diagnosis confirmed by abdominal X-ray.
- Laparotomy, resection of atretic segment, and end-to-end anastomosis.
- Stomas if there is peritonitis or concern regarding viable intestine's blood supply.

Hirschsprung's disease
- Incidence 1:5,000.
- Aganglionic bowel segments due to arrest of cranio-caudad migration of neural crest cells into the intramuscular and submucosal plexus of distal bowel.
- Results in functional bowel obstruction with delayed passage of meconium.
- Usually involves a short segment of the sigmoid colon and rectum.
- Associated with trisomy 21.
- Confirmed by suction rectal biopsy.
- Surgical options:
  - Resection of aganglionic segments and stoma formation, with later pull-through procedure.
  - Single-stage resection of aganglionic segment and endorectal pull-through procedure.

Anorectal malformation

- Incidence 1:5,000 with absence of normal anal opening.
- Associated with other anomalies, e.g. VACTERL.
- Presents as intestinal obstruction.
- Low malformations:
  - Rectum close to the skin and not associated with fistula formation.
  - Treated by primary anoplasty.
- High malformations:
  - Rectum located high in the pelvis; may be associated with fistulas to bladder, vagina, or urethra.
  - Treated by initial defunctioning colostomy; followed by posterior sagittal anorectoplasty (PSARP) or laparoscopically assisted anorectal pull-through (LAARP).

Malrotation and midgut volvulus

- Incidence 1:500.
- 50% occur in neonates.
- Occurs anywhere in GIT.
- Results from incomplete or abnormal rotation of the gut around its pedicle during embryological development.
- May be an incidental finding.
- Presents as intestinal obstruction; may develop into bowel ischaemia and infarction.
- Usually associated with Ladd's bands (anomalous peritoneal fibrous bands), which may aggravate obstruction.
- Confirmed by upper GI contrast study.
- Associated with abdominal wall defects, CDH, and their associated malformations.
- Surgery: Ladd's procedure, in which Ladd's bands are resected and mesentery is widened, bowel is derotated and positioned in normal site, and appendicectomy is performed.

Intussusception

- Incidence 1–4:2,000.
- Invagination of a portion of intestine into another, leading to obstruction and later to infarction.
- Commonest in infants; rare >5 years old.
- Risk factors in older child:
  - Meckel's diverticulum
  - Intestinal polyp
  - Henoch–Schönlein purpura
  - CF
  - Lymphoma.
- Present with intermittent pain, palpable abdominal mass, and bloody diarrhoea (redcurrant jelly stool). Signs and symptoms may be vague and intermittent.
- Ensure adequate fluid resuscitation prior to any intervention.
- Contrast or air enema used to aid diagnosis and as first line of treatment to reduce intussusception.
- Laparotomy if failure to reduce or signs of peritonitis.

Meconium ileus

- Obstruction of the distal ileum and colon with meconium.
- Presents as bowel obstruction.
- Strong association with CF (investigate postoperatively).
- Half present with a complicated form associated with volvulus, perforation, or atresia.
- Gastrografin® contrast enema confirms diagnosis; can act as a laxative and relieve obstruction.
- Surgery is indicated if there is a risk of perforation and when solubilizing enema fails to evacuate meconium. An enterotomy is formed to relieve the obstruction by expressing the meconium through the enterotomy or milking it distally. This is followed by saline irrigation and closure of the enterotomy with or without bowel segment resection.

Reversal of stoma

- Performed to restore bowel continuity and normal function.
- The optimal timing of closure of stomas unclear and depends on patient parameters and local protocols. It may be delayed >8–10 weeks after stoma formation or until child has gained weight >2kg to provide adequate time to recover from previous surgery and effects or prematurity.
- Stomas are associated with:
  - Inadequate absorption of nutrients
  - Metabolic disturbances: fluid and electrolyte derangements
  - Increased risk of strictures, prolapse, and retraction
  - Skin excoriation and wound breakdown.
- Above problems are commonest with jejunostomies and therefore may benefit from early closure.
- Early closure may ↓ stoma-related problems, but procedure may be associated with increased risk of anaesthetic and surgical complications.
- Systemic review shows no difference in surgical complications between early (<8 weeks after stoma formation) or delayed closure.

Anaesthesia for neonates undergoing laparotomy

Preoperative assessment

- Stabilize and optimise patient's condition as much as possible.
- Standard assessment, with additional focus on problems relevant to the proposed surgery, associated comorbidities, and effects of prematurity.

Preoperative preparation

- Check availability of age-appropriate anaesthetic equipment
- Blood products checked and available in theatre.
- Underbody forced air warming device, e.g. Bair Hugger
- ↑ theatre temperature to 25–27°C
- Warmed IV fluids.

Anaesthesia

- Induction on operating table.
- Routine non-invasive monitoring as per AAGBI standards.

- Preferably both pre-ductal and post-ductal SpO_2.
- NGT aspiration and continued low-grade suction.
- IV or inhalational induction as preferred. Note:
  - Signs of haemodynamic instability may be masked; prepare for rapid decompensation, i.e. resuscitation drugs should be prepared.
  - May be significant aspiration risk; consider RSI. This may be challenging because:
    —Pre-oxygenation is difficult in an uncooperative child.
    —Cricoid pressure may make laryngoscopy difficult and need to be removed.
    —To ↓ risk of desaturation, hand ventilation is continued whilst waiting for muscle relaxant to work.
- Insert second IV cannula.
- Indications for arterial line (22 G 5 cm):
  - Anticipated haemodynamic instability
  - Significant cardiorespiratory comorbidities
  - Significant bleeding expected
  - Need for inotropic support
  - Where surgical manoeuvres may compromise CO, e.g. closure of abdomen in the presence of raised IAP
  - Anticipated major fluid shifts with need for frequent blood gas analysis and lab sampling
  - If NIBP unreliable.
- Indications for CVP line (4 Fr double-lumen or 4.5 Fr triple-lumen):
    —Difficult venous access
    —Assessment of intravascular volume status
    —As an indicator of raised IAP
    —Inotrope infusion
    —Venous blood gases where arterial line is not used
    —Venous SaO_2 to assess adequacy of end-organ perfusion.
- Urinary catheter for UO monitoring as required.
- Maintenance using a combination of O_2/air and volatile anaesthetic.
- Ventilation can be challenging; aim to minimize barotrauma.
- Aim for SpO_2 in mid 90s and avoid high FiO_2.
- Fluid and glucose management:
  - Isotonic IV fluids for maintenance and to correct deficits.
  - Infusion of 8–10 mL/kg/h is normal, but to compensate for ongoing losses 15–20 mL/kg/h or more may be required.
  - Premature infants, newborn children in first days of life, and those on TPN are at risk of hypoglycaemia; use 5% or 10% glucose infusion if isotonic solution with 1% glucose is not available.
    —Avoid hyperglycaemia.
    —Hypotonic solution can lead to hypoNa⁺.
  - 0.9% saline or colloids (4.5% albumin, Gelofusine®) boluses for volume expansion.
- Consider blood transfusion if:
  - Estimated blood loss is >10–15%. Aim for Hb >120 g/L.
  - If >30 mL/kg of crystalloid infused and there is ongoing need for fluid resuscitation.

- Maximal allowable blood loss (MABL) reached:

  MABL = [(starting Hct −target Hct) ÷ starting Hct]

  x Estimated blood volume (80 −100mL / kg)

- Consider platelets and cryoprecipitate if clinically indicated or when one whole blood volume transfused.

Analgesia
- IV paracetamol (7.5 mg/kg up to 44 weeks gestational age)
- Opioids as continuous infusion; careful bolusing owing to risk of bradycardia
- Remifentanil 0.05–0.2 mcg/kg/h
- Fentanyl 2–5 mcg/kg/h
- Morphine 20–50 mcg/kg/h
- Opioid boluses at regular intervals:
  - Fentanyl 0.5–2 mcg/kg
  - Morphine 25–100 mcg/kg.
- LA block performed at beginning or end of procedure; often best to choose technique once extent of the surgery is known. Also, if performed at the end, the duration of a single-shot LA technique is maximized. Comorbidities, e.g. prematurity or complicated surgery, may benefit from a catheter technique, whereas a single-shot LA technique may be more appropriate for a full-term healthy baby having uncomplicated surgery.
  - Caudal: single-shot or catheter
  - Epidural: single-shot or catheter
  - Unilateral or bilateral TAP block
  - Unilateral or bilateral lower thoracic PVB.

Postoperative management
- Extubate if stable and surgery uncomplicated. Admit to ward or HDU.
- SpO_2 and apnoea monitoring (risk of apnoea).
- If cardiorespiratory support required, then transfer to PICU with appropriate sedation and ventilatory management.
- Analgesia depends on severity of surgery and comorbidities of neonate:
  - Regular IV paracetamol
  - PR codeine or PO morphine (if not NBM) if NCA considered inappropriate
  - NCA
  - Continuous LA technique
  - IV fluids.

Abdominal wall defects: gastroschisis and omphalocele (exomphalos)

Gastroschisis overview

- Herniation of bowel loops through a full-thickness defect of abdominal wall (usually right of the umbilical cord).
  - Organs, e.g. stomach or liver, rarely herniate into the sac.
  - No covering membrane. Bowel loops exposed to amniotic fluid in utero becoming thickened and covered with an inflammatory exudate (peel), making it hard to separate them.
  - Umbilical cord is separate from the defect and normal.
- Incidence 0.4–3:10,000.
- Higher incidence if maternal age <20, exposure to certain environmental toxins, smoking, and alcohol and drug abuse.
- Diagnosed on antenatal US and elevated maternal serum alpha-fetoprotein.
- Aetiology unclear. Possibly due to ischaemia in the region supplied by omphalo-mesenteric artery or umbilical vein or rupture of a previous exomphalos.
- Up to 25% associated with other GIT anomalies (complex gastroschisis), including intestinal atresia, volvulus, or compression of the mesenteric vascular pedicle. These cases are at increased risk of short-bowel syndrome, prolonged TPN, chest infection, prolonged ICU and hospital stay, and mortality.
- Not associated with other congenital malformations or chromosomal abnormalities.
- Increased risk of oligohydramnios, fetal death, IUGR, and prematurity.
- A surgical emergency because:
  - Exposure of viscera leads to heat and fluid loss.
  - Risk of injury to exposed bowel loops and infection.
  - Risk of vascular compromise if abdominal defect is very small or there is twisting of the mesenteric vascular pedicle.

Omphalocele overview

- A large central abdominal wall defect at the base of the umbilicus, with herniation of bowel loops and other organs, e.g. liver, in an umbilical sac.
- Sac is made of peritoneum and amniotic membrane with Wharton's jelly in between.
- Umbilical cord is inserted into the sac, which helps differentiate from gastroschisis when sac is ruptured.
- Possibly due to failure of the intestine to return into the abdominal cavity by 10th–12th week of embryogenesis owing to incomplete infolding of the embryonic folds.
- Incidence 1.5–3:10,000.
- Higher incidence if maternal age >30, and associated with fetal death, IUGR, and prematurity.
- Classified as giant exomphalos if defect is large and contains most of liver in sac.

- Occurs early in embryogenesis and hence other anomalies are common (50–70%).
  - Chromosomal anomalies (20%): trisomy 13, 14, 15, 18, and 21. Higher incidence in small exomphalos with liver not in sac.
  - Multiple associated anomalies are common in central exomphalos with no associated chromosomal defects.
  - Syndromes: Beckwith-Wiedemann syndrome (macroglossia, hypoglycaemia, organomegaly, and omphalocele) in 10% of cases.
  - Cardiac defects (30–50%): VSD, ASD.
  - Neural tube defects: meningomyelocele.
  - GIT: TOF, colonic atresia, imperforate anus.
  - Musculoskeletal - sacrovertebral and limb anomalies.
  - Renal: bladder dystrophy.
- Contents of sac and comorbidity often depend on location of defect:
  - Supraumbilical defect can occur with anterior diaphragmatic hernia, sternal cleft, cardiac (ectopia cordis, septal defects, TOF) and diaphragmatic pericardial defects (pentalogy of Cantrell).
  - Infraumbilical defect can occur with exstrophy of bladder or cloaca, genitourinary and anorectal malformations, meningomyelocele and vertebral anomalies.
  - Giant exomphalos is associated with lung hypoplasia.
- Malrotation and Meckel's diverticulum common in both defects.
- Diagnosed antenatal US and elevated maternal serum alpha-fetoprotein.
- Elective surgery unless sac is ruptured, when it is treated similarly to gastroschisis.

Surgery
- Reduction of bowel and other organs into abdominal cavity and closure of defect. If the defect is small, then this is done as a single procedure. If this is not possible, then it is completed in a staged manner by attachment of Silastic membrane (a silo) to the edges of the defect and reduction over a few days. The defect may need to be enlarged to reduce strangulation and allow inspection of contents. Ladd's bands if present are divided to prevent duodenal obstruction.
- In cases of exomphalos, excision of the sac and primary closure is attempted. If this is impossible, a silo is attached to the abdominal defect edges and reduced over time. The sac may be left intact and reduced over time, or silver sulfadiazine may be applied on the sac to encourage epithelialization and an elective hernia repair performed at a later date.

Immediate management
- The mode of delivery does not influence outcome, but should occur in a tertiary centre with neonatal ICU and surgical services.
- Delivery should be planned around 37 week's gestation in cases of gastroschisis to minimize injury to the exposed bowel from the inflammatory peel.
- In cases of giant exomphalos, consider elective caesarean section.
- BLS, airway management, and ventilation as required.

- Limit heat and fluid loss:
  - Exposed bowel of gastroschisis is covered in sterile plastic bag or drape. It may be necessary to place the lower part of the child in the plastic bag to provide adequate protection.
  - Overhead heaters or heated incubators.
- IV fluids: exposed bowel leads to increased fluid loss.
- In cases of exomphalos with an intact sac, fluid loss is lower but is still considerably greater than normal:
  - Fluid resuscitation to correct any fluid deficit: 0.9% saline boluses as required.
  - Maintenance fluid requirements may be 2–3 times normal: isotonic fluid with glucose and electrolyte supplementation.
  - Aim for UO of 1–2 mL/kg—avoid overhydration, since this is associated with increased morbidity and mortality.
  - Blood transfusion to maintain Hb >10 g/dL.
  - Maintain glycaemic status and electrolyte balance
- Minimize ischaemia and damage to bowel loops:
  - Support bowel loops in midline and prevent them from falling to one side to avoid kinking of the mesenteric vascular pedicle.
  - Patient may need to be nursed in right lateral decubitus position.
  - Bowel decompression with NGT and evacuation of meconium from rectum.
- ↓ risk of infection: IV antibiotics.
- ↓ risk of bleeding: vitamin K.

Preoperative assessment
- Evaluate risks of prematurity and associated defects.
- Review airway and ventilator management, venous access and monitoring, fluid resuscitation status, and management of associated comorbidities.
- Investigations:
  - ECHO
  - X-ray of chest and abdomen
  - Renal US scan
  - FBC, clotting, U+E, and blood gas
  - Chromosomal studies.

Anaesthetic technique
- As per neonatal anaesthesia (➲ Chapter 13).
- A clear plan for safe transfer from PICU to theatres.
- Minimize temperature loss:
  - ↑ theatre temperature to 25–27°C.
  - Warmed IV fluids.
  - Humidify and warm anaesthetic gases.
  - Forced air warming devices.
- Monitoring:
  - Small defects in stable neonates: use routine non-invasive monitoring.

- Large defects (>4 cm), significant comorbidities, ongoing or anticipated cardiorespiratory instability, or excessive fluid loss: use invasive monitoring:
    —Arterial and central venous lines, preferably in femoral vessels.
    —A surgical tunnelled central venous catheter may be inserted before the abdominal procedure to provide postoperative TPN; this can be used intraoperatively.
- SpO_2 monitoring on lower limb may help detect vascular compromise.
- Urinary catheter to monitor UO and decompress bladder.
- Aspirate NGT.
- High risk of aspiration—consider RSI.
- Induction as preferred. Avoid insufflating stomach.
- Endotracheal intubation after bolus of rapid acting non-depolarizing muscle relaxant; use nasal route if risk of prolonged postoperative IPPV.
- Vascular access preferably in upper limbs. Umbilical vessels can be cannulated for resuscitation, but need to be removed before surgery.
- Maintenance:
    - Avoid N_2O.
    - If extubation likely, use desflurane and remifentanil.
    - Adequate muscle relaxation to aid surgeon to reduce bowel loops.
    - Maintain thermoneutral environment.
    - Continued correction and maintenance of fluid and electrolyte balance : may need 10–15 mL/kg of isotonic IV fluids or blood as necessary.
    - Maintain normoglycaemia.
- Intraoperative management:
    - Reduction of abdominal contents and attempted closure of the defect may lead to increased IAP, resulting in:
        —Diaphragmatic splinting compromising ventilation.
        —IVC compression precipitating a ↓ CO.
        —Reduced perfusion of intra-abdominal organs may lead to NEC.
        —↓ renal blood flow–common when IAP >20 mmHg.
        —Tense suture lines leading to dehiscence.
    - Predictors of successful primary closure:
        —Peak ventilatory pressures remain <25 cmH_2O to maintain adequate V_T and normocapnia, or does not ↑ >10 cmH_2O on trial closure of abdomen.
        —Normal SpO_2 value and trace on a lower limb (no signs of congestion).
        —No evidence of acidosis, hypoxia, hypercapnia or increasing lactates.
        —Maintenance of UO >1 mL/kg/h.
        —Intragastric and intravesical pressures remains <20 mmHg (normal 5–7 mmHg).
        —CVP does not ↑ > 4mmHg (this correlates to intragastric pressure >20 mmHg and reflects increased intrathoracic pressure impeding venous return).
        —Splanchnic perfusion pressure (MAP − IAP) if measured remains >45 mmHg.

- Analgesia:
  - Regular IV paracetamol.
  - IV opioid boluses intraoperatively and postoperative infusion or NCA.
  - If aiming for extubation, perform TAP blocks, caudal or epidural (single-shot or catheter) at the end of surgery.
  - PR codeine (regular postoperative if not on NCA/morphine infusion).

Postoperative care

- Healthy children who have been stable intraoperatively and who have had small defects successfully closed should be extubated.
- If the patient is unstable or the defect cannot be reduced, they are transferred to the PICU, sedated, and ventilated. The aim is to reduce the silo on PICU over the next few days.
  - Lower limb perfusion, UO and ABGs are closely monitored; if there are signs of increased IAP, the wound is reopened.
  - Once reduction is complete, the child is returned to theatre for removal of silo and secondary closure.
- Decreased gut motility is common, requiring TPN for several days.

Congenital diaphragmatic hernia (CDH)

Overview
- A failure (of unknown aetiology) of fetal diaphragm to fuse, leading to herniation of abdominal organs, e.g. intestines, into the thoracic cavity.
- Results in pulmonary hypoplasia and pulmonary vascular abnormalities:
  - Severest on ipsilateral side, but can also involve the contralateral airway, lung parenchyma, and vascularity.
  - Leads to persistent pulmonary hypertension and respiratory failure; this can be aggravated by hypoxia, acidosis and IPPV at birth.
  - Degree of pulmonary hypoplasia is significant indicator of outcome.
- Incidence 1:3,000.
- Survival 60–90%; better outcomes and less need for ECMO in term babies with weight >3.1 kg. Poor prognosis with right-sided defects and if liver is intrathoracic.
- Types:
  - Majority posterolateral (Bochdalek's hernia, usually left-sided).
  - May be anterior (Morgagni's hernia).
  - Central or bilateral cases are rare.
- About 50% of cases have associated congenital anomalies:
  - Chromosomal defects: trisomy 13, 18, and 21; isochromosome 12p; 47XX or XY.
  - Cardiovascular: septal defects, tetralogy of Fallot, transposition of great arteries, truncus arteriosus.
  - CNS: myelomeningocele, spina bifida.
  - GIT: abdominal wall defects, malrotation.
  - Musculoskeletal: vertebral and limb anomalies, hypoplastic ribs.
  - Urogenital anomalies.
- Diagnosed by antenatal US in approximately 60% of cases
  - Fetal lung:head ratio after 24 weeks gestation is a good prognostic indicator, <1.0 associated with poor survival
- Postnatal diagnosis:
  - Signs of neonatal respiratory embarrassment with a scaphoid abdomen.
  - Auscultatory findings include displaced heart sounds, peristaltic sounds in chest, reduced breath sounds.
  - X-ray of chest and abdomen confirms diagnosis—NGT position.
  - A small percentage present later in life with respiratory or GIT manifestations.
- In specialist centres, fetal interventions are performed to improve pulmonary hypoplasia, though survival is unchanged compared with standard care. An example is fetoscopic endoluminal tracheal occlusion (FETO):
  - Endoscopically placed balloon plugs trachea above the carina. The balloon is deflated at 34 weeks gestation or as an EXIT procedure
  - Complications include premature labour, feto-maternal haemorrhage and unexplained fetal death

Immediate management

- Consensus statement from the European CDH Consortium recommends standardized treatment to improve outcomes:
  - Planned delivery or caesarean section >37 weeks gestation.
  - Utilize experienced tertiary centre able to manage IPPV and pulmonary hypertension.
  - Immediate placement of large-bore NGT to prevent bowel distension and urinary catheter to monitor UO.
  - Elective intubation and IPPV after birth, avoiding gastric insufflation.
  - Appropriate sedation and analgesia. A high threshold for use of muscle relaxants.
- Previously the IPPV strategy used hyperventilation with high FiO_2, aiming for normal SpO_2 and CO_2 levels; this is associated with increased morbidity and mortality.
- Aim to minimize ventilator-induced lung injury:
  - FiO_2 adjusted to target pre-ductal SaO_2 80–95% and post-ductal SaO_2 >70%:
    —Usually difference between pre- and post-ductal SaO_2 should not be >10%.
    —If >10%, then interventions to treat pulmonary hypertension are commenced.
  - Permissive hyperCO$_2$ of up to 8 kPa.
  - Limit peak pressures to 25 cmH$_2$O.
  - Surfactant not recommended (↑ mortality).
  - Avoid muscle relaxants; SV improves outcome.
  - Consider HFOV if:
    —Need peak inspiratory pressures >28 cmH$_2$O to maintain CO_2.
    —Minimal acceptable ABGs not achieved with conventional IPPV.
- Circulation:
  - Aim for normotension with appropriate use of fluid bolus and/or vasoactive agents.
  - Aim for MAP >50 mmHg for adequate end-organ perfusion.
  - Serial ECHO to assess pulmonary pressures and right heart function.
  - Arterial line and CVP line.
- Management of pulmonary hypertension:
  - Leads to RV dysfunction with shunting of deoxygenated blood from the right to the left side, resulting in hypoxia and poor end-organ perfusion reflected by preductal SaO_2 <80%, acidosis, and ↑ lactate level.
  - Inhaled NO as first-line treatment (not shown to influence outcomes).
  - Consider alprostadil infusion to maintain duct patency in cases of severe RV dysfunction.
- ECMO in appropriate cases (adequate amount of lung parenchyma) where there is sustained hypoxaemia, inadequate tissue perfusion, and persistent metabolic acidosis.
  - Surgery on ECMO has been reported.
  - Associated with increased mortality and morbidity compared with conventional treatment.

Surgery
- Not an emergency; consider only after a period of physiological stability.
- Open procedure:
  - Transverse abdominal or subcostal incision.
  - Reduction of herniated abdominal organs.
  - Closure of defect.
  - Prosthetic patch repair used for large defects or where closure of the abdominal wound leads to increased IAP and reduced lung compliance.
- Thoracoscopic repair (commoner in older children):
  - Possible for posterolateral defect where malrotation is excluded and liver is intra-abdominal.
  - Decreased postoperative pain and pulmonary dysfunction.
  - Decreased risk of incisional hernia.
- In neonates, repair is not associated with immediate postoperative improvement in gas exchange and respiratory compliance.

Preoperative assessment
- Check ventilator settings and inotropic support.
- Assess the need for HFOV, inhaled NO, or ECMO and plan how this will be continued intraoperatively.
  - If on HFOV, then arrange for second HFOV ventilator to be ready for immediate connection to the child on arrival from PICU.
  - If on inhaled NO and unfamiliar with circuit, have appropriate personnel available.
  - If on ECMO (rare), ensure appropriate personnel are available, including paediatric cardiac anaesthetist and perfusionist.
- Ensure patient is haemodynamically stable with adequate end-organ perfusion.
- Review recent CXR, ECHO, and blood results, including ABG.
- Blood loss is not usually an issue; group and save should suffice.
- A plan for transfer to theatres is discussed with all staff concerned.
- Combined management with PICU consultant may be useful in rare and challenging cases.

Anaesthetic technique
- As per neonatal anaesthesia; see ⊃ Chapter 13.
- Aspirate NGT and leave on free drainage.
- If patient is not intubated, take care not to insufflate the stomach at induction; avoid high-pressure ventilation through face mask.
- Induction as preferred; intubate as quickly as possible after bolus of rocuronium.
- Monitoring:
  - Pre-ductal (right hand) and post-ductal (lower limb) SpO_2.
  - Arterial (preferably right hand to reflect preductal SaO_2) and central venous pressures.
  - Regular ABGs.
  - Temperature and UO.
  - Optional: NIRS.
- Positioning: supine for open surgical procedures.

- Maintenance of GA:
  - Commence or continue PICU sedation and analgesia (commonly midazolam and fentanyl); increase according to clinical response.
  - Ensure patient is paralysed: regular boluses or infusion of non-depolarizing muscle relaxants.
  - Antibiotics as per local guidelines.
- IPPV: continue PICU ventilator management.
- Maintain normotension and end-organ perfusion (assess capillary refill time, UO, ABG—pH and lactate) by:
  - Isotonic IV fluids (fluid loss is not excessive).
  - Adding or ↑ inotropes as required.
- Measures to avoid pulmonary hypertension include:
  - Reduction of sympathetic stimulation by use of opioids.
  - Maintaining normothermia.
  - Maintaining normal blood pH and normoCO$_2$.
  - Adequate fluid balance.
- Intraoperative interventions:
  - HOFV adjustments to improve respiratory parameters:
    —To manipulate ETCO$_2$, alter frequency, amplitude, or bias flow.
    —To manipulate SaO$_2$, alter FiO$_2$, MAP, or inspiratory time.
  - Management of hypotension or reduced end-organ perfusion:
    —Consider differential diagnosis of hypovolaemia, cardiac dysfunction, or pulmonary hypertension; an ECHO may aid diagnosis.
- Give 10 mL/kg bolus of 0.9% saline or colloid:
  1. If adequate response, ↑ maintenance fluid and consider blood transfusion to maintain HB >12 g/dL.
  2. If unresponsive, add or ↑ inotropes (a combination of dopamine, adrenaline (epinephrine) or noradrenaline (norepinephrine) may be required) to ↑ BP to suprasystemic levels.
  3. If no improvement, consider treatment for pulmonary hypertension
     - Management of pulmonary hypertension:
     —A difference in pre- and post-ductal SpO$_2$ of >10% may indicate pulmonary hypertension due to R–L shunting of blood, but this difference may not be seen in cases where shunting happens at patent foramen ovale instead of the duct.
     —Ensure adequate ventilation, systemic BP, and intravascular filling.
     —Commence inhaled NO 10–20 ppm.
     —A suprasystemic pulmonary hypertension may necessitate commencing alprostadil to open the duct to ↓ RV dysfunction secondary to ↑ afterload.

Postoperative care

- PICU where ventilation weaning protocol is followed.
- Long-term problems include GORD, chronic lung disease, neurodevelopmental delay and growth failure (Box 18.1)

Box 18.1 Understanding HFOV ventilator settings

- Mean airway pressure (MAP)
  - Usually set +3–5 cmH$_2$O over PIP on conventional ventilation.
  - ↑ improves SaO$_2$ by recruiting and maintaining lung volume.
  - Hyperinflation increases dead space and decreases SaO$_2$.
- Frequency (f)
  - Set in Hz: 1 Hz = 60 breaths/min. Normal value is 6–15 Hz.
  - Increasing frequency decreases V$_T$ and increases ETCO$_2$.
- Power (p) or amplitude:
  - Increasing power increases amplitude of oscillation and increases V$_T$.
  - In neonates, set at 30–35.
  - Reflected by 'wobble'—ideally should be to mid-thigh region for optimum lung expansion.
  - CXR should show lung expansion to 8 ribs.
- Inspiratory time (Ti):
  - 33% equivalent to I:E ratio of 1:2.
- Bias flow:
  - FGF over oscillating membrane. Normally set at 20 L/min.
  - ↑ will raise MAP and ↓ EtCO$_2$.

Oesophageal atresia (OA) and tracheo-oesophageal fistula (TOF)

Overview

- Congenital defect resulting in a blind proximal pouch with absence of a normal connection to the stomach, and in the majority a tracheal fistula too.
- Incidence 1:3,000–4,000.
- Unknown aetiology; failure in separation of trachea and oesophagus from the embryonic foregut diverticulum.
- Gross classification (anatomical basis):
  - OA without TOF (8%):
    —CXR: NGT curled in the upper oesophagus and no gastric air bubble.
    —May be a large gap between upper and lower oesophageal segments.
  - OA with proximal TOF (1%):
    —Proximal pouch TOF.
  - OA with distal TOF (85%):
    —Proximal oesophageal atresia, distal TOF usually about 1 cm above carina.
    —Unable to pass NGT.
    —CXR: NGT curled in proximal oesophageal pouch. There is a gastric air bubble.
  - OA with proximal and distal TOF (2%):
  - TOF without OA (H-type fistula) (4%):
    —Often a late and difficult diagnosis.
    —Recurrent chest infections.
- Various scoring systems used to stratify risks and outcomes of surgery (Waterstone, Spitz, Okamoto). With advanced technology and improved management, the survival outcomes are very good (>95%).
- Associated comorbidities in >50% of cases. Commonest in isolated OA and uncommon in H-type TOF. Can be part of a syndrome or associated defects:
  - Prematurity (20–30%) and low birth weight.
  - Chromosomal defects (10%): trisomy 18, 21, and 13.
  - Syndromes: DiGeorge, Opitz, Goldenhar, CHARGE, Pierre Robin, polysplenia.
  - Cardiac (30%): VSD, tetralogy of Fallot, coarctation of aorta, ASD, PDA, right-sided aortic arch.
  - Respiratory: tracheobronchomalacia, pulmonary hypoplasia.
  - GIT: abdominal wall defects, CDH, anorectal malformations, duodenal atresia, imperforate anus.
  - Renal: dysplasia, polycystic or horseshoe kidney, hydronephrosis, posterior urethral valves, vesicourethral reflux, hypospadias, bladder dystrophy.
  - CNS: tethered cord, spina bifida, meningomyelocele, hydrocephalus.
  - Musculoskeletal: scoliosis, radial anomaly, polydactyly, hemivertebrae, lower limb defects.

- Other midline defects: cleft lip and palate
- VACTERL – presence of three or more vertebral, anorectal, cardiac, tracheo-oesophageal, renal, and limb defects. One-third of TOF children have three or more of these associated defects.
- Diagnosis (usually postnatal):
  - Antenatal US: polyhydramnios and absence of stomach air bubble.
  - Increased salivation, vomiting, coughing, and choking on feeds, with respiratory distress and cyanosis.
  - Distension of abdomen with crying.
  - Failure to pass NGT.
  - CXR:
    —NGT curled up in mediastinum: if high in the mediastinum, this indicates a short proximal pouch and possible proximal TOF.
    —Air in stomach: distal TOF.
    —Absent air in stomach in OA with no distal TOF or fistula is occluded.
  - Combination of other defects should raise suspicions.

Immediate management

- Nurse head-up.
- Replogle tube is inserted into the upper pouch for continuous low-negative-pressure suction of secretions that collect in the pouch. It is double-lumen, the large lumen (8 or 10 Fr) has side perforations close to a blind end for suctioning, and the smaller lumen (coloured) acts as an air vent.
- ETT and IPPV only if clinically indicated. IPPV may ↑ gastric distension, worsening pulmonary function and risking gastric rupture.
- NBM; start IV fluids.
- Investigations for associated comorbidities:
  - ECHO: a right-sided aortic arch may require a left instead of right thoracotomy.
  - Chest and abdominal X-ray.
  - Renal, cranial, and vertebral US.
  - ABGs.
  - Routine FBC, U+E, G+S.
- Broad-spectrum IV antibiotics.

Surgery

- Stabilize and complete necessary investigations prior to surgery. Only an emergency if ventilation compromised.
- Bronchoscopy to confirm number and location of fistulas and to define any airway issues.
- Then right posterolateral thoracotomy: skin incision at tip of scapula and then access through 4th–5th intercostal space.
- Extra-pleural approach to expose trachea and oesophagus in posterior mediastinum.
- Fistula identified, ligated, and then divided.
- Saline instilled in operation site and PEEP applied to check for air leak.
- Distal end of oesophagus opened and a suction catheter passed into stomach and contents drained.

- Proximal pouch opened and anastomosed to distal end of oesophagus.
  - Gentle pressure applied to a stiff catheter placed in proximal pouch to aid surgeon.
  - Trans-anastomotic tube (TAT): 6 or 8 Fr NGT introduced by anaesthetist and passed across anastomosis by surgeon under direct vision before completion. This is fixed securely and labelled (for postoperative feeding and gastric drainage).
- When primary anastomosis is not possible (i.e. long gap OA):
  - Fistula ligated, gastrostomy for feeding and proximal oesophagostomy to bring out proximal pouch for toileting. Oesophageal replacement by gastric pull-up or colonic pull-through at later date.
  - Various surgical and non-surgical techniques for oesophageal elongation have been described.
- A chest drain may be inserted.
- Chest closed.
- H-type fistula may need supraclavicular cervical incision and ligation of fistula:
  - Combined bronchoscopy and oesophagogram may be required to confirm diagnosis.
- Laparoscopic procedure: better visualisation of fistula, reduced musculoskeletal sequalae (scoliosis, asymmetry of chest walls, winged scapula), and less painful, but takes longer and needs necessary surgical skills and equipment.
  - Confirmation of fistula by bronchoscopy.
  - Left lateral semiprone position.
  - Three or four thoracic ports used with trans-pleural approach to locate fistula.
  - Insufflation to 5–6 mmHg to deflate lung on operative side.
  - Fistula ligated and divided.
  - Proximal and distal ends mobilized and anastomosed.

Preoperative assessment
- Issues of prematurity and low birth weight.
- Associated comorbidities.
- Complications of TOF:
  - Effects of aspiration from upper pouch and stomach via distal TOF: pneumonia, respiratory distress, and sepsis.
  - Gastric distension causing diaphragmatic splinting and atelectasis.
  - NBM: fluid and electrolyte imbalance and glycaemic status.

Anaesthetic technique
- As per neonatal anaesthesia (➜ Chapter 13).
- Monitoring:
  - Standard non-invasive monitoring.
  - Arterial line recommended, especially if child unstable or small with associated comorbidities. Lung retraction to expose trachea and oesophagus may compromise both ventilation and CO.
  - CVP not required unless haemodynamically unstable or difficult venous access.
  - Temperature monitoring.

- Induction
  - Aim to ensure intubation without:
    —Soiling of airway by aspiration of secretions from proximal pouch or gastric contents from distal fistula.
    —Compromising ventilation or gastric distension by passage of gases into the TOF following path of least resistance.
  - Suction Replogle tube prior to induction and if necessary use large-bore orogastric suction tube.
  - Induction as preferred.
  - Limb anomalies may make venous access and arterial cannulation difficult.
  - Gentle mask ventilation to avoid gastric distension via TOF.
  - Bronchoscopy:
    —Traditionally a rigid ventilating bronchoscope.
    —Flexible fibreoptic bronchoscopy (FOB) has recently replaced this technique. In a stable child, this can be performed via an LMA whilst maintaining SV. Change to ETT for main operation.
    —Proximal fistula may be missed; an LMA avoids this problem.
    —Increased ventilator pressures may be requires to ventilate; this may ↑ gastric distension.
  - Endotracheal intubation:
    —Facilitated by muscle relaxant.
    —Or under deep volatile anaesthesia ± LA to cords; maintain SV. Negative intrathoracic pressures generated can ↓ deviation of gas flow to TOF.
  - Measures to minimize gastric distension:
    —ETT position: case series examining position of distal fistula by FOB has demonstrated fistula in up to one-third of cases to be near carina (11%) or <1 cm (22%) from carina.
    —FOB confirmation of optimum ETT tip position to prevent intubation and ventilation of fistula.
    —Consider left endobronchial intubation if gastric distension makes ventilation difficult, though maintaining oxygenation may be challenging.
    —Rotating the ETT so the bevel faces anteriorly may help.
    —Maintain SV until fistula ligated.
    —Consider limiting gas flow through TOF by placement and inflation of bronchial blocker catheter or Fogarty balloon catheter in fistula during bronchoscopy.
    —Active measures to decompress gastric distension:
      1. Percutaneous needle gastric aspiration.
      2. Emergency gastrostomy: may divert the ventilator gases owing to low-resistance pathway in TOF, leading to further compromise of ventilation.
      3. Emergency thoracotomy and trans-pleural ligation of fistula may be required.
  - In majority, gentle IPPV suffices to prevent gastric distension and maintain ventilation

- Positioning:
  - Left lateral position with right arm extended—ensure access to IV lines.
  - Pressure points padded.
  - Consider reconfirming ETT position with FOB.
  - Place a stiff oral catheter that can be used to identify the proximal pouch intraoperatively, and a 6 Fr NGT that will be advanced later as the TAT.
- Intraoperative management:
  - Maintenance with O_2/air and volatile anaesthetics.
  - Temperature control: warmed IV fluids, active warming blankets.
  - Bleeding or excessive fluid loss usually not a problem.
  - Lung retraction may ↓ CO and compromise ventilation:
    —Hand-ventilate to maintain SpO_2; allow permissive hyperCO_2.
    —May be necessary to interrupt surgery and release retractors.
    —High degree of suspicion of ETT displacement into fistula or bronchi if there is a sudden change in parameters.
  - IVC may drain into heart via azygous vein. It may need to be ligated; this may ↓ CO.
- Analgesia:
  - IV paracetamol.
  - Regional anaesthesia:
    —US PVB: single shot or catheter at T6–7.
    —Thoracic epidural block at T6–7: single shot or catheter.
    —Caudal catheter positioned at T6–7; confirmed by US.
    —Surgically inserted PVB catheter at end of procedure.
    —Others: intercostal block, LA infiltration.
  - Opioids as described for laparotomy.

Postoperative care

- Extubate if surgery uncomplicated and child stable with minimal comorbidities.
- May be surgical preference to keep sedated and IPPV, especially if anastomosis is tense.
- If long-term IPPV planned, change oral to nasal ETT.
- Transfer to HDU or PICU.
- Traditionally nursed with head in the midline and neck slightly flexed for 3–5 days to minimize tension on anastomosis.
- NGT-fed or TPN for 5–7 days until contrast study confirms anastomotic integrity.
- Complications:
  - Missed or recurring fistula.
  - Anastomotic leak or breakdown: usually treated conservatively.
  - Stricture.
  - Tracheobronchomalacia (10%): may need aortopexy.
  - Recurrent laryngeal nerve injury.
  - GORD (40%): >50% of symptomatic cases require fundoplication.

Pyloric stenosis

Overview

- Obstruction to gastric outlet secondary to hypertrophied pyloric muscles.
- Incidence 2–4:1,000, M4:F1.
- Presents at 3–5 weeks of age with projectile non-bilious vomiting after feeds, resulting in dehydration and failure to thrive.
- Signs of shock may be present, depending on severity, including:
  - Lethargy
  - Sunken fontanelle
  - Reduced skin turgor
  - Dry mucous membrane
  - Increased capillary filling time
  - Thready pulse
  - Decreased UO.
- Diagnosis by history, visible peristalsis, and olive-sized mass palpable above and to the right of umbilicus. US confirms thickened and elongated pyloric canal.
- Metabolic disturbance includes hypoCl⁻, hypoK⁺, hypovolaemia, metabolic alkalosis associated with varying degree of hyper- or hypoNa⁺.
  - Vomiting leads to loss of Na⁺, Cl⁻ and H⁺, causing alkalosis and dehydration.
  - Renal compensation leads to HCO_3 excretion along with Na⁺ as preferential cation to conserve Cl⁻. With time, Na⁺ loss is replaced by K⁺ and H⁺ excretion, leading to paradoxical aciduria and further hypoK⁺.
  - In addition, CO_2 retention (respiratory compensation).

Immediate management

- Basic assessment of ABC.
- Fluid resuscitation and correction of electrolyte imbalance preoperatively:
  - Fluid deficit replaced with 0.9% saline boluses.
  - NGT inserted and placed on free drainage.
- Following resuscitation, maintenance fluid is commenced and alkalosis corrected:
  - 0.45% saline + 5% glucose infusion at 150 mL/kg/day until alkalosis is corrected
  - KCl 10 mmol/L added to the infusion to correct hypoK⁺ once urine is being passed.
  - If plasma hypoNa⁺ use 0.9% saline + 5% glucose.
  - Once alkalosis corrected, ↓ maintenance fluid infusion to 100 mL/kg.
  - 4-hourly NG aspirates replaced with 0.9% saline.
  - Aim for UO >1 mL/kg/h.
  - Blood gases (usually capillary) every 12 h.
  - Daily U + E.
  - Once alkalosis corrected, blood gases daily (usually morning) and U + E every 48 h.
  - Check local protocol.

Surgery
- Not an emergency.
- Surgery performed as early as possible following stabilization.
- <1 hour duration.
- Open procedure:
  - Semicircular incision in the supraumbilical skin fold.
  - Linea alba divided and peritoneum opened.
  - Pylorus is delivered through the opening and a longitudinal submucosal incision from antrum of stomach to duodenum is made.
  - Air-leak test may be performed to test integrity of mucosa.
  - Pylorus replaced in abdominal cavity and abdomen closed.
- Laparoscopic procedure:
  - Similar advantages to other laparoscopic procedures, including better pain relief, reduced PONV, early feeding, and shorter hospital stay.

Preoperative assessment
- Usually ASA 1.
- Ensure adequate correction of alkalosis, fluid, and electrolyte balance:
  - UO >1mL/kg/h.
  - Normal pH, HCO_3, and base deficit.
  - Cl^- level >100 mmol/L (95–112 mmol/L) and normal K^+ levels
  - Persistent alkalosis increases risk of postoperative IPPV.

Anaesthetic technique
- As per neonatal anaesthesia (➔ Chapter 213).
- Aspirate NGT to minimize risk of aspiration. Aspiration is performed whilst turning the infant through both lateral quadrants, supine and prone head-down positions. Success can be assessed with US.
- Routine non-invasive monitoring applied before induction.
- Induction as preferred.
- Modified RSI as per local protocol with immediate endotracheal intubation after administration of non-depolarizing muscle relaxant. IPPV
- Maintenance with desflurane in O_2/air.
- Fluid loss usually not an issue; continue isotonic maintenance fluid.
- For laparoscopic procedure, anaesthetic considerations are similar to those for other intra-abdominal laparoscopic procedures.
- Analgesia:
  - IV or PR paracetamol.
  - Bilateral rectus sheath block performed pre-incision.
  - Bilateral TAP block performed pre-incision.
  - LA infiltration at end of procedure.
- Remove NGT unless concerns regarding when feed will be commenced.
- Extubated awake.

Postoperative care
- SpO_2 and apnoea monitoring for 12 h.
- Regular paracetamol.
- PRN codeine PR.
- Maintenance IV fluids until feeds established.
- Discharge home after feeds established.

Torsion of testes

- Reduction in testicular blood supply due to twisting of testes and spermatic cord. Causes pain and tenderness and leads to testicular necrosis.
- Emergency and requires urgent scrotal exploration.
- Common around puberty, but may occur in neonates.
- Other causes of acute scrotum include:
  - Torsion of appendage of testes: most common finding, usually occurs at younger age.
  - Acute epididymitis.
  - Trauma.
  - Incarcerated hernia, appendicitis.

Surgery

- Manual de-torsion may be attempted awake, but is difficult and even if symptoms improve, surgery is still required.
- Testes exteriorized through scrotal incision, untwisted, and examined for viability.
- If perfusion improves, the testes are fixed; if a testis is non-viable, it is removed.
- Contralateral testes are fixed at the same time.

Preoperative assessment

- Usually ASA 1.
- May be unfasted; however, do not delay surgery.

Anaesthesia

- Induction as preferred; RSI.
- Maintenance as preferred; IPPV.
- Maintain a deep plane of GA, since traction on testes may cause significant vagal response.
- Antiemetic.
- Analgesia:
  - IV paracetamol
  - 50 mcg/kg morphine
  - LA infiltration to incision site

Postoperative care

- Regular PO paracetamol and NSAID.
- PRN PO morphine.

Maxillofacial, craniofacial, and cleft surgery

Ed Carver and Doug Johnson

Elective maxillofacial surgery

Overview

- Includes correction of mandibular hypoplasia, alveolar bone grafts to correct bony defects in cleft patients, and midface advancement procedures in patients with faciocraniosynostoses (for more detail see the section on craniofacial surgery), as well as straightforward oral surgery.
- May be associated with difficult airway, e.g. in Treacher Collins syndrome.
- Bone grafts may be taken from the iliac crest; a trephine rather than open osteotomy is less painful.
- Costochondral rib grafts may be used; beware pneumothorax.
- With midface advancement procedures, grade of laryngoscopy may paradoxically ↑ postoperatively.
- Midface advancement often involves osteotomies followed by the application of a RED frame—rigid external distraction—in order that correction can occur gradually. Presence of the frame will limit access to the airway; therefore, tools must always be with the patient for quick removal and the anaesthetist must have a plan for alternative airway management, i.e. LMA rather than facemask.
- Jaws may be wired together during surgery to achieve dental occlusion, but it is unusual for this to continue into the postoperative period; this should be verified at team brief.

Preoperative assessment

- Particular attention is paid to the airway in the context of associated syndromes.
- Review any comorbidity, e.g. CHD in associated syndromes.
- Patients may have associated breathing problems, e.g. OSA, and may need a review by a respiratory physician for advice on preoperative investigations, e.g. sleep studies and perioperative care.

Anaesthetic technique

- Most cases will require an ETT. Discuss surgical access at team brief and decide on oral or nasal approach.
- If using a nasal ETT, a topical vasoconstrictor, use of a soft tube or a presoftened (using warm sterile water) tube will help ↓ nasal trauma and bleeding. Advancing the ETT over a suction catheter or via a fibreoptic scope may help to avoid damage.
- In certain circumstances, an elective tracheostomy may be performed first.
- In the case of a difficult airway, discuss at team brief the plan for induction, extubation, and postoperative airway management (➔ Chapter 9)
- Maintenance: volatile or TIVA approach. Remifentanil will ↓ volatile requirements and help with cardiovascular stability.
- Haemorrhage can be significant, especially with maxillary surgery. Ensure adequate IV access, and have cross-matched blood in theatre suite.
- A throat pack should be placed by the surgeon, documented, included in the swab count, and removal confirmed.
- Bradycardia can result from traction on the maxilla via the trigeminal–vagal reflex arc.

Postoperative care

- May need HDU or continued intubation in ICU.
- An elective tracheostomy must be cared for on HDU/ICU, since loss of airway can be catastrophic.
- Oral intake may be limited: consider continuing IV fluids.
- Pain from bone or cartilage graft sites can be severe: use LA infiltration at surgery and a postoperative wound catheter for continued analgesia.
- Prescribe regular paracetamol, an NSAID, plus an opioid (NCA, PCA, or morphine sulfate solution PRN as appropriate).
- Prescribe antiemetics, especially if opioids are required or jaws are wired together.

Emergency maxillofacial surgery

Overview

- Roughly 70% of facial trauma in children is soft tissue, 25% dental, and 5% facial fractures.
- Lip laceration is common in preschool children; if it needs GA, place on next trauma list.
- MUA of nasal fracture is done on elective basis after swelling subsides, 2–7 days post injury.
- Mandibular fractures are rare. The commonest causes are cycling accidents and falls, with assault more common >12 years of age. Younger children have a higher incidence of condylar fractures, often treated conservatively. Body and angle fractures are more common in >12-year-olds and are more likely to need operative fixation.
- Midface fractures are very rare, classified as Le Fort 1–3, depending on the extent of bony injury. They are indicative of considerable trauma; therefore, seek out associated injuries, e.g. skull fracture, traumatic brain injury. Airway compromise may result from swelling, bleeding, and mobile segments of the facial skeleton.

Preoperative assessment

- Assess for airway compromise and potential for difficult airway management. Trismus usually resolves on induction of GA, but swelling and mobile segments of mandible can make intubation difficult.
- Assess for associated injuries, need for brain and spine imaging, and adequacy of resuscitation.
- Most facial fractures do not need immediate fixation and can be done electively once swelling and haematoma is starting to resolve.

Anaesthetic technique

- Inhalational induction if there is doubt regarding airway control or difficult intubation.
- Consider bone fragments, loose teeth, foreign bodies, and the potential for airway obstruction.
- Flexible LMA for lip lacerations.
- Nasal fracture: MUA is usually a short procedure where a facemask is sufficient; occasionally, an LMA will be required. Beware fresh postnasal bleeding.
- Facial and mandibular fracture fixation will need an ETT. Armoured may be useful. Surgeons may request a nasal tube to assess and achieve dental occlusion. Operative treatment is typically ORIF and postoperative intermaxillary fixation is unusual; therefore, the patient should be able to open their mouth.
- A throat pack should be placed by the surgeon. Include in swab count, document, and confirm removal.
- Maintenance: volatile or TIVA technique.
- Fentanyl or morphine boluses for analgesia in addition to paracetamol and NSAID.
- LA infiltration or dental blocks by surgeon.
- IV dexamethasone 0.1–0.15 mg/kg reduces swelling, analgesic requirements, and PONV.

Postoperative care

- Observe for developing airway compromise. Consider HDU care or continuing intubation on ICU.
- Oral intake may be limited due to pain/mouth opening. Continue IV fluid as needed.
- Regular simple analgesics plus morphine sulfate solution are usually adequate.
- If jaws wired together, prescribe regular antiemetics, e.g. ondansetron plus dexamethasone.

Craniofacial surgery

Overview

- Craniosynostosis is premature closure of cranial sutures resulting in dysostoses with abnormal bone growth. Incidence 1:2,000 live births (80% non-syndromic, 20% syndromic).
- Resulting abnormalities and sutures involved include scaphocephaly (sagittal suture), brachycephaly (bicoronal sutures), trigonocephaly (metopic suture) and anterior plagiocephaly (unicoronal suture). Posterior plagiocephaly is much rarer, with lambdoid synostosis accounting for 1% of cases.
- Posterior positional plagiocephaly is caused by simple moulding of the skull in infants who favour one side when lying supine and does not need surgical treatment.
- The faciocraniosynostoses are rare and more complex syndromic conditions with abnormalities of the skull and facial development (particularly midface hypoplasia). There may be multiple suture involvement with significant limitation of skull growth, raised ICP if untreated, and a need for repeat surgery to allow ongoing skull and brain growth. Syndromes include Apert, Crouzon, and Pfeiffer, and can have ocular malposition, pseudoproptosis and respiratory difficulties, e.g. severe OSA. There may be associated congenital abnormalities, e.g. syndactyly in Apert.
- In syndromic craniosynostoses:
  - ICP may be chronically raised in untreated cases, especially if multiple sutures are involved.
  - Pseudoproptosis due to midface hypoplasia can lead to exposure keratitis and loss of vision. This can be treated by lateral tarsorrhaphy, but may need early bony surgery to allow more orbital protection.
  - There may be preoperative respiratory problems in the faciocraniosynostoses. Respiratory function must be optimized preoperatively, e.g. treatment of choanal atresia. An early tracheostomy may be needed.
- Surgery is performed to relieve raised ICP, ↑ cranial volume, correct deformity, and cosmesis.
- Fronto-orbital advancement and remodelling (FOAR) reshapes the forehead and increases the volume of the cranial vault to allow growth of the brain. Facial advancement techniques are used for midface hypoplasia.
- A variety of approaches exist to manage isolated sagittal synostosis, e.g. total calvarial remodelling, spring-assisted cranioplasty.
- Simple cases usually undergo surgery in the first 2 years of life and typically do not need further calvarial surgery.
- In complex cases, an operation on the frontal and cranial part of the malformation is usually performed between 4 and 12 months of age. Occasionally, a posterior augmentation of the skull is performed by a distraction/augmentation technique to ↑ cranial volume. Any facial retrusion is corrected later, typically after final dentition appears, around 12 years of age; however, some element of midface advancement may be performed at an early age to treat severe OSA or impending visual loss due to exposure of the eyes.

- Blood loss may be large, and the oculocardiac reflex may be triggered by orbital dissection.
- There is a significant risk of air embolism due to the extensive dissection of skin and bone.

Preoperative assessment

- Thorough airway assessment is essential and involves a detailed history, including feeding difficulties, failure to thrive, sleep disturbance, daytime somnolence, and developmental difficulties.
- A team approach to optimize ENT and respiratory care, including overnight sleep studies to assess upper airway obstruction with or without OSA is required in patients with maxillary hypoplasia.
- Preoperative improvement of the airway using choanal dilation with or without bony dissection, nasal stenting, NPA, and nocturnal nasal CPAP is often required in the faciocraniosynostoses.
- Tracheostomy may be needed in those with severe airway problems to provide a patent airway and provide time for growth before planned surgical intervention. Most complex children will have had GA for preoperative procedures, e.g. MRI, and the records will give useful information about any difficulties with the airway or venous access.
- Evidence suggests that minor subclinical air-embolic events occur in most patients having transcranial surgery. The presence of CHD with structural abnormalities connecting left and right circulations creates a high risk for paradoxical air embolus and stroke. Careful assessment of any cardiac lesion is required and surgical plan adjusted accordingly.
- FBC and coagulation screen. Cross-match blood—ensure checked and immediately available in theatre blood fridge.

Anaesthetic technique

- Sedative premedication can be given if there is no respiratory compromise or ↑ ICP.
- An inhalational induction may be preferred in the younger child, if there are airway problems, or when limb anomalies, e.g. syndactyly, make venous access difficult.
- Children with maxillary hypoplasia may develop airway obstruction after induction, and their facial anatomy may make it difficult to form a seal with the facemask. An inverted face mask or two-handed technique may help.
- Anticipate and plan for possible difficult intubation in syndromic cases. Many cases with good mouth opening are managed with indirect video laryngoscopy techniques but fibreoptic intubation may be needed.
- ETT and IPPV are necessary. The type of ETT depends on the surgery, but it is usually either armoured or preformed. An armoured ETT may mitigate or decrease tube kinking during intraoperative head and neck repositioning. Secure fixation of the ETT is essential and for maxillary osteotomies mandibular intradental wiring is the most secure method. A throat pack is needed for facial procedures.
- For major procedures, two large-bore cannulas, arterial and central venous lines (femoral or internal jugular), and a urinary catheter are needed.

- Start active warming during induction.
- Positioning may be difficult and it is important to avoid cerebral venous congestion by excessive neck rotation. Pressure area care must be meticulous and may require a foam/gel mattress. Great care is required for eye protection in prone patients, especially if proptotic; eye shields may be helpful.
- A moderate head-up position is often employed. Beware of air embolism, which may be signalled by a sudden ↓ in $ETCO_2$, oxygenation, and BP. It may be difficult to differentiate this from sudden massive haemorrhage,; however, the initial management should be the same: fluids, head-down position and flooding the surgical field, vasopressors, and external cardiac massage if indicated.
- A prone or sphinx position may be used for certain approaches to the vertex or posterior skull.
- A balanced anaesthetic technique to provide cardiovascular stability includes a combination of opioid and volatile agent or TIVA. A remifentanil infusion 0.1–0.5 mcg/kg/min or intermittent fentanyl boluses are typically used in the UK.
- Infiltration with LA and adrenaline (epinephrine) improves haemostasis, but is insufficient alone for postoperative analgesia.
- Raised ICP may be occult in syndromic cases. Attention must be given to maintain an appropriate MAP to ensure adequate CPP prior to craniotomy.
- Prepare for the possibility of massive haemorrhage. Careful scalp dissection limits blood loss. As craniotomies are often extensive, there may be continuous oozing from bone edges during this period. Sudden rapid loss can occur from venous anastomoses or tears of cerebral venous sinuses. Be alert to the development of hypovolaemia, indicated by increased variability of the arterial pressure trace with IPPV.
- Antifibrinolytics, e.g. tranexamic acid, ↓ blood loss in craniofacial surgery: bolus 10 mg/kg followed by 5 mg/kg/h infusion.
- Cell salvage may reduce perioperative transfusion, but donor blood is commonly needed.
- Most cases are managed with packed red cells ± cell saved blood alone. The routine use of FFP does not confer any benefit in the absence of coagulopathy. Platelet transfusion is required in a minority of cases, according to local protocols, e.g. to maintain platelet count $>100 \times 10^9$/L.
- Coagulopathy may develop in massive blood loss, monitor with TEG/ROTEM. Hypofibrinoginaemia occurs first and may need treatment with cryoprecipitate or fibrinogen concentrate in the context of ongoing bleeding.
- Beware of sudden rises in serum K^+ during rapid transfusion, particularly when using older or irradiated blood.
- Approximately 1 h from the end of surgery, give 100–150 mcg/kg of IV morphine, IV paracetamol, and an antiemetic.

Postoperative care

- Most patients are extubated and nursed in HDU. In some patients, a period of IPPV is required, especially after facial surgery.
- Prescribe maintenance fluids.

- After major procedures, blood loss may continue into the postoperative period and babies may lose 10% of their blood volume into a drain or head bandages. For these cases, regular assessment of the cardiovascular system is required and a series of FBCs is performed. Blood is transfused if indicated—typically when Hb <70–80 g/L.
- Analgesia: a combination of paracetamol plus an opioid (NCA or regular morphine sulfate solution). An NSAID is added when bleeding is no longer a concern.
- PONV is common despite the use of prophylactic antiemetics.
- Considerable facial swelling/bruising may develop and limit eye opening in the first 48–72 h.

Cleft lip and/or palate

Overview

- Commonest congenital abnormalities of the orofacial structure.
- Embryological failure of fusion or breakdown of fusion between the nasal and maxillary processes and the palatine shelves at 6–9 weeks of gestation. The lip forms between 4–7 weeks gestation.
- A diverse group:
  - Cleft lip and palate 1:700 live births.
  - Isolated cleft palate 1:1,000 live births.
  - Considerable racial variation. More common in Asians > Caucasians > African Americans.
  - Isolated cleft palate has similar prevalence in different populations.
- Isolated cleft palate (45%), unilateral cleft lip and palate (23%), unilateral cleft lip (22%), bilateral left lip and palate (10%).
- Cleft palate ± cleft lip may be:
  - Submucous (occult) mildest form: no visible cleft, non-union of palatal muscles.
  - Incomplete: soft palate cleft.
  - Complete: soft and hard palate cleft. May include the alveolar portion of the maxilla.

Aetiology

- Complex and multifactorial.
- Clefts occur in a number of single-gene syndromes with autosomal-dominant inheritance.
- Where no diagnosed syndrome has occurred, and there is no family history of cleft, the recurrence risk in subsequent offspring is <5%.
- Multiple environmental factors have been identified: maternal smoking, IDDM, infection, drugs (benzodiazepines, anticonvulsants), alcohol excess, and folic acid deficiency.
- Cleft lip and palate occurs as part of >100 syndromes, including:
  - Pierre Robin sequence
  - Stickler syndrome
  - Velocardiofacial syndrome
  - Fetal alcohol syndrome
  - Down syndrome
  - Hemifacial microsomia (Goldenhar syndrome)
  - Treacher Collins syndrome
  - Klippel–Feil syndrome.
- Associated with:
  - CHD (16%)
  - Musculoskeletal abnormalities
  - Urogenital tract anomalies
  - URTI and chronic otitis media
  - Subglottic stenosis.

Treatment

- Goals are cosmesis, normal speech, and normal dental development.
- The optimal timing of repair remains debatable.

- Cleft lip is repaired at 3–4 months, allowing time to diagnose other congenital conditions.
- Cleft palate is repaired at 6–12 months (prior to speech development).
- Cleft lip repair is often combined with repair of the front of the palate.
- Exact type of repair depends on the extent of available tissue, and usually involves advancement of a skin, muscle, and mucosal flap.
- Operation involves mobilization of lateral tissue to allow midline closure. This includes apposition of the levator palati muscles, which are required to elevate the soft palate, occluding the nasopharynx and preventing nasal speech. Large defects may require stepped procedures.

Preoperative assessment

- Associated conditions may affect conduct of GA.
- Isolated cleft palate is associated with other anomalies in 50% of cases.
- If there is evidence of recent or incipient respiratory infection, the procedure is deferred, since the airway may be marginal postoperatively.
- Chronic airway obstruction or OSA ↑ the risk of postoperative airway problems. Overnight SpO_2 can be measured preoperatively. If episodes of hypoxia occur, then refer for a formal sleep study.
- There may be physiological anaemia at 3–6 months of age. Blood is grouped and saved, although significant blood loss is rare.

Anaesthetic technique

- Sedative premedication is uncommon.
- Inhalational induction.
- ETT and IPPV are required. This is usually uneventful, but occasionally techniques for management of the difficult airway and intubation are required (➲ Chapter 9). A south-facing preformed ETT (RAE) or reinforced ETT is usually used.
- A throat pack should be placed by the surgeon. Include in swab count, document, and confirm removal.
- A balanced technique is used, with volatile in O_2 and air with bolus fentanyl or morphine. Remifentanil reduces volatile requirements and promotes rapid emergence.
- TIVA is preferred in older patients.
- In some centres, a 10–15 mg/kg bolus of tranexamic acid is administered.
- Intraoperative analgesia:
  - Infiltration with LA and adrenaline (improves haemostasis, but insufficient alone for postoperative analgesia).
  - Morphine 100–150 mcg/kg or fentanyl 2–4 mcg/kg IV.
  - Infraorbital nerve block for cleft lip repair. The infraorbital nerve is a terminal branch of the trigeminal nerve. It supplies sensory innervation to the skin and mucous membrane of the upper lip and lower eyelid, to the skin between them, and to the side of the nose. The nerve is blocked at the level of the infra-orbital foramen, which is palpated adjacent to the alar of the nose in the mid-pupillary line. The needle enters intraorally through the buccal mucosa and is advanced towards the foramen until bony resistance is felt. The needle is then withdrawn slightly and 1–2 mL of 0.5% bupivacaine ± 1:200,000 adrenaline is injected after performing a negative aspiration test. The needle should not enter the infraorbital foramen.

- In some centres, intraoperative NSAID administration is controversial— discuss with surgical team.
  - Paracetamol 15 mg/kg IV.
- Maintenance fluids. Volume replacement if required.
- Broad-spectrum antibiotics ↓ postoperative complications.
- Dexamethasone 0.1–0.4mg/kg may ↓ airway oedema.
- Hypothermia is not usually a problem; however, temperature should be monitored (rectal or skin) and facilities to warm the patient must be available.
- For cleft palate repair:
  - A mouth gag is used. It is important to check for kinking/obstruction of the ETT while this is being positioned. Communicate with surgeon to attain a mutually satisfactory position.
  - A roll or bolster placed under the shoulders extends the neck and improves surgical access.
  - A tongue suture is sometimes placed to be used postoperatively to pull the tongue forward and relieve airway obstruction.
  - 10% develop some evidence of airway obstruction, especially if the repair is tight or the palate has been lengthened. Surgeon may place an NPA at the end of surgery. Combined lip and front-of-palate repairs may precipitate blocked nasal airways.
  - Gentle suction under direct vision is performed without damaging the repaired palate.
  - Aim for smooth emergence and extubation. Crying and agitation may precipitate bleeding.
  - Awake extubation avoids some risks of airway compromise.

Postoperative care

- Regular observation and SpO_2 without supplementary O_2 (unless required) to detect airway obstruction.
- Maintenance fluids until feeding (often very early in the postoperative period).
- A combination of paracetamol, NSAID, and oral morphine is usually prescribed.
- Postoperative complications commonest with isolated cleft palate patients and in those patients with other anomalies. They include:
  - Haemorrhage—rarely requires exploration.
  - Upper airway obstruction secondary to upper airway narrowing, blood clot, tongue swelling from retraction by the mouth gag, or inadequate mouth breathing.
- Airway obstruction may require an NPA or ETT and IPPV. Patients at high risk of postoperative airway obstruction, e.g. severe Pierre Robin syndrome, may be admitted to ICU intubated for ventilation for 24–48 h until oedema and swelling have resolved.
- Cleft lip patients, if comfortable, usually feed early. Cleft palate repairs are more variable.
- Early feeding promotes general comfort, ↓ agitation, and ↓ crying from hunger. There is no evidence of increased complications with early feeding. NG feeding is used to aid early feeding in some centres.

Medical specialties

Naveen Murali

Gastroenterology

Overview

- Endoscopic procedures are mainly performed on day-case lists in remote theatre locations or endoscopy suites. Emergency endoscopies are usually performed in emergency theatre.
- Unlike adults, most children will need a GA or deep sedation to enable a safe and effective examination.
- Majority are diagnostic procedures in healthy children.

Therapeutic endoscopies

- Polypectomy.
- Foreign body retrieval.
- PEG insertion/removal.
- Banding or injection of bleeding varices.

Diagnostic endoscopies

- OGD and colonoscopy ± biopsy.
- Wireless capsule endoscopy.
- Double-balloon enteroscopy (small intestine).
- MR enteroclysis (small intestine).
- ERCP.

Contraindications

- Absolute: intestinal perforation or peritonitis.
- Relative: severe coagulopathy or recent GI surgery.

Preoperative assessment

- Patients are often anxious—may need premedication.
- Beware of dehydration, especially if patient has had bowel prep.
- Assess severity of reflux and consider prophylaxis.
- Blood tests for coagulation and liver dysfunction if there are associated medical conditions.
- Associated comorbidities.
- Diagnostic blood tests are often performed under GA.
- Risk of hypoglycaemia, especially in metabolic disorders. Need special care and planning, e.g. first on the list.
- Antibiotic prophylaxis as per guidelines (AHA or ASGE).
- Emergency OGD for variceal bleeding or coagulopathy—prepare for potential transfusion.

Oesophagogastroduodenoscopy (OGD)

- Significant ↑ in demand due to an ↑ in presentation and diagnostic abilities of gastroenterologists.
- Common indications: GOR, eosinophilic oesophagitis, inflammatory bowel disorders (IBD), follow-up of GVHD.

Anaesthetic technique
- IV or inhalational induction.
- Intubation facilitated by lidocaine 1% spray to vocal cords, or alfentanil 5 mcg/kg, or propofol 1–2 mg/kg IV bolus.
- ETT is secured to the left side to facilitate passage of endoscope from the right.

- LMA: useful alternative for older children in absence of significant reflux.
- IPPV or spontaneous ventilation, with volatile or TIVA maintenance.
- Left lateral position. A bite block is usually placed.
- Paracetamol IV.
- Awake extubation in left lateral position.

Percutaneous endoscopic gastrostomy

- Children unable to feed orally or needing enhanced nutrition can be assisted via:
  - Nasogastric tube
  - Nasojejunal tube
  - Percutaneous endoscopic gastrostomy (PEG)
  - Percutaneous endoscopic jejunostomy tube (J-PEG).

Indications
- Obstructive pathologies: oesophageal stricture and tumours.
- Neurological disorders affecting swallow, e.g. neurodegenerative disorders.
- Supplementing nutrition:
  - Malignancies, chemo- or radiotherapy
  - Short-bowel syndromes
  - Malabsorption pathologies
  - Malnutrition
  - Burns
  - Sepsis
  - EB.

Advantages
- Minimal discomfort compared with NGT.
- Easy to use and maintain on an ambulatory basis.
- Longer term: >6 weeks without changing.
- J-PEG can be used in children with severe reflux.

Procedure
- PEG is inserted using a modified Seldinger technique.
- J-PEG is inserted under direct vision into the jejunum.

Complications

- Major complications of the procedure i.e. PEG/JPEG <1%.
- Complications of endoscopy <0.01%.
- Cellulitis or fasciitis.
- Pneumoperitoneum.
- Ascites.
- Peritonitis.
- Oesophageal rupture.
- Major haemorrhage.

Anaesthesia
- Consider comorbidities.
- Inhalational or IV induction.
- Secure IV access.
- ETT ± lidocaine to cords.
- Paralysis (rocuronium 0.5mg/kg or atracurium 0.3 mg/kg) is useful since it reduces gag reflex and relaxes the abdominal wall for insertion.

- Paracetamol IV and LA infiltration by surgeon is sufficient.
- Extubate awake in lateral position after reversal of muscle relaxant.
- Postoperative analgesia provided by paracetamol and NSAIDs.

Colonoscopy

- Common indications: juvenile polyps (most common cause of bleeding), IBD, lower GI bleeding (haematochezia), abdominal pain, or diarrhoea.
- Risks: colonic perforation (0.3%), bleeding (2.5%).

Bowel preparation

- Individualized for child's age and tolerability. No standard regimen available.

Anaesthetic technique:

- Similar to OGD.
- LMA can be used, since not sharing airway.
- ETT if significant risk of aspiration.
- Paracetamol IV.

Capsule endoscopy (CE) or wireless CE

- Suitable technique for children >2 years.
- Indications: evaluation of small-intestinal pathologies, unexplained GI bleeding.
- Crohn's disease, tumours, and polyps of small intestine.
- Capsule is usually placed with a gastroscope (attached to the tip of the scope) in children, needing deep sedation or GA.
- Complications: retention of capsule, bowel obstruction.

Endoscopic retrograde cholangiopancreatography

- Safe in children >1 year or >10 kg.
- Common indications:
  - Biliary indications: bile duct calculi, choledochal cysts, bile leak post surgery or trauma, cholestasis, and sphincter of Oddi dysfunction.
  - Pancreatic disorders: chronic pancreatitis, pancreas divisum, and pancreatic trauma.
- Complications: perforations, haemorrhage, acute pancreatitis, cholangitis.
- Common interventions:
  - Papillotomy
  - Removal of common bile duct (CBD) stones.
- Avoids need for surgical exploration of CBD or intraoperative cholangiogram.
- Advances in radiology, e.g. magnetic resonance cholangiopancreatography (MRCP), have reduced the need for diagnostic ERCP.

Preoperative assessment

- Assess severity of liver dysfunction, e.g. coagulopathy.

Anaesthesia

- IV or inhalational induction.
- ETT plus IPPV.
- Avoid opioid analgesics, to minimize sphincter spasm.
- TIVA is ideal.
- Extubate awake and recover in lateral position.

Ingestion of caustic substances
- May be accidental or deliberate (self-harm in teenagers).
- Common substances:
  - Alkali: bleaches, hairsprays, and dishwasher tablets—oesophageal injury.
  - Acids: cleaning solutions (rare)—gastric injury.
- Alkalis cause more extensive and deeper burns.
- Solid preparations cause more damage to oral and oesophageal mucosa.
- Early management as per burns resuscitation guidelines (See CH 25).
- Acute decompensation may occur owing to perforation.
- Gastrointestinal burn manifests as vomiting, haematemesis, salivation, dysphagia, and associated orofacial burns.

Role of endoscopy
- Immediate management (first 12–24 h):
  - OGD <24 h of ingestion, irrespective of symptoms.
- Delayed management (2–3 weeks):
  - Monitor changes
  - Therapeutic procedures: dilation of strictures or pyloric stenosis.
- OGD usually avoided between 5 and 15 days owing to perforation risk.

Anaesthesia
- Careful assessment, including airway burn, other associated burns, risk of difficult airway, decompensated cardiovascular status, and need for ICU postoperatively.
- Emergency OGD must be performed in a theatre setting, with full resuscitation equipment available.
- Difficult airway secondary to a burn may need surgical backup.
- ETT (or tracheostomy in severe oropharyngeal burns).
- Inhalation or TIVA technique.
- Decision regarding IPPV postoperatively based on the severity of airway and inhalation injury.

Common ingested foreign bodies
- Coins and toys (may contain neodymium magnets—with risk of perforation, fistula, and obstruction).
- Batteries (oesophageal necrosis and fistula formation).
- Sharp objects (perforation).
- Emergency endoscopy if suspicion of ingestion of neodymium magnet, even if asymptomatic.

Anaesthesia
- Consider possibility of aspiration.
- Vomiting or salivating child may be difficult to assess and/or pre-oxygenate pre-induction.
- IV induction preferable.
- RSI with propofol & IV suxamethonium 2 mg/kg or IV rocuronium 1 mg/kg.
- ETT plus IPPV, with volatile or TIVA maintenance.
- Awake extubation in lateral position after reversal of neuromuscular block.
- Close monitoring postoperatively.

Oncology

Overview

- About 1,500 new cases of childhood cancer are diagnosed yearly in the UK.
- 30% are leukaemias—acute lymphoblastic leukaemia (ALL) and acute myeloid leukaemia (AML); 20% involve the CNS; 7% are neuroblastomas; 6% non-Hodgkin's lymphoma; 6% Wilms' tumour (nephroblastoma); 5% Hodgkin's lymphoma.
- GA is required for many procedures, e.g. tumour biopsy/resection, vascular access, LP, intrathecal chemotherapy, bone marrow aspiration, and imaging. This is at a time of extreme physiological and emotional stress for parents and child.
- Significant anaesthetic input is required for acute, chronic, and palliative care pain management.
- Patients are often immunosuppressed. Presentation of infections may be subtle and atypical. Avoid suppositories, owing to risk of bacteraemia.
- There is often a thrombocytopenia: avoid IM injections, and carefully consider need for epidural.

Leukaemia

- Commonest form is ALL (80% of leukaemias and 25% of all childhood cancer). Highest incidence is 2–3 years of age. 30% more frequent in boys than girls. AML comprises 15% and chronic myeloid leukaemia <4% of cases.
- Clinically: lethargy, fever, malaise, signs of marrow failure, and pain due to marrow infiltration. Anaemia, neutropenia, and thrombocytopenia may be present.
- Management: treat symptoms and signs of the disease; treat the leukaemia and the complications of therapy. Three phases:
  - Induction (of remission): lasts approximately 4 weeks. High rate of tumour cell death (tumour lysis syndrome).
  - Consolidation: involves additional prolonged treatment ± intrathecal chemotherapy ± cranial radiotherapy
  - Maintenance: comprises pulses of chemotherapy (over 2–3 years) to continue remission and eradicate the leukaemia.
- Survival: ALL 5-year survival is around 80%. Acute non-lymphocytic leukaemia is around 55%, increasing to 67% with bone marrow transplantation (BMT).

Lymphomas

Non-Hodgkin's lymphoma (NHL)

- Diverse group of lymphocytic cancers; accounts for 60% of paediatric lymphomas.
- Proliferation of immature lymphoid cells outside bone marrow is common.
- 30% are T-cell lymphoblastic lymphomas (very similar to ALL).
- 50% are B-cell lymphomas.
- 20% are large-cell lymphomas (originating from T cells, B cells, or indeterminate).

- T-cell NHL tends to manifest in the anterior mediastinum and is associated with airway compression, pleural effusions, and large-vessel vascular compression (SVC syndrome).
- B-cell NHL manifests most commonly in the abdomen, leading to pain, distension, ascites, and intestinal obstruction.
- Treatment is similar to ALL. Remission in 90% of children. 5-year survival is approximately 80%.

Hodgkin's lymphoma
- Incidence rises from 2 years of age, peaking between 15 and 30 years. Firm cervical or supraclavicular lymphadenopathy is typical (up to 60% will also have enlarged mediastinal nodes).
- Staging 1–4 depends on sites of lymphadenopathy (1 = single region, 2 = two regions on same side of diaphragm, 3 = spread across diaphragm, 4 = disseminated) plus 'A' for asymptomatic or 'B' for symptomatic (night sweats, fever, weight loss).
- Treatment: chemotherapy and radiotherapy.
- Survival: 5-year survival in grade 1A is 90–95%; grade 4 is 65%.

CNS tumours
- Commonest solid tumours.
- Around 40% are astrocytomas (usually low grade) and medulloblastomas. Ependymomas and gliomas comprise most of the remainder.
- Clinical presentation: depends on tumour location. Infratentorial tumours may present with signs of ↑ ICP (headache, nausea and vomiting, nystagmus, ataxia, or cranial nerve lesions). Supratentorial lesions may present with seizures, hemiparesis, and ↑ ICP.
- Treatment: includes surgery (biopsy, excision, debulking, and shunt insertion), chemotherapy, radiotherapy, and occasionally molecular or immunotherapy.

Chemotherapy
- Anthracyclines (doxorubicin) causes cardiac side effects, e.g. acute atrial and ventricular dysrhythmias, and cardiac failure.
- Bleomycin can cause interstitial pneumonitis and fibrosis.
- Cisplatin is nephrotoxic.
- Mucositis: 40–75% incidence. Often reported as most debilitating aspect of treatment. Usually oral but may extend throughout GIT.
  - Treatment: cautious oral debridement, decontamination (nystatin, clotrimazole, chlorhexidine), prevention of trauma and bleeding (maintain platelets >20,000/mm³).
  - Pain management: oral care and rinses help. May require NCA or PCA. Adjuncts maybe necessary, e.g. ketamine, gabapentin, and clonidine. NSAIDs are relatively contraindicated.
- Tumour lysis syndrome:
  - Spontaneous or on commencement of chemotherapy (especially first 5 days)
  - Most commonly seen with Burkitt's lymphoma.

- Trigger factors include surgical manipulation and steroid administration.
- Intracellular contents released into the circulation: $\uparrow K^+$, PO_4, and uric acid. Precipitation in the renal tubules may cause renal impairment: $\downarrow Ca^{2+}$ (bound with phosphate)—tetany, hyperK$^+$—dysrhythmias.
- Treatment: hyperhydration therapy aiming for UO >100 mL/m^2/h. Such a volume load may lead to severe tissue or pulmonary oedema. Allopurinol or rasburicase to treat hyperuricemia. Aluminium hydroxide and diuretics for hyperphosphataemia
- Hyperviscosity syndrome:
  - Defined as white cell count (WCC) >100 $\times$ 10^9/L. Severity of symptoms is proportional to WCC and proportion of blast cells in blood. High blood viscosity results in stasis and poor blood supply to organs, leading to cerebral infarction, cerebral haemorrhage, renal failure, hypoxia, or ventilatory failure
  - Treatment includes starting chemotherapy early, hyperhydration therapy, leucopheresis, and exchange transfusion. Avoid any factors that $\uparrow$ viscosity, e.g. dehydration and blood transfusion

Immunocompromised child

- Assume all children with haematological tumours or undergoing chemotherapy/radiotherapy are immunocompromised.
- Congenital abnormalities, e.g. Fanconi's anaemia, may coexist.
- Infections, e.g. EBV or CMV, may further compromise immunity.
- General considerations:
  - Strict hand hygiene.
  - Staff with infections must not contact patient.
  - Avoid infective cases prior to the child.
  - Standard infection control measures.
  - Handle indwelling tunnelled lines with care.
  - Central blocks and continuous catheter techniques are generally avoided.

Haemopoietic stem cell transplant

- Used to treat various conditions, mainly acute leukaemia and NHL.
- Autologous (patient's own stem cells) or allogenic (donor stem cells).
- High morbidity and mortality.
- Complications include sepsis, pulmonary oedema, respiratory failure and graft-versus-host disease (GVHD).
- GVHD:
  - Acute (<5 weeks) or chronic.
  - High morbidity and mortality.
  - Organs affected include skin (rash, skin loss, and ulceration), GIT (mouth ulcers, vomiting, diarrhoea, and ileus), and liver dysfunction.
  - Treatment is support to organs, and aggressive immunosuppression with high-dose IV steroids (methylprednisolone) and mycophenolate, or serotherapy, e.g. rituximab.

Lumbar puncture, intrathecal drugs, bone marrow aspiration, and trephines

- Lumbar puncture (LP) may be diagnostic or therapeutic.
- Many children tolerate, even prefer, conscious sedation over GA using midazolam, ketamine, or propofol.

Preoperative assessment
- Examine for evidence of toxic side effects:
  - Cardiac: cyclophosphamide, doxorubicin (dysrhythmias, cardiac failure), radiation (cardiomyopathy).
  - Respiratory: respiratory tract infection is common (fever may not be evident), bleomycin, cyclophosphamide, methotrexate (pulmonary toxicity).
- Most children and parents have a preference for the method of induction; facilitate this unless there is a clinical contraindication.
- FBC ± U+E are checked preoperatively.
- In leukaemia, a normal platelet count may not mean normal function. There is no consensus as to a safe level for LP. If <50,000/mm³, a platelet infusion may be needed.

Anaesthetic technique
- Patients frequently have indwelling vascular access: use an aseptic non-touch technique for induction. For anything other than a brief procedure, a peripheral cannula is inserted to ↓ handling of the indwelling venous access. If an indwelling central line is accessed, it must be flushed with the locally agreed heparin solution.
- Face mask or LMA.
- Maintenance is with volatile in O_2 and air or N_2O.
- LP performed by oncology staff. The anaesthetist should not be involved as both operator and anaesthetist.
- Anaesthetists do not perform intrathecal injections of chemotherapeutic drugs. There is a local register of staff permitted to prescribe, check, and administer intrathecal chemotherapy drugs and procedures to avoid incorrect administration. Fatalities have occurred after errors, e.g. intrathecal vincristine.
- Intrathecal drugs: cytarabine, methotrexate, thiotepa, gentamicin, vancomycin, and hydrocortisone.
- Antiemetic, e.g. ondansetron IV, if intrathecal chemotherapy given.
- Bone marrow aspirates and trephines are usually taken from the posterior superior iliac region with the patient lateral or semiprone. Postoperative pain is moderate. LA infiltration to aspiration sites.
- Patients receiving maintenance therapy are treated as day cases. There is an incidence of post-LP headache, especially in older children, which may require bed rest and oral analgesics.

Insertion of portacath or Hickman line

- The biggest groups are patients with cancer requiring chemotherapy and intestinal failure requiring TPN. Haemophiliacs usually have a portacath inserted for daily administration of factors.

- Many children undergo multiple procedures because of changes in their clinical condition or loss of catheters to infection (25%), thrombosis, wound infections (15%), or systemic bacterial or yeast infections that colonize the catheters.
- For more details, ➲ Chapter 18.

Bone marrow harvest
- Performed to obtain stem cells to treat:
  - Haematological tumours, e.g. leukaemia, Hodgkin's lymphoma.
  - Solid tumours, e.g. Wilms' tumour.
  - Fanconi syndrome.
- Bone marrow (autologous from the patient or allogenic from a suitable donor) is harvested, frozen, stored, and then reinfused (after high-dose chemotherapy) to re-establish cell production.

Preoperative assessment
- For an autologous harvest, the patient must be well enough to be anaesthetized safely and undergo the procedure. FBC and U+E results must be acceptable. For allogenic donation, consent from adults is straightforward. When the donor is a child (often a sibling), there is the ethical quandary of exposing the donor child to risk with no personal benefit in order to treat another child.

Anaesthetic technique
- Usually performed in prone position, takes 60–90 mins.
- ETT and IPPV.
- Maintenance as preferred.
- Up to 10% of bone marrow is harvested, potentially rendering donor hypovolaemic and anaemic. Fluid replacement is required. If blood transfusion is required, this must be delayed until the harvest is complete or there will be contamination.
- Multiple punctures are made. Give paracetamol, LA infiltration and an opiate, e.g. morphine or fentanyl IV, as well as an antiemetic e.g. ondansetron.
- Postoperative care consists of IV fluids until oral intake resumes. PO paracetamol, morphine and a NSAID if no contraindications.

Wilms' tumour
- Commonest intra-abdominal malignant tumour in children.
- Incidence 0.8:100,000.
- Mean age at presentation is 3.5 years, and 90% present before 8 years.
- Aetiology:
  - Sporadic gene mutations account for 90%.
  - 1.5% of cases are familial.
  - 10% are associated with syndromes, e.g. Beckwith–Wiedemann, isolated hemihypertrophy, trisomy 18, Denys–Drash, WAGR (Wilms' tumour, aniridia, GU malformation, mental retardation)
- Presentation:
  - Painless abdominal/flank mass
  - Abdominal pain
  - Haematuria (30%), anaemia
  - Fever

- Anorexia
- Nausea and vomiting
- Hypertension in 50% of cases (↑ renin produced by renal cortex trapped within tumour or compressed adjacent to it, acts on angiotensinogen (angiotensin I, converted in lungs to angiotensin II, results in vasoconstriction, polydipsia, and hypertension).
- Investigations:
  - Abdominal US
  - CT or MRI of abdomen and chest to look for: IVC or atrial thrombosis, vascular extension of tumour, or pulmonary metastases
  - Intravascular tumour extension (renal vein, IVC, right atrium) is assessed further by angiography and ECHO. May warrant preoperative chemotherapy to shrink the tumour and ↓ operative complications. Consider cardiopulmonary bypass.
- Treatment:
  - Treatment is staging and surgical resection followed by chemotherapy and radiotherapy.
  - Preoperative chemotherapy is only given where masses are bilateral, extending into vascular structures, or unresectable.
- Staging is carried out during laparotomy and resection (Table 20.1).
- Staging and histology determine the chemotherapy regimen.
  - Stages I and II with favourable histology: 18 weeks of vincristine and dactinomycin.
  - Stage II unfavourable (anaplastic) histology and stage III: 24 weeks of vincristine, dactinomycin, and doxorubicin (cardiotoxic).
  - Stage IV: chemotherapy + radiotherapy to abdomen ± chest
  - Stages II to IV (with poorest histology): 24 weeks vincristine, doxorubicin, cyclophosphamide, and etoposide + radiotherapy
- Cure rate in Stage I disease is >85%.
- 5% are bilateral (each is staged independently). After initial staging and 6–8 weeks of chemotherapy to shrink tumours (one side may disappear completely), a definitive operation is performed aiming for resection of the tumour with minimal loss of function. 5-year survival is 70% (risk of renal failure).

Preoperative assessment
- Chemotherapy history.
- Sites of previous vascular access.

Table 20.1 Staging during laparotomy and resection

Stage I	Limited to kidney, completely resected
Stage II	Extrarenal extension, completely resected
Stage III	Residual non-haematogenous tumour, confined to abdomen (or stage II with intraoperative capsule rupture or tumour spillage)
Stage IV	Haematogenous metastasis
Stage V	Bilateral tumours

- ACE inhibitors (captopril) and the angiotensin II antagonist saralasin may be used to treat hypertension.
- Renal function, FBC, and cross-match.
- Coagulation screen (up to 10% have an acquired von Willebrand's disease with platelet dysfunction and coagulopathy). If present, seek haematological advice regarding preoperative cryoprecipitate and/or FFP.
- Polycythaemia is occasionally seen due to ↑ erythropoietin.
- Review CT and, in the case of IVC or atrial extension, review angiography and ECHO.

Anaesthetic technique
- IV induction if possible. Consider an RSI because of the large upper abdominal mass.
- ETT and IPPV are necessary.
- Maintenance is with volatile in O_2 and air. An infusion of remifentanil 0.1–0.25 mcg/kg/min reduces volatile requirements and helps maintain cardiovascular stability.
- Two wide-bore peripheral IV cannulas, preferably in the upper limbs. IVC compression from the tumour mass or surgical manipulation may ↓ venous return.
- Most cases require arterial and central venous lines. BP is often labile during surgery owing to contracted intravascular volume, LVH, and IVC compression (acute hypertension during handling of the tumour is uncommon). Hypertension that is labile or severe (similar situation to phaeochromocytoma and neuroblastoma) with contraction of intravascular volume and LVH may require intraoperative phenoxybenzamine, phentolamine, or sodium nitroprusside.
- Urinary catheter and NGT inserted.
- Blood loss is usually replaced with colloid, and blood transfused if necessary.
- This may be lengthy abdominal (retroperitoneal) surgery. Meticulous thermoregulation and fluid balance are essential. Monitor central temperature.
- Analgesia is best provided by a thoracic epidural. The incision is transverse across the upper abdomen so that the contralateral kidney can be examined. Epidural veins are often dilated by IVC compression, but the benefits are usually considered to outweigh the risks.
- Alternatively, give IV morphine/fentanyl.
- IV paracetamol.
- No NSAIDs in view of potential haemorrhage and renal impairment.

Postoperative care
- Usually HDU.
- O_2 may be required because of diaphragmatic splinting.
- Maintenance fluids plus colloid/blood to maintain fluid balance and UO.
- Epidural or NCA/PCA required for 48 h.
- Regular paracetamol avoid NSAIDs.
- Check FBC and U+E.
- BP may take several weeks to return to normal.

Neuroblastoma

- Malignancy of primitive neural crest cells of the adrenal medulla and sympathetic ganglia.
- Commonest malignant neoplasm in <1-year-olds.
- >70% are abdominal (one-third retroperitoneal sympathetic chain and two-thirds adrenal medulla), 20% thoracic, and 5% cervical.
- 50% are diagnosed at <2 years of age and 75% <4 years.

Aetiology

- Usually caused by a sporadic gene mutation.
- 1–2% are familial.

Presentation

- Abdominal mass ± pain.
- Hypertension (compression of renal vasculature or secretion of catecholamines).
- Diarrhoea (secretion of vasoactive intestinal peptide).
- Respiratory distress (5% of posterior mediastinal masses cause tracheal compression or deviation).
- Thoracic or abdominal tumours may invade the epidural space, causing back pain or spinal cord compression.
- Metastases present in >50% at diagnosis. Tend to invade surrounding structures (nephroblastoma and hepatoblastoma tend to grow without local invasion, compressing neighbouring tissue).
- Associated with von Recklinghausen's neurofibromatosis, Hirschsprung's disease, and Ondine's curse.

Investigations

- MRI, CT.
- 85% of cases produce catecholamines, detected in 24-h urine collection as vanillylmandelic acid and homovanillic acid.
- mIBG (meta-iodobenzylguanidine) scan.
- Excess catecholamine exposure may induce cardiomyopathy, LVH, and cardiac failure: full cardiac assessment, including ECHO.

Treatment

- Surgery for localized tumours without distant metastases. Where the tumour has spread, preoperative chemotherapy is used.
- Postoperative chemotherapy if unfavourable histology.
- Radiotherapy for disseminated disease.

Staging

- Fully resected localized tumours have a >80–90% cure rate. Much lower for metastatic disease unless age <1 year (Table 20.2).

Preoperative assessment

- Chemotherapy history.
- Sites of previous vascular access.
- Renal function, FBC, U+E, cross-match.
- There may be airway compression with posterior mediastinal masses.
- Preoperative BP control allows re-expansion of the intravascular compartment, can reverse catecholamine-induced myocardial

Table 20.2 Tumours

Stage I	Localized tumour, completely excised
Stage IIA	Localized tumour, incompletely excised
Stage IIB	Localized tumour, incompletely excised; local lymph nodes
Stage III	Tumour crosses midline; regional bilateral nodes
Stage IV	Distant metastases
Stage IVS	<1 year old; localized tumour; metastasized to liver, skin, or marrow

dysfunction, and reduces the incidence and severity of intraoperative hypertensive events (➔ 'Phaeochromocytoma' for BP management).
- Although hypertension is common at presentation, intraoperative hypertensive crises during tumour manipulation are rare compared with phaeochromocytoma (relatively fewer intracellular catecholamine storage granules, a mix of cholinergic and adrenergic cells in the tumour, and a relative lack of the enzymes necessary to convert dopamine to noradrenaline (epinephrine) and noradrenaline (norepinephrine) to adrenaline in neuroblastoma cells). However, BP surges can occur.

Anaesthetic technique
- Similar to nephroblastoma and phaeochromocytoma.
- ETT and IPPV. NGT and urinary catheter.
- Maintenance as preferred. An infusion of remifentanil reduces volatile requirements and helps maintain cardiovascular stability.
- Two wide-bore peripheral IV cannulas.
- In most cases, arterial and central venous lines are inserted. BP is sometimes labile intraoperatively, may require phenoxybenzamine, phentolamine, or sodium nitroprusside to control.
- Meticulous thermoregulation and fluid balance. Measure central temperature. Use a warming mattress, warming blanket, and fluid warmer.
- For abdominal tumours, analgesia is best provided by a thoracic epidural.
- Alternatively, a bolus of morphine.
- IV paracetamol plus NSAID if no contraindications.

Postoperative care
- Nursed in HDU. O$_2$ may be required because of splinting of the diaphragm. FBC and U+E are checked. Maintenance fluids plus colloid or blood if required to maintain fluid balance and urine output.
- An epidural or PCA/NCA usually required for 48 h.
- Regular paracetamol can be prescribed. NSAIDs if no contraindications.

Phaeochromocytoma
- Originates from chromaffin tissue of the adrenal medulla and sympathetic ganglia (around aortic bifurcation, GI tract, bladder, and in the chest).
- If functional, can secrete large amounts of noradrenaline, adrenaline, and dopamine.
- Rare: 2–8 cases/million population annually.

- Most are teenagers, rare <8 years old.
- In children, compared with adults:
  - Malignancy is less common.
  - Bilateral and extrarenal or multiple sites are commoner
  - Noradrenaline is the predominant catecholamine in most cases.
  - Increased incidence of multiple endocrine neoplasia (MEN): hyperparathyroidism, medullary carcinoma of thyroid, and phaeochromocytoma.
  - Associated with neurofibromatosis and tuberous sclerosis.

Presentation
- Symptoms of sympathetic overdrive:
  - Nausea, vomiting
  - Fatigue
  - Abdominal pain
  - Sweating
  - Headaches
  - Palpitations
  - Hypertensive crisis with possible cerebrovascular haemorrhage, pulmonary oedema, or cardiac failure.

Investigations
- 24-h urine collection for catecholamine metabolites.
- CT (95% accuracy) and/or MRI (99% accuracy) to locate tumours and plan resection.
- mIBG scan can be used (radiolabelled isotope taken up by neural cells: 80% sensitivity).

Treatment
- Laparoscopic surgery becoming more common (associated with less surgical stimulation and better postoperative recovery).

Preoperative management
- Assessment of end-organ hypertensive damage.
- Cardiac effects include LVH, cardiomyopathy (dilated or obstructive), dysrhythmias, ischaemia, and heart failure. ECG and ECHO required.
- Cardiac dysfunction precludes the use of perioperative beta-blockers (negative inotropic effects—pulmonary oedema, hypotension). Cardiac dysfunction is usually reversible and treatment reduces intraoperative morbidity and overall mortality. There may be pulmonary oedema, renal impairment, biochemical changes ($\uparrow$ Ca^{2+} (hyperparathyroidism), $\downarrow$ K^+ ($\uparrow$ renin (secondary hyperaldosteronism), and/or hyperglycaemia (alpha-receptor stimulation in pancreas ($\downarrow$ insulin).
- Preoperative alpha-receptor blockade to reverse the effects of excess catecholamines. Phenoxybenzamine, a selective α_1 antagonist (with some α_2 blockade), forms a non-competitive alkylated bond with the receptor. It is long-acting and so can act into the postoperative period, resulting in resistant hypotension (until new alpha receptors are produced). Start at 0.25–1.0 mg/kg/day orally, increasing dose until control is achieved (may take weeks). Criteria for adequate blockade include: normal BP; orthostatic hypotension; and a $\downarrow$ haematocrit of around 5% due to plasma expansion.

- Preoperative alpha-receptor blockade has reduced mortality from 50% to 3%.
- Beta blockade to treat reflex tachycardia from unopposed alpha blockade is rarely required.

Anaesthetic technique
- Minimize adrenergic responses and catecholamine release.
- Sedative premedication, e.g. midazolam.
- IV induction in older children.
- ETT and IPPV. Attenuate the pressor response to laryngoscopy using a bolus of remifentanil or fentanyl ± topical lidocaine to cords.
- Two wide-bore IV cannulas.
- Maintenance as preferred. An infusion of remifentanil reduces volatile requirements and helps maintain cardiovascular stability.
- Standard monitoring plus arterial and central venous line, urinary catheter, and temperature.
- For open procedures, a thoracic epidural provides good analgesia, but will not prevent release of catecholamines during handling of the tumour. For laparoscopic procedures, a bolus of morphine/fentanyl is given towards the end of surgery if an infusion of remifentanil is used or at the start if not.
- Intraoperatively BP may be labile. Volatile anaesthetics provide a rapidly titratable vasodilator effect. Short-acting vasodilators and pressors should be available (once the adrenal vein is ligated, there may be precipitous hypotension). Most commonly used are:
  - Sodium nitroprusside 0.5–4 mcg/kg/min, a direct vasodilator with quick onset and offset. Tachyphylaxis and cyanide toxicity (only if rate >10 mcg/kg/min) are possible problems.
  - Phentolamine 5–50 mcg/kg/min, a short-acting alpha antagonist. Tachycardia and tachyphylaxis occur.
  - Esmolol 0.5 mg/kg over 1 min or 25–200 mcg/kg/min, a short-acting beta-blocker.
  - Magnesium sulfate 50 mg/kg reduces catecholamine release from the adrenal medulla and sympathetic nerve endings, blocks adrenergic receptors, has a direct vasodilator effect, and is an antidysrhythmic.
- Hypotension post resection is treated initially with fluid boluses. Thereafter use:
  - Phenylephrine 2–10 mcg/kg, an alpha agonist
  - Noradrenaline 0.02–0.1 mcg/kg/min.
- Measure glucose hourly until the adrenal vein is ligated, then more frequently.

Postoperative care
- HDU.
- Check FBC and U+E.
- Maintenance fluids plus colloid if required to maintain fluid balance and UO.
- Hypotension may be due to bleeding or residual preoperative alpha blockade.
- May be transient hypoglycaemia: monitor regularly and infuse 10% glucose if necessary.

- Epidural or PCA/NCA usually required for 48 h.
- For laparoscopic procedures, a PCA/NCA overnight is adequate.
- Regular paracetamol and NSAID.
- Patients may remain hypertensive for several weeks.
- Laparoscopic procedures provide faster resumption of feeding and discharge.

Mediastinal tumours

- The mediastinum is the interpleural space situated between the lungs. It is subdivided into superior and inferior (further divided into anterior, middle, and posterior) by an imaginary line drawn at the sternal angle.
- Most are symptomatic and a third are malignant.
- Symptoms vary depending on tumour origin, compressive effects (varying size), invasive effects, neuroendocrine effects, and malignant nature or systemic effects of a malignant neoplasm.
- Common symptoms include cough, haemoptysis, hoarseness, dysphagia, SVC syndrome, failure to thrive, fatigue, fever, and sepsis.

Diagnosis

- CXR: 90% of tumours identified.
- CT scan (identify nature of tumour).
- MRI (better structural differentiation).
- Biochemical markers.
- Tissue biopsy (gold standard for diagnosis): mediastinoscopy, anterior mediastinoscopy, transbronchial biopsy, EBUS, or VATS thoracoscopy.

Types of tumours

- Lymphomas, e.g. ALL, NHL, and Hodgkin's lymphoma.
- Germ cell tumours, e.g. teratoma (most common).
- Thymic tumours.
- Vascular tumours (e.g. haemangioma), double aortic arch, LV aneurysm.
- Neurogenic tumours, e.g. ganglioma, ganglioneuroma, and neuroblastoma. Mostly posterior mediastinal tumours.
- Cysts, e.g. enteric cysts and bronchogenic cysts.
- Others, e.g. mediastinal lymph nodes.

Anaesthesia for anterior mediastinal mass (AMM) biopsy

- Significant risk of airway obstruction and cardiovascular collapse.
- Careful planning with MDT involving oncologist, radiologist, and surgeon.
- If severe obstructive symptoms, consider pretreatment with corticosteroids (5 days).
- Biopsy may be performed under LA ± sedation in older children.

Preoperative assessment

- High-risk factors:
  - Signs of airway obstruction, e.g. stridor, wheeze, or orthopnoea
  - Venous obstruction—SVC syndrome
  - Tracheobronchial obstruction on imaging
  - Pericardial effusion
  - Ventricular dysfunction.
- Review imaging CT/MRI to gain a clear picture of the mass.

- Establish onset/resolution of symptoms with positional changes.
- High-risk consent, frank discussion, including LA option.
- ICU or HDU postoperatively.
- Correct any coagulopathy and arrange adequate blood products.
- Ensure cardiothoracic surgical availability.

Anaesthetic
- Resuscitative equipment ready and additional senior anaesthetic help present.
- Selection of smaller-sized and reinforced ETT, and rigid bronchoscope available.
- Sedative premedication generally not advised.
- IV cannula before induction.
- Slow IV or inhalation induction with sevoflurane in 100% O_2.
- Maintain SV until the airway is secured.
- Volatile or TIVA are equally effective.
- Consider topical LA to vocal cords and trachea.
- Consider alternative strategy of IV ketamine, face mask, and LA.
- Wide-bore IV access secured in preparation for major haemorrhage.
- Standard monitoring is sufficient in most cases.
- Consider invasive arterial monitoring in unstable patients with significant cardiac compromise.
- Analgesia: LA, plus paracetamol.
- Awake extubation and re-establish adequacy of ventilation in theatre in presence of surgical assistance.

Critical events during procedure
- Airway collapse on induction:
  - CPAP plus 100% O_2
  - Position lateral or prone.
- Difficult intubation:
  - Fibreoptic or GlideScope
  - Smaller-sized ETT
  - Rigid bronchoscope.
- Cardiovascular collapse/cardiac arrest:
  - Fluid bolus
  - Resuscitation drugs
  - Positional changes to relieve compression
  - Open chest compressions
  - ECLS (mostly unsuccessful).
- Haemorrhage.
  - Blood products.

Postoperative care
- HDU or ICU, since delayed respiratory or cardiovascular compromise may occur.
- Simple analgesics.

Radiotherapy

Overview

- GA usually requested for children <5–6 years of age, or older children who cannot cope with the planning, preparation, and execution of radiotherapy.
- With adequate preparation, older children usually manage without GA.
- Usually daily treatment for several weeks (rarely twice daily—hyperfractionated).
- 6 weeks course for CNS tumours, 2–3 weeks for abdominal tumours, 1 week for total body irradiation (TBI).

Indications

- CNS tumours.
  - Conformal irradiation of tumour bed:
    —High-grade astrocytoma
    —Low-grade glioma.
  - Whole craniospinal irradiation:
    —Medulloblastoma.
- Hyperfractionated radiotherapy:
  - Metastatic medulloblastoma.
- Wilms' tumour, neuroblastoma.
- Others.
  - Pretransplant conditioning for relapsed leukaemia (TBI).
  - Palliation of symptoms: bone pain or soft tissue tumours, spinal compression.

Toxic effects of radiation

- The child's clinical condition may change during the course of treatment. Side effects of radiotherapy may develop: hair loss, skin damage, nausea, fatigue.
- Acute reactions include mucositis, myelosuppression, and localized skin reactions resembling sunburn.
- Late effects include hormonal deficiencies, infertility, hypertension, cataract, and secondary tumours.

General considerations

- Remote site, often in another hospital, almost always with limited facilities for induction, maintenance, and recovery from GA.
- There may be transport issues for patients and staff to the location.
- Must be overseen by consultant anaesthetist if remote site.
- There may be intercurrent problems, especially respiratory infections or psychological effects of daily GA and fasting.
- A 'Key worker' is assigned, who acts as a liaison nurse to coordinate multispeciality involvement.
- 'Play therapist' may help in the management of anxiety and in providing some continuity of care.
- GA is initially required for planning and simulation, followed by treatments.

- Patient must be alone in radiotherapy room while being treated; cameras are used to observe and monitor the patient.
- Actual treatments are short—each field to be irradiated may only be exposed for 30–90 s, although there may be several fields to treat.
- Prior to therapy, the fields are marked after plotting. The usual sequence for CNS tumours involves constructing a unique plastic 'shell' from a plaster cast of the head (which may extend over the neck and upper chest), upon which marks are made to guide the focused radiation beam. This is used for every treatment, and is used in conjunction with imaging to simulate the radiotherapy prior to actual exposure.
- Simulation: numerous images of the tumour and surrounding tissue are used to form a 3D 'model' of the patient's anatomy (computer based). This is used to ascertain the best approach to the tumour, with minimal injury to surrounding organs and tissue. Different approaches are tried until a plan is constructed for actual radiotherapy.

Anaesthetic technique
- Preferably first case in morning to limit fasting and to minimize disruption to radiotherapy suite and anaesthetic activity.
- Radiotherapy must be planned carefully. Interruptions in treatment are not favourable. Children may need to be anaesthetized when they are ill in order to complete the course.
- Anaesthetic machine usually uses cylinders rather than piped gases.
- As it is often a remote location, there may be limited stocks of drugs and equipment. Appropriate checks are performed.
- Ensure easy access to self-inflating bag and emergency airway equipment.
- Patients often have a Hickman line or portacath with Gripper needle in place.
- Patients may arrive from home once a routine is established. Alternatively, they may be transported from the oncology ward.
- The ideal anaesthetic is rapid-onset, short-duration, reproducible, safe, maintains a patent airway in all positions, and provides immobility and prompt recovery.
- Induction often takes place in the treatment area.
- Induction is usually inhalational to minimize infection risk to long-term lines. Children are usually quite adapted to gas induction and generally prefer inhalational route.
- Usually LMA with SV (supine or prone positions) and maintenance as preferred.
- Analgesia is not required.
- Analgesics need to be continued if already on them.
- Administer an antiemetic.
- Once recovered, patients are often discharged home.

Respiratory procedures

Overview
- Bronchoscopies can be diagnostic or therapeutic.
- Performed in remote locations or ENT theatres.
- Shared airway with operating surgeon.
- Advanced bronchoscopic procedures are performed in tertiary centres.
- Child may present with significant respiratory compromise and coexisting disorders.

Rigid bronchoscopy
- Diagnostic indications:
  - Congenital stridor (most common)
  - Laryngeal web
  - Recurrent laryngeal nerve palsy—CHD (double aortic arch)
  - Vocal cord paralysis
  - Subglottic stenosis
  - Failed extubation
  - Tracheomalacia.
- Therapeutic indications:
  - Tracheal dilations
  - Vocal cord injections
  - Foreign body (FB) aspiration
  - Laser treatment of polyps/cysts.
- Contraindications:
  - Acute respiratory or cardiac instability
  - Unstable cervical spine
  - Severe coagulopathy
  - Limited mouth opening.
- Equipment:
  - The Karl Storz endoscope is a hollow aluminium tube with bevelled and narrowed distal end. The proximal end has ports for connection of light source and ventilation circuit. There is a main working channel, for the introduction of endoscopes, forceps, suction, or laser.
  - Available in various sizes.
  - Concentric tube with the lighting system (Hopkins rod-lens system) can be introduced into the outer Storz endoscopic tube for visualization and capturing images. The Hopkins rod can be used alone to examine the airway, since it is narrow and more manoeuvrable.

Foreign body (FB) removal
- Usually infants and toddlers.
- Aspiration deaths usually occur pre hospital.
- Rigid bronchoscopy is the gold standard for FB removal.

General considerations
- Coughing, gagging, complete airway obstruction, and collapse may follow sudden choking on an FB.

- Normal CXR does not exclude an FB. It is important to note any lung collapse, air trapping, or mediastinal shift suggesting distension or collapse of the affected side.
- Late presentation: haemoptysis, pneumonia, bronchiectasis, or chronic cough.
- Acute airway obstruction leading to compromise requires emergency removal. Subacute and delayed presentations may be treated in a planned manner.
- Need an experienced team in a tertiary level set-up.

Anaesthetic considerations
- Careful assessment is crucial, noting airway patency and adequacy of oxygenation.
- Review CXR.
- IV access is usually secured on presentation; if not, ensure adequate senior help during induction.
- Inhalation induction is preferred to assess the airway and breathing.
- At laryngoscopy, check to see if FB visible; if so, remove with Magill forceps.
- Otherwise, spray vocal cords and trachea with lidocaine 1–2%.
- Airway is not intubated at this stage and SV is maintained with facemask or LMA.
- NPA can provide a channel for insufflating O_2 during some stages in bronchoscopy.
- Close monitoring and communication with the operating surgeon is essential.
- An ETT of appropriate size plus stylet is kept ready.
- Once the bronchoscope is introduced into the trachea, the anaesthetic circuit is connected to the inferior ventilating port to insufflate O_2 and inhalational gases.
- The surgeon may need more than one attempt.
- Adequate preparation must be made for critical events.
- TIVA is a suitable alternative and equally effective.

Complications
- Failure to remove, fragmentation, or dislodgement of the FB.
- Trauma to the airway and bleeding.
- Inadequate oxygenation, bronchospasm, and laryngospasm.
- Perforation of trachea leading to pneumomediastinum or pneumothorax.
- Bradycardia or cardiac arrest.

Flexible fibreoptic bronchoscopy (FOB)

General considerations
- Patient usually has a degree of respiratory compromise and may have associated congenital disorders, e.g. cystic fibrosis.
- Preoperative assessment must include respiratory reserve, baseline saturation, O_2 requirements.

Diagnostic indications
- Bronchogram.

- Bronchoalveolar lavage (BAL): diagnostic and therapeutic.
- Brushed bronchial biopsies.
- Transbronchial biopsies.
- Transbronchial needle aspiration.

Therapeutic indications
- Removal of FB.
- Tissue debridement.
- Balloon bronchoplasty.
- Endobronchial stenting.

Complications
- Coughing.
- Bronchospasm, laryngospasm, and desaturations.
- Bleeding into airway.
- Pneumothorax.

Equipment
- Conventional fibreoptic bronchoscopes are made of carefully packed fibreoptic bundles. Images are viewed at the proximal eyepiece. They also have a suction port and a separate working channel. A variety of sizes are available.
- Disadvantages of the older scopes include high maintenance costs, breakage of fibreoptics leading to distorted images, and comparatively poor-quality images.
- Newer scopes are essentially 'videoscopes'. A true-colour chip placed at the distal tip records the images and transmits it to the eyepiece or any other viewing platform. Fibreoptic cables are still used to transmit light. They are lighter and provide superior-quality images.
- Flexible bronchoscopes may be adult or paediatric, with interchangeability based on the requirement of the operator. They can also be classed as diagnostic or therapeutic scopes. Therapeutic scopes have a larger external diameter and a larger working channel, and thus a greater risk of discomfort and mucosal damage.

Anaesthetic considerations
- Aim of GA is to maintain SV, avoid coughing, and maintain adequate oxygenation.
- Establish basic monitoring prior to induction.
- Secure an IV cannula either before or after gas induction.
- Gas induction with O_2 + sevoflurane is preferred
- Laryngoscopy is performed, after achieving sufficient depth of anaesthetic
- Topical spray of lidocaine 1% or 2% (maximum dose of 4 mg/kg) to vocal cords and trachea. In some institutions, this is avoided for BAL because lidocaine (bacteriostatic) may contaminate the specimen, preventing bacterial yield.
- LMA with absent epiglottis bars provides a smooth channel for the bronchoscope.
- A swivel adaptor attaches to the LMA; it allows continued ventilation via the anaesthetic circuit and has a port for entry of the bronchoscope.

- SV with O_2 + sevoflurane to maintain anaesthesia.
- CPAP 5 cmH$_2$O prevents desaturation during bronchoscopy.
- ETT may be used in children needing much smaller scopes and higher ventilatory support.
- PICC line inserted for children needing long term medications or bloods at home.
- Recover in lateral position to prevent aspiration.
- NBM for 1 h post LA spraying of cords.
- Basic monitoring continues in the ward or HDU for apnoea and hypoxemia.

Novel bronchoscopic techniques
- Navigational bronchoscopy: bronchoscopy assisted by interventional radiology (CT-guided).
- Virtual bronchoscopy.
- Endobronchial ultrasound (EBUS): transbronchial biopsies.

Rheumatology

Overview

- Inflammatory arthritis is the commonest chronic disease in children, leading to long-term morbidity and disability.
- Juvenile idiopathic arthritis (JIA) is defined as:
  • Persistent joint pain, stiffness, and joint swelling
  • Duration >6 weeks
  • Age of onset 16 years.
- JIA is subclassified based on the number of joints involved, sacroiliac joint involvement, and systemic effects into:
  • Oligoarticular JIA (peak 2 years; females predominate 5:1):
    —Involves <5 joints.
    —Usually involves the knee.
    —Uveitis common.
  • Polyarticular JIA (peak 3 years):
    —Involves >5 joints in the first 6 months.
    —Commonly involves small joints; symmetrical distribution.
    —Cervical spine involved in up to 70%; may present with torticollis.
    —Bilateral TMJ involvement may limit mouth opening and mandibular development, leading to micrognathia.
    —Systemic manifestations are usually mild, e.g. fever, anaemia, rash.
    —Two subgroups: seronegative or positive for RhF.
    —RhF +ve are usually female, >8 years old, more destructive disease.
    —Rh F −ve have a less destructive and asymmetrical disease, especially involving the TMJ and neck.
  • Systemic JIA or Still's disease:
    —Involves >5 joints.
    —Associated with fever, macular rash, bone marrow disturbances, and hepatosplenomegaly.
    —Any joint can be involved, especially TMJ and cervical spine.
    —Serious manifestations include uveitis (commonly girls, ANA+, oligoarticular JIA > 80%), pleuritis, and pericarditis.
    —Complications:
      ○ Growth retardation.
      ○ Severe osteomalacia.
      ○ Macrophage activation syndrome: persistent fever and consumptive coagulopathy.
  • Spondyloarthropathies:
    —Involve sacroiliac joint, enthesopathy, psoriasis, and bowel disease.
    —Subclassified: juvenile spondylitis, psoriatic arthritis, and arthritis of IBD.
    —Positive for HLA-B27.

Treatment of JIA

- Goals are to alleviate clinical symptoms, ↓ inflammation, arrest disease progression, prevent deformity, and prevent blindness (uveitis).
- Patients present for various non-disease-related procedures, e.g. MRI, CT, arthrograms, EUA eyes (yearly for uveitis), vascular access, and joint injections.

- NSAIDs while second-line agents (methotrexate, ciclosporin, sulfasalazine, gold salts, and penicillamine) take effect.

Anaesthesia for joint injections

- Commonly performed as day case under GA or conscious sedation for:
  - Children <8 years
  - Multiple joint injections
  - Small-joint injections (painful).
- In children >8 years, consider non-sedative topical analgesic methods, e.g. EMLA™ (lidocaine/prilocaine) cream, lidocaine injection, or ethyl chloride spray.

General considerations:

- Children may be very anxious and need premedication
- Airway assessment for TMJ (limited mouth opening) or cervical spine (limited neck movement) involvement. May need radiological investigation for atlanto-axial subluxation. There may also be cricoarytenoid joint involvement presenting with hoarseness, stridor, and dysphagia.
- Laryngoscopy may be difficult. Fibreoptic intubation may be necessary.
- Systemic manifestations of JIA may result in pericardial and pleural effusions assess preoperatively with ECG, CXR, or ECHO.
- Assess for side effects of medications used in treatment of JIA, e.g. immunosuppression, renal, respiratory, hepatic, and bone marrow dysfunction.

Anaesthetic technique

- Preoperative paracetamol.
- Usually on an NSAID—avoid redosing.
- IV (be careful holding the patient's hand if these joints are affected) or inhalational induction.
- Careful consideration of N_2O and concomitant use of chemotherapeutic agents.
- Careful handling of cervical spine, especially if intubating.
- LMA with SV.
- Maintenance as preferred.
- Positioning may be difficult owing to contractures, and all pressure points must be carefully padded to avoid any pressure-related injuries.
- Handle indwelling tunnelled lines with strict aseptic technique and ensure any residual drugs are flushed.
- Recover in lateral position.
- Postoperative morphine sulfate solution prescribed.

Further reading

Oduro-Dominah L, Brennan LJ. Anaesthetic management of the child with haematological malignancy. *Contin Educ Anaesth Crit Care Pain* 2013;13:158–64.

Lin TK, Barth BA. Endoscopic retrograde cholangiopancreatography in paediatrics. *Tech Gastrointest Endosc* 2013;15:41–6.

Weigert A, Black A. Caustic ingestion in children. *Cont Educ Anaesth Crit Care Pain* 2005;5:5–8.

Thorp N. Basic principles of paediatric radiotherapy. *Clin Oncol* 2013;25:3–10.

Evans P, Chisholm D. Anaesthesia and paediatric oncology. *Curr Anaesth Crit Care* 2008;19:50–8.

Roy S, Basañez, I, Alexander RE. Rigid bronchoscopy. In: Hagberg CA (ed). *Hagberg and Benumof's Airway Management*, 4th edn, 2018: 517–524 (Chap 28).

Friedt M, Welsch S. An update on pediatric endoscopy. *Eur J Med Res* 2013;18:24.

Baddour LM, Wilson WR, Bayer AS, et al. Diagnosis, Antimicrobial Therapy, and Management of Complications: A Statement for Healthcare Professionals from the Committee on Rheumatic Fever, Endocarditis, and Kawasaki Disease, Council on Cardiovascular Disease in the Young, and the Councils on Clinical Cardiology, Stroke, and Cardiovascular Surgery and Anesthesia, American Heart Association—Executive Summary: Endorsed by the Infectious Diseases Society of America. *Circulation* 2005;111:3167–84.

Kasapcopur O, Barut. K. Treatment of juvenile rheumatoid arthritis and new treatment options. *Turk Ped Ars* 2015;50:1–10.

Kelly A, Ramanan AV. The principles of pharmacologic treatments of juvenile idiopathic arthritis. *Paediatr Child Health* 2011;21:563–68.

Schrag SP, Sharma R, Jaik NP, et al. Complications related to percutaneous endoscopic gastrostomy (PEG) tubes. A comprehensive clinical review. *J Gastrointestin Liver Dis* 2007;16:407–18.

Neurosurgery

Elizabeth Wright

Introduction

- Neuroanaesthesia requires an understanding of cerebral physiology and intracranial pathology. Key elements are perioperative control of ICP and avoidance of hypotension.
- Patients often require repeated procedures.
- Significant comorbidities are common, especially cerebral palsy and epilepsy.

Preoperative assessment

- Clinical signs of ↑ ICP:
  - Headache and vomiting
  - Seizures
  - Cranial nerve palsies (especially 6th nerve)
  - Papilloedema
  - Agitation, drowsiness
  - Behavioural changes
- Altered conscious level—refer to baseline neurological assessment.
- Possibility of aspiration during episodes of decreased GCS.
- Absence of airway protective reflexes (bulbar dysfunction).
- Assessment of hydration and electrolyte balance as result of:
  - Mannitol administration
  - Prolonged vomiting
  - Diabetes insipidus (common with midbrain tumours).
- Seizure history: type, frequency, anticonvulsant therapy. Presence of vagal nerve stimulator (beware of cautery, defibrillators, and MRI).
- Review CT/MRI: intracranial tumour, haemorrhage, or AVM. Assess site, size, and vascularity of lesion.
- Ensure blood cross-matched
- Continue regular medication, especially baclofen, steroids, and antiepileptics.

General principles

- Avoid further rises in ICP:
  - Maintain cerebral tissue oxygenation.
  - Control $PaCO_2$.
  - Avoid direct vasodilation by drugs, volatile agents >1 MAC, and N_2O.
  - Maintain CPP; avoid hypotension.
  - Avoid premedication in emergency cases as may lead to ↑ in CO_2.

Induction

- IV induction is preferable when intracranial compliance is low; however, a smooth inhalational induction is often more realistic.
- If inhalational induction is necessary in acutely unwell patients (raised ICP or decreased GCS), ensure that a second anaesthetist is available to establish IV access quickly and give half the induction dose of propofol or thiopental to rapidly achieve the correct level of anaesthesia.
- The sympathetic response to laryngoscopy may be attenuated with a bolus of short-acting opioid, e.g. fentanyl.
- Intubation is required; consider using a microcuff tube in younger children, especially if prone. Check for bilateral lung expansion with the head in the intended surgical position—important when a degree of cervical flexion may result in endobronchial intubation. Secure well with tape. A mouth pack supports the ETT and absorbs secretions to prevent tapes loosening.
- There are few indications for SV or LMA.

Maintenance

- Aim for normocapnia or mild hypocapnia (4.5–4.8 kPa).
- Hyperventilation is reserved for acute rises in ICP.
- Maintenance with volatile (sevoflurane or desflurane 1 MAC) in O_2 and air or TIVA.
- TIVA with BIS monitoring is indicated when electrophysiological monitoring is planned, e.g. brainstem lesions, epilepsy surgery, and spinal procedures. Volatile agents and long-acting muscle relaxants can only be used at induction.
- Avoid N_2O for craniotomy (potential ↑ in CBF and intracranial air spaces).

Positioning

- Check all pressure areas; consider using a pressure-relieving mattress.
- Moderate head-up position; check jugular vessels are free from compression.
- Beware of hyperflexion of the neck.
- When prone, ensure the abdomen is not compressed, since this will adversely affect venous pressure and ventilation.
- Protect eyes and orbits.

Fluids

- Fasting deficit and maintenance fluid replaced with isotonic crystalloid, e.g. Hartmann's or Plasma-Lyte.
- IV antibiotics as per local policy.

Analgesia

- Intraoperative analgesia for craniotomy is usually provided by remifentanil infusion (0.1–0.3 mcg/kg/min). Posterior fossa procedures are more painful.
- Wound infiltration with LA ± adrenaline (epinephrine) for analgesia and haemostasis at start of the procedure. If used at the end of surgery for postoperative analgesia, be aware that dural closure may be incomplete, allowing LA to pass directly into the CSF.
- Patients for elective craniotomy may require a bolus of morphine (100–200 mcg/kg) towards the end of the case.
- Other procedures may require fentanyl 1–2 mcg/kg or increments of morphine. Opiates may need to be reduced or omitted (LA infiltration is often adequate), especially in ex-premature infants weighing <5 kg.
- IV paracetamol.
- Exercise caution with opiates in emergency cases, e.g. blocked shunts, intracranial haematoma. If preoperative GCS is compromised, it may not return to normal at the end of the procedure, despite a theoretical reduction in ICP.

Postoperative care

- Care from experienced paediatric neurosurgical nurses.
- Access to PICU beds if needed.
- Regular neurological observations for first 24 h, continued until stable.
- Preterm babies and those with neural tube defects require apnoea monitoring.
- Postoperative analgesia consists of:
  - Regular IV or PO paracetamol
  - Ibuprofen (avoid in <44 weeks PGA, and in first 24 hr post craniotomy)
  - Morphine PO
  - Morphine or fentanyl PCA/NCA for craniotomy.
- Regular antiemetics may be required, particularly following posterior fossa surgery.
- Maintenance fluids until oral intake resumes.
- Patients at risk of complex fluid and electrolyte disturbances need accurate fluid balance and regular serum and urine sampling for electrolytes and osmolality.

Elective procedures

- Insertion of ICP monitor.
- Treatment of ↑ ICP:
  - VP shunt
  - Endoscopic third ventriculostomy.
- Craniotomy:
  - Tumour/epilepsy/AVM
  - Posterior fossa decompression (Arnold–Chiari malformation).
- Endovascular:
  - Embolization of AVM.
- Spasticity:
  - Insertion of baclofen pump
  - Selective dorsal rhizotomy.
- Spinal:
  - Untethering of spinal cord
  - Spinal tumours.

Emergency procedures

- Head injury, including initial resuscitation and management.
- Control of acute ↑ in ICP:
  - ICP monitor
  - External ventricular drain
  - Revision of VP shunt
  - Craniotomy for evacuation of haematoma/elevation of depressed fracture
  - Craniotomy for drainage of abscess/empyema
  - Decompressive craniotomy.
- Closure of myelomeningocele (to prevent infection).

Ventriculo-peritoneal (VP) shunt insertion

- Hydrocephalus is an abnormal accumulation of CSF within the cranium.
  - It results in dilatation of the ventricles, ↑ ICP and brain damage.
  - In neonates and infants, gradual changes in ICP may be accommodated by expansion of sutures, resulting in an ↑ head circumference and bulging anterior fontanelles. Classic 'setting sun' eyes is a late sign.
  - Intracranial pathology in neonates may present with apnoea ➔ 'General principles'.
  - Neonates rarely need emergency surgery, because the unfused sutures give some protection from acute rises in ICP.
- Many patients with hydrocephalus have complications associated with prematurity.
- Diagnosis is confirmed by CT, MRI, or an ICP monitor.

Aetiology

- Obstruction to CSF flow:
  - Non-communicating hydrocephalus secondary to obstruction to the CSF flow within the ventricular system (third ventricle, aqueduct, or fourth ventricle) or from external pressure on the system:
    —Congenital:
      o Aqueduct stenosis
      o Myelomeningocele
      o Arnold–Chiari syndrome.
    —Acquired:
      o Infection
      o Neonatal intraventricular haemorrhage
      o Tumour.
  - Communicating hydrocephalus: CSF flows between the ventricles into the subarachnoid space, but is obstructed distally because of an inability to absorb CSF, e.g. following meningitis.
- Excess secretion of CSF: e.g. choroid plexus papilloma (rare).

Treatment

- Surgical diversion of excess CSF from the lateral ventricles to the peritoneum via a shunt. Shunts have three components:
  - Ventricular catheter placed into the ventricle through a burr hole ± a dome-shaped self-sealing reservoir (may be used to sample CSF).
  - A valve attached in series to the catheter ensures unidirectional CSF flow and prevents over-drainage with change of posture. Valves are available with various opening pressures and some are programmable (which need checking post MRI).
  - Silastic tubing connected to the valve distally and tunnelled subcutaneously. The distal end is placed into the peritoneal cavity through a small incision in the abdominal wall. If the abdomen is soiled or is unable to absorb CSF, the distal end may be positioned in the right atrium via the internal jugular vein or into the pleural space.

- Raised ICP may be temporarily controlled by removing a small volume of CSF from the shunt reservoir.
- Endoscopic third ventriculostomy is an alternative treatment for non-communicating hydrocephalus. A small hole is created in the floor of the third ventricle so that CSF can flow directly into the subarachnoid space and bypass the aqueduct. This may ↓ the risk of infection and blockage.

Shunt malfunction

- Blockage is relatively common and requires either revision of one component or replacement of the whole system. Most commonly, the proximal ventricular catheter is obstructed with cells, choroid plexus, or debris. There may be kinking of the tubing, disconnection or fracture of components, or migration of the distal end.
- Shunts also fail because of infection, usually during the first 3 months following insertion. Infection rates are highest in neonates.
- Premature babies with hydrocephalus resulting from intraventricular haemorrhage have a high incidence of early failure from infection or obstruction by resolving blood products. Alternative management options are insertion of a ventricular access device (Rickham or Ommaya reservoir) for repeated ventricular taps or a subgaleal shunt. Once they reach term, a VP shunt is less prone to fail.
- Shunt malfunction usually presents with dilated ventricles on CT or MRI scan, but it can occur in children with small or normal-size ventricles. Clinical symptoms overrule scan findings.

Perioperative management

- ➔ 'General principles'.
- Difficult to predict duration of the procedure. It may be possible to replace the ventricular end without re-tunnelling the catheter. Replacing the whole shunt may take 1–2 h.
- Position the patient so there is anatomical alignment of the planned shunt route from the burr hole site, down the neck, across the chest, and into the abdomen. Ensure the patient is physically stable and the neck veins are unobstructed. Positioning maybe difficult because of anatomical deformities, e.g. spina bifida.
- Antibiotics according to local policy. Strict asepsis is vital to ↓ the incidence of infection.
- Minimal blood loss; invasive monitoring is not required.
- Additional analgesia (fentanyl) is often required during subcutaneous tunnelling.

Endoscopic third ventriculostomy

- A short catheter is inserted into the lateral ventricle through a burr hole. An endoscope is introduced via the catheter through the foramen of Munro into the third ventricle, which may be irrigated with warmed isotonic fluid.
- Ensure the patient is immobile, since the basilar artery lies just below the floor of the third ventricle.
- If bleeding occurs or the CSF is cloudy, large volumes of irrigation fluid may be used.

- Potential problems:
  - Cooling of irrigation fluid will result in a ↓in brain temperature; therefore, run the fluid through a blood-warming coil situated close to the patient's head
  - A low-pressure infuser device pumps fluid through the endoscope into the ventricles. The irrigation fluid escapes by flowing back up the ventricular catheter outside the scope. If the outflow of fluid is impeded, there is a rise in ICP and a Cushing's response. Management is withdrawal of the scope so that excess irrigation fluid may drain.

Craniotomy

Elective

- Most common indication is tumour resection.
  - CNS tumours are the second most common malignancy in children.
  - 40% of tumours are in the posterior fossa.
  - Astrocytomas are commonest, followed by medulloblastoma, then ependymoma.
  - Peak incidence is 1–8 years of age.
- Other indications include epilepsy and vascular lesions.

Emergency

- For control of acute ↑ ICP by removing:
  - Haematoma (extradural, subdural or intracerebral)
  - Contused brain
  - Abscess/empyema.

Perioperative management

Induction

- ⊃ 'General principles'.
- Blood checked and in theatre suite.
- Two large peripheral lines.
- Arterial line.
- CVP line essential in:
  - Babies and young children
  - Prone position
  - Expected large blood loss
  - Risk of diabetes insipidus (DI), e.g. suprasellar tumours
- Internal jugular lines may partially obstruct cranial venous outflow, creating raised venous pressure in the cerebral circulation, leading to an ↑ risk of bleeding and difficult surgical access. The femoral route is more comfortable for the child, but has increased risk of DVT.
- Urine catheter for long cases, especially if:
  - Mannitol has/may be given.
  - High UO anticipated postoperatively (craniopharyngioma).
  - Significant bleeding expected.
- NGT if bulbar dysfunction present or expected postoperatively.
- Orogastric tube where base of skull fracture is possible or if previous trans-sphenoidal surgery.
- Temperature probe: oesophageal or rectal.

Intraoperative

- The head is fixed in position using external pins. Insertion of pins causes a marked haemodynamic response, which must be anticipated and attenuated by an ↑ in the rate of remifentanil infusion.
- Pins are not used in infants <12 months, since they may penetrate the bony table.
- The sitting position is rarely used because of concern regarding venous air embolism. However, it does have many advantages, e.g. better anatomical orientation, less bleeding, lower ICP, and lower incidence of

postoperative cranial nerve damage. Postural hypotension is rare, but patients should still be moved gradually to the full sitting position over a few minutes.

- Consider dexamethasone for reduction of brain swelling. Patients may be receiving regular dexamethasone; if so, continue and/or give a supplementary dose. Consult with surgeon.
- Antibiotics as per hospital protocol.
- Vigilance required when the proposed bone flap is close to a venous sinus. Occasionally the sinus is partially de-roofed as the bone is lifted, leading to rapid haemorrhage. In neonates and infants, consider having blood checked and run through drip before bone flap is turned. Sinus bleeding is difficult to control, since it cannot be clipped like a normal vessel.
- Hypertension and sudden changes in HR may result from direct surgical stimulation of cardiovascular centres in the brainstem. Resist the temptation to treat a bradycardia with atropine or glycopyrronium bromide. Inform the surgeon of haemodynamic changes. Acute cardiovascular changes are a useful monitor of brainstem wellbeing.
- Haemorrhage is difficult to assess accurately, since:
  - CSF is constantly produced and aspirated.
  - Surface of brain is repeatedly flushed with saline to prevent drying.
  - It is impossible to weigh small neuro swabs.
- Transfusion is guided by clinical assessment, UO, serial measurements of haematocrit and ABGs.
- Children <10 kg usually require a blood transfusion.
- Cell saver is usually contraindicated for trauma or tumour cases.
- Use isotonic fluids, e.g. Hartmann's or Plasma-Lyte. Avoid glucose-containing fluids, since hyperglycaemia is associated with worse neurological outcome.
- However, neonates and children with a history of prolonged vomiting are more prone to hypoglycaemia; close monitoring of blood glucose guides administration of glucose solutions.
- A degree of fluid restriction (50% of normal maintenance) is usual to avoid cerebral oedema in craniotomy for trauma. Despite this concern, the priority is to maintain adequate circulating blood volume for cerebral perfusion. Inotropes may be required.
- Mannitol (0.5 mg/kg) may be given if the brain is particularly tight. Some surgeons routinely request mannitol.
- Patients with suprasellar tumours may have additional hormonal influences on fluid handling during surgery. It is unusual to see DI intraoperatively—it generally occurs 12–18 h postoperatively.

At end of surgery

- The aim is to wake all patients even if GCS is predicted to be suboptimal. Close neurological observation following small fluctuations in GCS will give more useful clinical information than keeping the patient intubated. Repeated CT scans cannot assess function.
- Possible reasons to keep patients intubated and ventilated:
  - Major trauma and associated bone injury, which will require significant analgesia
  - Major blood transfusion

- Significant preoperative neurological insult, i.e. pupils dilated for a length of time
- Aspiration
- Unstable cardiovascularly/brainstem intraoperatively.
- Discuss with surgeon and organize transfer to PICU.

Postoperatively
- Regular neurological assessment by experienced neurosurgical nurses in HDU or PICU.
- CVP line left in for the first 24 h for blood sampling/CVP monitoring and/or infusions of anticonvulsants if seizure activity becomes a problem.
- Postoperative analgesia: Consider NCA/PCA. Posterior fossa procedures are painful and require IV analgesia for at least 24 h.
- Vomiting is often related to site and extent of surgery rather than GA. Support with regular antiemetics, reassurance, and hydration.
- Cerebral oedema in response to brain handling starts at the time of surgery and reaches a peak 24–48 h postoperatively before subsiding. Patients may be less responsive on the first postoperative day. Improvement usually occurs after 48 h. If any doubt, rescan.
- Lower cranial nerves are also involved in postoperative swelling. Swallowing and sensation may be normal immediately postoperatively, but patients may have sudden onset of bulbar dysfunction up to 2 days later. Maintain close observation. Older children can be kept NBM and fed via NGT, but this may prove impossible in the very young.
- Suprasellar tumour excision may promote mishandling of water and electrolytes. Posterior pituitary function switches on and off episodically as a result of localized oedema and hypoperfusion. Keep an accurate fluid balance, send regular paired urine and serum for U+Es and osmolality, and be alert for SIADH and DI.
- Watch for new or altered seizure activity.

Intraoperative MRI

- Neuronavigation (based on a preoperative scan) is used routinely for accurate location of intracranial lesions.
- The navigation image becomes increasingly inaccurate as tissue is removed.
- Engineering and software developments have enabled intraoperative MRI scanning with automatic registration to be carried out at multiple points during surgery to give instantaneous updated images.
- The MRI scanner is located within the theatre or in a room immediately adjacent.

Benefits

- Complete resection of tumour is achievable in a single procedure with immediate confirmation of results before closure of the wound.
- Routine postoperative tumour resection MRI sequences may be done at the end of surgery, thereby avoiding the need for a further GA in a small child up to 48 h later.

Essential considerations

- MRI safety check lists must be completed at various stages, in addition to WHO checklists.
- Potentially long cases, with issues of fatigue in anaesthetists, theatre staff, and surgeons.
- Positioning:
  - The head-holding frame incorporates a solid receiver coil and the titanium pins; it is fixed to the operating table and has minimal potential for adjustment.
  - The patient must be manoeuvred carefully into position.
- Access to ETT in prone patients will be restricted by the lower plate of the inner coil.
- Tape pilot balloon of ETT cuff to the breathing circuit filter so that it does not distort the MR image
- Patient ear protection: apply ear defenders before skin preparation.
- Pressure-relieving measures needed.
- Monitoring:
  - Standard monitoring equipment may be used in theatre but must be changed to MRI-conditional for scanning.
- Infusion pumps: MRI-conditional pumps tend to be simple volumetric pumps without programmable infusion regimes.
- Prior to draping, ensure all metal has been removed from the operating table—scissors, laryngoscope and blades, razors, and Magill forceps will become lethal missiles within the magnet.
- Prior to transfer into the magnet, remove all attached metal, e.g. temperature probes, conventional ECG electrodes and monitoring wires, diathermy plates, charging leads for MRI-conditional pumps, blood warmers, BIS, and neurophysiological monitoring wires

- Safety:
  - There should be a further safety check list before moving the patient into the magnetic field.
  - If the magnet is in the operating theatre, there must be a safety protocol for all members of staff coming into theatre, i.e. removal of phones, bleeps, metal in pockets, etc.
- Transfer into scanner and scan may take up to an hour.

Epilepsy surgery

- Considered when epilepsy is drug-resistant or where high doses of anticonvulsants affect cognition and quality of life.
- Targeted resection of carefully identified lesion causing focal epilepsy, or disconnective surgery to prevent epileptiform activity spreading to both hemispheres.
- Preoperative assessment may include:
  - Videotelemetry to confirm that EEG abnormality coincides with observed seizure activity
  - Neuroimaging to accurately identify abnormal area
  - Neuropsychiatric assessment.

Treatment

- Temporal lesionectomy, corpus callosotomy (disconnection surgery), or hemispherectomy. Perioperative management is as for standard craniotomy.
- A two-stage surgical procedure is required if there is need for intraoperative cortical mapping by EEG to identify focus with greater accuracy and/or monitor motor function.

Perioperative management for two-stage surgery

- Clear seizure medication plan written in notes prior to first surgery. Anticonvulsant dose often reduced or omitted to encourage seizure data collection. Rescue medication plan should be documented.
- Avoid benzodiazepine premedication (may reduce seizure incidence).
- Set up as standard craniotomy
- TIVA required; avoid muscle relaxants.
- Depth electrodes (placed via burr hole) or grids are laid on the surface of the brain via craniotomy. May be bilateral.

Postoperatively

- Patient returns to ward for continuous EEG monitoring.
- Consider clonidine patch for analgesia (less sedation than NCA).
- IV antibiotics for duration of monitoring.
- Once seizure mapping has been achieved, patient is returned to theatre for second surgery to remove grids ± cortical resection. TIVA not needed for second procedure.

Arteriovenous malformation (AVM) embolization

- Age of child at presentation usually indicates the size of the AVM.
- Neonates and infants present with large malformations, which may precipitate high-output cardiac failure.
- Infants may have seizures or increasing head size from hydrocephalus.
- Older children present with neurological deficit from the effect of vascular steal.
- AVMs may rupture spontaneously, causing sudden loss of consciousness.
- Some lesions are associated with high mortality and morbidity, e.g. aneurysm of the vein of Galen.
- Interventional radiology and embolization is the treatment of choice.
- Emboli of various substances, e.g. coils, glue, or onyx, are positioned in one or more feeding arteries or vessels. Several sessions may be needed.
- Partial embolization of lesions may be useful before planned surgical excision to ↓ the risk of haemorrhage during surgery.
- Risks of the procedure include:
  - Intracerebral bleeding from rupture of the AVM
  - Bleeding from inadvertent puncture of vessels during manipulation of the intravascular catheters
  - Dislodging of the embolus, resulting in CVA or PA emboli.
- Procedures are technically demanding and may be prolonged.

Perioperative management

- Patient may be on maintenance aspirin or antiplatelet therapy, usually continued.
- Angiography suite often has limited space for anaesthetic equipment, subdued lighting, and a cool ambient temperature. It is not an ideal place for induction of infants and insertion of invasive monitoring. It may be preferable to anaesthetize small children in a safer location and then transport them to the angiography suite.
- Setup as for craniotomy.
- Blood checked and available in the theatre suite.
- ETT and IPPV.
- Limited patient access requires long extensions for IV access and ventilator tubing.
- Maintain normocapnia.
- Avoid hypotension.
- Avoid dehydration. Keep the patient warm, well-filled, and vasodilated to maintain maximum vessel patency to help with the passage of intravascular catheters.
- The procedure is usually performed via an angiography catheter inserted into a femoral vessel. Catheters are relatively large in small children.
- Repeated flushing of the angiography catheter may result in hypervolaemia, especially in infants

- There may be cardiovascular instability with hypertension and tachycardia as a result of dramatic alterations in blood flow within the malformation when key vessels are embolized. Inform the radiologist.
- Sudden hypertension may occur in response to an intracranial vessel perforation.
- IV contrast media is iodine-based and carries a small risk of allergic-like reactions. The recommended maximum dose of contrast media is 2–3 mL/kg. Newer contrast agents are iso-osmolar; however, there is a need for caution in patients with poor renal function.

Postoperative care
- Postoperative assessment is directed to detection of new neurological deficit.
- Maintain good hydration. Monitor fluid balance and electrolyte status resulting from flush and contrast media.
- Regularly observe femoral puncture site for bleeding, and assess perfusion of the leg.
- May require admission to PICU for a brief period of IPPV, especially if the child has hypothermia or has been transported between hospitals.

Posterior fossa decompression for Arnold–Chiari malformation

- Complex malformation, cause uncertain, defined by descent of the cerebellar tonsils below the level of the foramen magnum.
- The Arnold–Chiari type II lesion comprises a bony abnormality of the posterior fossa and upper cervical spine, with caudal displacement of the cerebellar vermis, fourth ventricle, and lower brainstem.
- Type II is associated with hydrocephalus and dysraphism/spina bifida.
- Medullary cervical cord compression may occur, with abnormal ventilatory responses to hypoxia and hypercarbia.
- Lower cranial nerves may become stretched, resulting in swallowing and upper airway reflex problems.

Treatment

- Directed towards increasing the space available for the compressed brainstem by removing the posterior rim of the foramen magnum and/ or the arch of the atlas. If bony decompression alone does not improve CSF flow, then the dura is also opened.

Perioperative management

- As for craniotomy.
- Postoperative management on HDU or PICU.
- Surgical decompression of the medulla and lower cranial nerves may result in acute postoperative swelling, leading to respiratory difficulties, stridor, or sudden loss of upper airway reflexes with risk of aspiration.

Baclofen pump insertion

- Motor spasticity arises from damage to the descending inhibitory control in the spinal cord and can be a major problem in cerebral palsy.
- Baclofen is an agonist at γ-aminobutyric acid (GABA) beta receptors and acts in the spinal cord to inhibit release of excitatory neurotransmitters. Used to ↓ muscle spasms and associated pain, and may delay the development of contractures.
- Oral baclofen improves spasticity, but clinical use is limited by systemic side effects, e.g. somnolence, confusion, ataxia, and urinary frequency.
- Intrathecal baclofen is effective at lower doses and has fewer side effects, and may significantly improve quality of life.
- Initial trial is performed to assess patient response. A thorough examination takes place under GA to assess the maximum achievable range of movement. A subarachnoid catheter is inserted and intrathecal baclofen administered as a bolus or infusion for 48–72 h.
- HDU care required.
- If the trial is effective in reducing dystonia and/or spasticity, a long-term pump is inserted.

Perioperative management

- Complex patients with multiple comorbidities.
- Elective procedure; therefore, patient must be as well as possible
- Endeavour to continue normal doses of baclofen intraoperatively via a PEG or NG tube. Omission of one dose may lead to a spastic crisis. Important to maintain normal PO baclofen doses following pump insertion, since the intrathecal baclofen may take 48 h to be effective.
- Lateral position. Most patients have severe cerebral palsy and require meticulous care, with padding of pressure points, positioning of contractures, and attention to temperature maintenance.
- A catheter is inserted percutaneously via a Tuohy needle into the subarachnoid space.
- An indwelling pump and drug reservoir system are placed in the lateral abdominal wall and connected to the catheter by subcutaneous tunnelling.
- The catheter and pump are primed according to local policy.

Postoperative care

- HDU indicated. Overdose of baclofen can present suddenly or insidiously and may be manifest as rostral progression of hypotonia, drowsiness, respiratory depression, or loss of consciousness.
- A ↓ in spasticity is usually noted within 24–48 h after starting the infusion.
- Abrupt withdrawal from PO or intrathecal baclofen may result in seizures, hallucinations, disorientation, dyskinesias, and itching, with symptoms lasting up to 72 h.
- The main complications are infection and catheter problems, e.g. disconnections or fracture.
- Pump malfunction is a risk. Subsequent MRI scanning may cause the pump motor to stall; therefore, patients must be closely monitored post scan.
- When the pump needs refilling, baclofen is instilled into the reservoir percutaneously. The system has external programming.

Selective dorsal rhizotomy (SDR)

- Lower limb spasticity is a common feature of cerebral palsy. SDR
  involves sectioning some of the lumbar sensory spinal cord nerve fibres
  that originate in the muscle and are responsible for increased muscle
  tone via the sensory–motor reflex arc.
- Intraoperative neurophysiological monitoring is used to identify the
  relevant sensory nerve rootlets, which are then divided.
- Physiotherapy is needed for months after the procedure in order to
  retrain muscle groups.

Perioperative management

- Ensure PO baclofen doses continued perioperatively.
- Gabapentin may be given the night before and for 3 months
  postoperatively.
- Physiotherapist assessment of range of movement once anaesthetized.
- Patient positioned prone as for laminectomy.
- TIVA; avoid volatile agents and muscle relaxants to allow use of
  neurophysiological monitoring.
- Consider Mg^{2+} infusion.
- Intraoperative IV morphine. Postoperative PO morphine, NCA if
  needed.

Untethering of spinal cord

- ETT and IPPV.
- Prone position.
- Continuous EMG monitoring with direct stimulation of lower sacral
  nerves; therefore, no need to avoid volatile agents and muscle relaxants.
- IV paracetamol.
- Consider LA infiltration.
- PO morphine postoperatively.
- More complex dysraphisms may require use of evoked potentials;
  therefore, use TIVA to avoid volatile agents and muscle relaxants.

Head injury: initial resuscitation and management

- Anaesthetists are involved in:
  - Resuscitation
  - Intra-hospital transfer, e.g. to CT
  - Inter-hospital transfer
  - GA for surgery
  - ICU.
- Head injury is the commonest cause of trauma death between 1 and 15 years of age.
- The commonest cause is road traffic accidents, followed by falls.
- In infancy, the commonest cause is non-accidental injury (NAI).
- Damage to the brain is caused by primary or secondary effects of the injury.
  - Primary damage includes:
    —Cerebral lacerations and contusions
    —Intracerebral haematoma
    —Dural tears
    —Diffuse axonal injury.
  - Secondary damage (consequences of the initial injury):
    —Ischaemia caused by inadequate cerebral perfusion as a result of ↑ ICP and/or hypovolaemia
    —Hyper/hypoperfusion due to impaired cerebrovascular autoregulation
    —Hypoxia due to airway obstruction or chest injuries
    —Hypoxia from hypoventilation caused by damage to the respiratory centre and loss of respiratory drive.
    —Cerebral oedema
    —Hypoglycaemia and loss of metabolic homeostasis, leading to cellular breakdown in cerebral tissues.
    —↑ cerebral metabolic rate, e.g. convulsions or fever.

Primary survey

- As per APLS or ATLS guidelines:
  - Airway with cervical spine control.
  - Breathing.
  - Circulation assessment and intervention if necessary.
  - Disability: examine pupils and assess level of consciousness (LOC).
  - The AVPU scale is a good rapid assessment tool in younger children:
    —A: Alert to voice
    —V: responds to Voice
    —P: responds to Pain
    —U: Unresponsive.

Secondary survey

- Examine the head for bruises, lacerations and skull fractures. Signs of a basal skull fracture: CSF leak from ears or nose, haemotympanum, 'panda eyes', or bruising behind the ears
- Conscious level is assessed using the GCS (Table 21.1). or the Children's Coma Scale if < 4 years (Table 21.2). A 'snapshot' assessment is obtained and repeated regularly to detect a trend.

Table 21.1 Glasgow Coma Scale (4–15 years)

Eye opening	
Spontaneously	4
To verbal stimuli	3
To pain	2
No response to pain	1
Best motor response	
Obeys verbal command	6
Localizes to pain	5
Withdraws from pain	4
Abnormal flexion to pain (decorticate)	3
Abnormal extension to pain (decerebrate)	2
No response to pain	1
Best verbal response	
Orientated and converses	5
Disorientated and converses	4
Inappropriate words	3
Incomprehensible sounds	2
No response to pain	1

- Examine fundi for papilloedema. Retinal haemorrhages are indicative of NAI, especially if there are other unexplained injuries.
- Limbs are examined for spontaneous movements, tone, and reflexes. Lateralizing signs may indicate the presence of an intracranial bleed.
- Care must be taken on transferring the patient from trolley to X-ray/ theatre table, since there may be associated spinal injuries. The patient must be log-rolled when necessary.

Investigations
- FBC, U+E, glucose, clotting screen, cross match, ABG.

Initial management
- Aim to prevent secondary brain damage.

Maintain ventilation and oxygenation
- If SV is inadequate, anaesthetize and intubate with manual in-line stabilization of the cervical spine. Induce with thiopental 2–5 mg/kg or propofol 2–4 mg/kg, and suxamethonium 1–2 mg/kg or rocuronium 1 mg/kg.
- IPPV mandatory. Capnography is essential and ABGs are checked to ensure low normocapnia (4.5–5.0 kPa).

Minimize ↑ ICP
- Ongoing sedation (midazolam 100 mcg/kg/h or propofol 100–300 mcg/kg/h) adjusted according to response.

Table 21.2 The Children's Glasgow Coma Scale (<4 years)

Eye opening	
Spontaneously	4
To verbal stimuli	3
To pain	2
No response	1
Best motor response	
Spontaneous or obeys verbal command	6
Localizes to pain or withdraws to touch	5
Withdraws from pain	4
Abnormal flexion to pain (decorticate)	3
Abnormal extension to pain (decerebrate)	2
No response to pain	1
Best verbal response	
Alert, babbles, coos, words to usual ability	5
Less than usual words, spontaneous irritable cry	4
Cries only to pain	3
Moans to pain	2
No response to pain	1

- Maintain paralysis.
- Analgesia, e.g. fentanyl.
- Positioned 20–30° head-up to improve venous drainage and ↓ ICP.
- Control generalized seizures, since they ↑ cerebral metabolic O_2 demand. The first-line therapy is benzodiazepines, e.g. diazepam 200–400 mcg/kg IV or lorazepam 100 mcg/kg IV (repeated if necessary). Persistent or prolonged seizures may require a phenytoin infusion (20 mg/kg over 30 min).
- If there are signs of ↑ ICP and there is a delay in definitive treatment, hyperventilate the patient to a $PaCO_2$ of 4.0 kPa, give mannitol 0.5–1 mg/kg IV, and consider furosemide up to 1 mg/kg IV (urinary catheter required).

Maintain circulation
- MAP to achieve an age-appropriate CPP (→ Chapter 1).
- An arterial line is useful, but must not delay treatment.
- Fluid resuscitation 20 ml/kg isotonic crystalloid or colloid repeated as required; avoid glucose-containing solutions.
- If normovolaemic, consider a vasopressor, e.g. noradrenaline (norepinephrine) 0.01–0.5 mcg/kg/min.

Imaging
- CT scanning is an essential baseline.
- Skull X-rays provide limited information; severe intracranial trauma may be present in the absence of a fracture.

Neurosurgical referral essential if:
- Deteriorating LOC
- Focal neurological signs
- Depressed skull fracture
- Penetrating head injury
- Basal skull fracture
- Coma score of <12/15.

Surgical options
- Include evacuation of an intracranial haematoma, insertion of a ventricular drain, or insertion of a bolt to measure ICP.
- Paediatric neurosurgery services are based in tertiary paediatric centres and an inter-hospital transfer is often required (➜ Chapter 28).

Myelomeningocele

- Secondary to a failure of fusion of the embryonic neural tube during the fourth week of gestation.
- Myelomeningocele refers to a lesion containing neural tissue.
- Meningocele contains CSF without neural tissue.
- Usually diagnosed antenatally by US. 75% of lesions occur in the lumbo-sacral region.
- Associated with varying degrees of neurological dysfunction below the level of the lesion.
- There may not be a covering of skin.
- Associated with an Arnold–Chiari type II lesion.
- High risk of infection: ideally defect should be closed within 24 h.
- Hydrocephalus will develop in 70–85% of neonates with myelomeningocele; therefore, they must be closely monitored for several weeks after the primary repair.

Perioperative management

- Nurse prone.
- Lesion is covered with an occlusive dressing to stop tissues drying out.
- Extensive defects often require a joint neurosurgical and plastic surgery team.
- Level and extent of the lesion affect duration of surgery and potential blood loss.

Induction

- The baby may need to be supported on a cushion or jelly ring to avoid pressure on the lesion. Lateral or semilateral may be the only option, depending on the exact anatomy.
- Position prone for surgery. Small rolls are placed under the shoulders and pelvis to allow free abdominal movement during ventilation.
- Surgeon may wish to stimulate nerves during the procedure. Discuss this before giving a long-acting neuromuscular blocker.
- Sensory level is usually unclear at this point, so analgesic requirements are variable. Administer IV paracetamol ± small increments of fentanyl (be guided by clinical response).
- Care is required during LA infiltration owing to potential for direct transmission into the CSF.
- If stable, extubate at the end of the procedure; however, tight closure of an extensive lesion may impair ventilation. A coexisting Chiari malformation may affect postoperative respiratory function; therefore, monitor postoperatively on an HDU.

Orthopaedic surgery

Naveen Raj

Operations on the hip and proximal femur

Conditions requiring orthopaedic intervention

Developmental dysplasia of the hip (DDH)

- Previously known as congenital dislocation of the hip. A spectrum of defects due to laxity of the hip capsule resulting in hip joint instability, ranging from mild dysplasia of the acetabulum to complete dislocation (may be irreducible).
- Incidence 1:1,000 or more.
- Common on left side; 20% bilateral. 3F:1M.
- Aetiology unclear. Commoner in Europeans, firstborn child, birth weight >5 kg, breech and footling positioning, twins, and oligohydramnios.
- Higher incidence in children with torticollis, foot metatarsus adductus, and calcaneovalgus.
- DDH is a dynamic disorder evolving over time: either spontaneously reducing with normalization of the hip or worsening with persistent dislocation and development of irreversible changes.
- Pathophysiology is thought to be due to changes occurring in the hip joint, in structures that have developed normally during fetal life, resulting in the femoral head sliding in and out of a shallow acetabulum associated with increased capsular laxity and abnormal labrum. If the normal relationship of the femoral head and acetabulum are not maintained, then the joint will not develop normally, and further changes in the soft tissues will worsen acetabular dysplasia, resulting in persistent dislocation.
- Clinical presentation and diagnosis depend on age. Early detection and hip reduction improves outcome. From birth to 3 months of age, it can be detected during routine clinical examination with positive Ortolani (reduce a dislocated femoral head) and Barlow (dislocate an articulated femoral head) hip stability tests. After 3 months of age, the dislocated hip may not be reducible and the Ortolani and Barlow tests may not be useful. A limited hip abduction when flexed to 90° and a positive Galeazzi sign (limb length inequality when both hip and knee are flexed to 90°) aids diagnosis. In cases of unilateral hip defects, asymmetric skin crease, shorter limb, and limited abduction in flexion on the effected side may be seen. Those of walking age will demonstrate a positive Trendelenburg gait and limited abduction in a fully flexed hip.
- Radiological investigations: US is useful up to 4 months of age, since the hip is cartilaginous; beyond this, X-ray will be required. If adequate information is not obtained, an arthrogram under GA is required.
- Treatment. If evidence of dysplasia but hips are stable, observation is recommended for 6 weeks. Treatment depends on age, the earlier the

treatment is initiated the better, since acetabular remodelling occurs during the first 3–6 months:

- 0–6 months:
  —If the hip is dislocated but reducible, then use a Pavlik harness to maintain joint in 100° flexion and considerable abduction. US examination. If after 2 weeks the hip is stable, continue harness for 6 weeks, then replace by part-time splinting until radiological evidence of stability
  —If there is a suspicion of instability, examine the hip under GA with arthrogram. Perform a closed reduction and apply a hip spica for 12 weeks, followed by part-time splinting. After 6 weeks, the spica may need to be changed to adjust for growth-associated changes.
  —If disability persists, pelvic osteotomy is required
- 6–18 months:
  —EUA performed to assess reducibility and stability. If closed reduction is feasible, then a hip spica is applied as described above. An adductor tenotomy and or psoas tenotomy is performed to aid reduction.
  —If the hip is irreducible or unstable, then open reduction should be performed before application of a spica and splinting.
  —If disability persists, pelvic osteotomy is required.
- 18 months to 3 years:
  —Open reduction followed by hip spica application should be attempted, with a need for pelvic and femoral osteotomies to correct deformities becoming common.
- >3 years:
  —There is no consensus about the upper age limit for surgical correction or the technique to be used.

Teratologic hip dislocation

- Fixed rigid dislocation due to abnormal development in utero.
- Associated with congenital anomalies and neuromuscular disorders: myelomeningocele, arthrogryposis, lumbosacral agenesis, diastrophic dwarfism, chromosome abnormalities.
- Hip is usually irreducible and different from those seen in DDH.
- Requires surgical correction, which includes anterior open reduction, and pelvic and femoral osteotomy.

Perthes' disease

- Disruption of femoral head blood supply. Unknown aetiology leads to avascular necrosis followed by revascularization, resorption, repair, and remodelling. Affects varying parts of the femoral head, with anterior parts being most commonly effected.
- 4M:1F.
- Usually 4–8 years of age.
- Bilateral 15%.
- Presents with painless limp.
- Association with ADHD, trisomy 21, and skeletal dysplasia.
- X-ray confirms diagnosis, monitors progress, assists in grading severity, and helps planning treatment.

- Treatment and prognosis depend on age at onset, stage of disease at presentation, and extent of femoral head deformity.
- There is a choice of non-surgical and surgical means of containing femoral head within acetabulum during disease process to maintain the spherical shape of the head:
  - In patients <5 years old, aim to provide adequate analgesia and maintain full range of joint movement. Abduction plasters (broomstick) applied if severe symptoms. May require EUA, arthrogram, and adductor tenotomy before application of hip cast (optimally abducted for femoral head containment)
  - Those >5 years old in whom there is >50% of epiphysis involved require femoral varus osteotomy and/or Salter's innominate osteotomy followed by hip spica.
  - In older children, salvage procedures including Chiari osteotomy or shelf acetabuloplasty (especially those with severe defects) are required.

Slipped upper femoral epiphysis (SUFE)

- Displacement of the femoral epiphysis on the metaphysis because of an increased shear force or a weak physis. The femoral head remains in the acetabulum, whilst the neck slips forward and outwards.
- Incidence 2:100,000.
- M>F, usually 12–15 years of age (slightly younger in females).
- Commoner on left side; bilateral in up to 50%.
- Obesity a risk factor.
- Classification:
  - Idiopathic or atypical:
    —Age–weight test assists in differentiating idiopathic from atypical, with patients <10 years or >16 years and weight >50 centile showing increased occurrence of atypical SUFE.
    —Atypical is associated with endocrine disorders, trisomy 21, and renal failure.
  - Weight-bearing: stable if able to mobilize and bear weight, and unstable if painful and unable to mobilize.
  - Onset: pre-slip (symptoms with no evidence of slip), acute (symptoms of sudden onset <3 weeks duration), chronic (>3 weeks duration of symptoms), and acute on chronic (symptoms >3 weeks with a sudden ↑ in pain and disability).
  - Direction of displacement: varus (posteromedial) is common, but valgus (posterolateral) occurs in 5%.
  - Radiological: Wilson grades 1–3, depending on the displacement of the physis as a proportion of the neck from less than one-third (mild) to more than two-thirds (severe).
    —Confirmed by classical history, presentation, and pelvic X-ray.
    —Increased incidence of avascular necrosis in unstable hip. Reduction by forced manipulation is associated with increased risk of avascular necrosis.
- Surgery:
  - Stable slip: pinning in situ (PIS). A cannulated screw is inserted across the growth plate under fluoroscopy through a small longitudinal

incision at the level of the head of the femur. In severe slip, proximal femoral osteotomy may be necessary
- Unstable: risk of avascular necrosis is high and currently there is no consensus on management, which varies from PIS with >1 cannulated screw combined with aspiration of the hip joint to an open reduction. Treatment within 24 h of diagnosis reduces risk of avascular necrosis
- Contralateral hip: no consensus on fixing contralateral hip in idiopathic SUFE, but this may be of benefit in atypical presentation.
- Delayed presentation or failed PIS: a corrective intertrochanteric osteotomy or hip arthroplasty may be indicated

Surgical procedures

Adductor tenotomy and psoas release
- Percutaneous or open tenotomy.
- In open tenotomy, a 3–4 cm transverse incision is made just distal to the groin crease, adductor longus, and pectineus tendons, and the gracilis is transected.

Open reduction of hip
- Indication: failed closed reduction.
- Medial approach —if <1 year old. A longitudinal incision is made parallel to the adductor longus 1 cm distal to the groin crease. An adductor tenotomy and psoas release is performed, the hip capsule opened, and the ligamentum teres removed.
- Anterior approach (Salter's osteotomy)—if >1 year old. A bikini-line incision is made, with dissection to expose the capsule, which is opened with a T-shaped incision. The ligamentum teres is removed, the joint reduced, and capsulorrhaphy performed as required.
- Finally a hip spica is applied.

Pelvic osteotomy
- Aim is to improve femoral head coverage, encouraging acetabular development, and to stabilize and minimize progressive degeneration of the hip joint.
- Classification:
  - Re-directional
    —Salter's innominate osteotomy. A bikini line incision is made 1–2 cm below the iliac crest, extending from the middle part of the iliac crest to the middle of the groin fold. The acetabulum is rotated anterolaterally and ilium bone grafts taken to hold the displacement in position; it is then fixed with K-wire. Normally performed when hip joint is congruent.
  - Reshaping osteotomies or acetabuloplasty:
    —Incomplete osteotomies that alter the volume and shape of acetabulum to achieve a congruent joint; require a reduced hip.
    —Pemberton acetabuloplasty—useful with anterolateral acetabular defects. The osteotomy is curvilinear, beginning between the anterior iliac spines and passing backwards and downwards to end above the posterior branch of the triradiate cartilage; an ilium bone graft is used to keep it open and tip the acetabulum.

- Salvage procedures:
  —Used in older children to improve femoral head coverage where this is inadequate or reduction is impossible.
  —Chiari osteotomy is a medial displacement osteotomy that improves posterior and lateral coverage. Performed through an oblique incision extending from a point 2 cm medial and below the ASIS to the junction of middle and posterior third of the crest. A shelf is created over the dysplastic hip.

Proximal femoral osteotomy (PFO)

- Aim is to maintain hip joint congruency and thus prevent long-term changes.
- Indications:
  - Dislocation or subluxation of hip in children with neuromuscular disability
  - Legg–Calvé–Perthes disease
  - DDH
  - Slipped upper capital femoral epiphysis.
- Types:
  - Intertrochanteric: varus, valgus, flexion or extension
  - Greater trochanter osteotomies: simple or double with femoral neck lengthening.
- Technique:
  - Patient supine; dynamic examination of hip under fluoroscopy ± arthrogram.
  - A lateral longitudinal incision is made from the tip of the greater trochanter extending into the proximal thigh parallel to the femoral shaft.
  - Soft tissue dissection, retraction, and periosteal elevation to expose proximal femur are performed.
  - A Steinman pin is inserted into the femoral neck to aid osteotomy and fixation.
  - A blade plate chisel is hammered into the femoral neck.
  - Osteotomy is performed and distal femur rotated as required.
  - A blade plate is inserted and fixed to the femoral shaft.

Preoperative assessment

- Patients range from infant to adolescent, and from ASA 1 to ASA 3. with significant neurodisability and associated comorbidities.
- Very difficult to assess respiratory and cardiac reserves in severely affected neurodisability patients. Enquire after ability to lie supine: if unable to do so, they may have marked VQ mismatch. How have they behaved during recent GA?
- Careful examination and documentation of neuromuscular signs must be undertaken, especially if nerve blocks are planned. Assess spine for scoliosis, since this will make a successful epidural less likely.
- Patients often have chronic hip pain. Explain to patient and family the proposed analgesia plan, including a Plan B. Discuss primary and rescue block, e.g. a lumbar plexus block for unilateral surgery if epidural impossible. Performing blocks may be challenging in patients with fixed

joint contractures and scoliosis, owing either to difficulties in positioning or to inability to feel landmarks or needle.
- Plan for postoperative care, including analgesic technique and where recovery will occur.
- Most recover well and return to a general ward, but an HDU bed may be required for those with significantly reduced cardiopulmonary reserve or requiring close monitoring.
- Consider preoperative chest physiotherapy to optimize pulmonary function and possible continuation postoperatively.
- Need plan to continue essential routine medications, e.g. antiepileptics perioperatively—may need to liaise with the medical team. If PEG fed, this is usually not a problem.
- Routine investigations, including FBC and ferritin, clotting, U+E, and CXR, must be reviewed. If iron-deficient, prescribe PO iron for 6–8 weeks before surgery.
- Blood products may need to be ordered, depending on local policies and planned procedure. For combined pelvic and femoral osteotomies, salvage procedures, or bilateral hip surgeries, cross-match blood and arrange cell saver and appropriate personnel.

Anaesthesia
- Most children require GA. Regional or local anaesthetic block with sedation is a safe alternative but is not common practice.
- If the patient is on baclofen and the surgery of such a length that a dose will be missed, ensure a double dose is given prior to coming to theatre.
- Induction as preferred. Note that IV access may be difficult owing to postural defects and if there is a history of prematurity.
- Usually ETT and IPPV. SV acceptable for short cases.
- Increased risk of aspiration in neuromuscular disability, warranting a RSI. ETT is often preferred with long-duration cases, and always if patient is prone or has reduced pulmonary reserve.
- Note the application of hip spica at the end of surgery may need the patient prone, necessitating intubation and control of ventilation.
- LMA can be used even in prolonged cases in older ASA 1 patients. Often the hardened Spica cast prevents compression of abdomen when prone, thereby maintaining adequate respiratory effort.
- Large-bore IV access in upper limbs—if access is difficult, use US to locate veins in upper arm or insert an internal jugular CVL.
- Monitoring:
  - Routine non-invasive monitoring.
  - Arterial line in those having redo or complex surgical procedures, which may be bilateral, and where bleeding is anticipated, or if there are severe comorbidities
  - Central venous line is indicated if inotropes are anticipated owing to significant comorbidity.
- Positioning may be difficult in those with significant scoliosis or contractures.
- Temperature: neurodisability patients are particularly at risk of hypothermia. Commence active measures before induction. Warm IV fluids and use forced air warming devices.

- Antibiotics given within an hour of commencement of surgery and repeated in prolonged cases.
- Maintenance as preferred. For severely neurodisabled patients, desflurane and remifentanil allow rapid emergence, but need to be managed carefully when used in conjunction with an epidural, owing to hypotensive effects.
- Tranexamic acid (as described for scoliosis surgery) in major hip surgery.
- Cell savers for combined bilateral femoral and pelvic osteotomies, salvage, and redo hip procedures.
- Monitor blood loss using ABGs.
- Analgesia:
  • Preoperative PO paracetamol and ibuprofen for minor hip surgery.
  • Moderate to major surgery: IV paracetamol ± PR diclofenac at end of surgery.
  • Magnesium 100 mg/kg.
  • Epidural:
    —Careful positioning, since bones are fragile in wheelchair-bound patients,
    —If scoliotic, US can assist by assessing degree of vertebral rotation.
    —Ideally insert at T11/12 (if spinal rods are present, use L4/5). Bolus 0.5 mL/kg of 0.25-0.5% levobupivacaine with 2 mcg/kg clonidine. The higher concentration helps diminish postoperative muscle spasms for major surgery.
    —Tunnel and glue catheter.
  • If insertion of epidural fails, a lumbar plexus block ± catheter is an alternative for unilateral surgery
  • Caudal is suitable for <2-year-olds having soft tissue releases.

Postoperative care

- Assessing pain and ensuring adequate analgesia can be challenging in young children and those with severe learning difficulties.
- Regular IV paracetamol and PO or PR NSAID. PRN PO morphine.
- Continued LA infusion. Epidural clonidine infusions may improve muscle spasms. Normally epidural is left in for 3 days for major surgery.
- If epidural is not providing adequate analgesia, start a ketamine infusion or a PCA/NCA for osteotomy patients.
- Muscle spasms are a problem. Ensure patient receives their baclofen and prescribe PRN (possibly regular) diazepam.
- Regular antiemetics may need to be prescribed.

Operations on the foot

Curly toes

- Congenital deformity commonly affecting the lateral three toes. Characterized by flexion varus deviation and lateral rotation of interphalangeal joints.
- May resolve spontaneously, but for fixed deformities that are uncomfortable, flexor tenotomy is performed with patient supine and an oblique incision on the plantar surface of the proximal phalanx of the involved toes.
- Metatarsal LA blocks or posterior tibial nerve block ± sural nerve block.

Hallux valgus

- Lateral deviation of great toe with a prominence of the first metatarsal head; can be primary (due to increased intra-metatarsal angle) and/or secondary (due to inappropriate footwear).
- Usually an adolescent female; can be bilateral.
- Increased incidence with CP, collagen storage disorders, and rheumatoid arthritis.
- Pain is main indication for surgery when conservative treatments fail. Corrective surgery involves dorsomedial incision over the surface of the bunion, excision of bony exostosis, osteotomy, tendon transfers, and soft tissue repair to correct the great toe valgus and metatarsal varus deformities. A below-knee POP cast is used to immobilize the foot.
- LA technique: superficial and deep peroneal nerve, and posterior tibial nerve blocks.

Overriding of fifth toe

- Familial deformity of the fifth metatarso-phalangeal joint resulting in the toe being extended, rotated and adducted to lie over the fourth toe. Usually bilateral.
- Surgery: Butler procedure, which involves racquet incision on both plantar and dorsal surfaces of the affected toe, division of the extensor tendon, and widening of the capsule to free the toe.
- LA technique: sural, superficial peroneal and posterior nerve block.

Club foot: congenital talipes equinovarus (CTEV)

- Commonly a congenital abnormality involving the lower leg and foot, with equinus and varus position of the rear foot, and adduction and inversion of the forefoot.
- Incidence 1:1000, 2M:1F.
- 50% are bilateral.
- Aetiology unclear.
- Classification:
  - Idiopathic
  - Neuromuscular: Charcot–Marie–Tooth, poliomyelitis, CP, and neural tube defects
  - Syndromic: arthrogryposis, myelodysplasia, amniotic band syndrome, Pierre Robin syndrome, diastrophic dwarfism

- Diagnosis by antenatal US or clinical examination. Severity graded using Dimeglio or Pirani classification; also aids monitoring and treatment.
- Mild defects respond to serial casting. Severe irreducible malformations require surgery.
- Associated with DDH; therefore US scan to exclude.
- Treatment:
  - Non-surgical:
    —Ponseti method of manipulation and serial above-knee POP casting used to sequentially correct cavus, abduction, varus, and equinus deformities.
    —Subsequently a foot abduction orthosis (Ponseti or Denis Browne braces) is worn 23 h a day for 3 months, and then when asleep for 2–4 years.
    —Decision for surgical intervention made at 3–4 months after commencement of treatment. Relapse treated with further serial casting or surgical interventions.
  - Surgery:
    —Achilles tendon lengthening by percutaneous tenotomy is required in 90% of cases to correct residual equinus deformity followed by a cast for 2 weeks before braces. May need to be repeated if relapses occur.
    —If conservative treatment fails or there is persistent residual deformity, surgery is tailored to individual cases. This is more common in severe deformity and cases associated with syndromes and neuromuscular conditions. Surgery is timed for the child to be able to walk and bear weight when the postoperative casts are removed and involves release of contractures with realignment of joints of the foot. Up to 2 years of age, soft tissue procedures suffice; beyond this age, additional bony osteotomies may be required.
    —Tibialis anterior tendon transfer to midfoot to correct adduction and supination deformity. Dorsal medial incision is made over the cuneiform bone, and the tendon is detached and mobilized. Lateral incision is made over the third cuneiform bone, and the tendon is passed through a hole drilled in the bone and fixed on the plantar aspect.
    —Posterior, medial, and lateral release for failure of conservative treatment or recurrence. Various incisions are made on foot and lower leg, and open Achilles tendon Z-plasty lengthening is performed. Ankle joint is released from posteromedial to posterolateral corners. On the medial side, the tendons of the posterior tibialis, flexor digitorum longus, and flexor hallucis longus are lengthened.
    —Triple arthrodesis if present >8 years of age.
    —Soft tissue release, tendon transfers, and distal tibial + midfoot + hindfoot osteotomies + external fixator (Ilizarov) in severe deformities presenting in older child or recurring deformities.

- Anaesthetic considerations:
  - Percutaneous Achilles tenotomy usually performed at 2–4 months of age.
  - Associated with prematurity.
  - Usually idiopathic, but can be associated with syndromes and systemic disorders.

Metatarsus adductus
- Adduction of the forefoot in relation to a normally aligned hindfoot of unknown aetiology, resulting in a bean-shaped foot, which can be a bilateral deformity. This can be associated with DDH and needs to be differentiated from CTEV.
- Can resolve spontaneously by 6 years of age or respond to serial POP casting and footwear.
- Surgery is indicated in cases of persistent deformity with pain and callus formation.
  - Longitudinal incision over the dorsal lateral surface and a closing wedge osteotomy of the cuboid to shorten the lateral column.
  - Longitudinal incision over the medial aspect of the foot and a medial cuneiform bone opening wedge osteotomy to lengthen the medial column is performed if the above procedure does not correct the deformity. The cuboid bone harvested from the lateral osteotomy is used as a wedge and a K-wire used for stabilization. A POP cast is applied after the procedure
- LA technique: saphenous nerve at level of adductor canal and popliteal sciatic nerve blocks, or ankle block.

Flat foot
- Congenital vertical talus (congenital flat foot).
  - Unknown aetiology. 50% associated with other congenital defects, e.g. spinal anomalies, neuromuscular disorders, malformations, or chromosomal defects. Results in rocker-bottom-shaped foot owing to vertical orientation of talus with dislocation of talonavicular joint and calcaneocuboid joints, abnormal displacement of peroneus longus and posterior tibial tendons, and shortening of Achilles tendon
  - Treatment is surgical, performed as an infant. Follows reverse Ponseti serial casting. Surgery includes Achilles tendon lengthening, posterior capsulotomy, dorsolateral extensor tendons lengthening, and reduction of calcaneocuboid joint on the lateral side and reduction and fixation of the navicular bone on the talus and reconstruction of calcaneonavicular ligament. A below-knee POP cast is applied after surgery
- Tarsal coalition
  —Abnormal bony, fibrous, or cartilaginous connection between bones of the foot; usually calcaneonavicular and talocalcaneal. Usually adolescents with pain and progressive flat foot with limited movements.
  —Surgery if conservative treatment (orthosis) fails. The coalition is resected with an appropriate dorsal medial or lateral incision, defect filled with soft tissue to prevent recurrence, and foot is

immobilized with POP cast. Surgery for talocalcaneal coalition is
more complicated and arthrodesis may be required
- Flexible flat foot
  - Increased ligamentous laxity resulting in a flattened medial arch
  combined with a tight Achilles tendon and gastrocnemius complex.
  - May be associated with Marfan, Ehlers–Danlos, or Down syndrome.
  - Surgery indicated in symptomatic older children. A lateral column
  lengthening calcaneal osteotomy is performed through an incision
  extending in an oblique and inferior direction from the dorsolateral
  aspect of the talonavicular joint to 2.5 cm inferior to the lateral
  malleolus (Ollier incision). The osteotomy is performed at the
  neck of the calcaneus, a bone graft is inserted to lengthen the bone
  and is fixed with a screw or plate, and the foot is immobilized in a
  cast. Achilles tendon lengthening ± gastrocnemius release may be
  required.
  - Medial column shortening with tightening of the posterior tibialis
  tendon and reduction in the talonavicular joint capsule ± medial
  cuneiform wedge closing osteotomy may be required (longitudinal
  incision on medial side extending from base of first metatarsal to tip
  of medial malleolus).

Pes cavus
- Abnormal elevation of longitudinal arch of foot, resulting in a
forefoot equinus deformity (simple) or associated with hindfoot varus
(cavovarus) or calcaneus (calcaneocavus) deformities.
- Classification:
  - Congenital: idiopathic; usually older children or adults.
  - Associated with neurodisability in more than two-thirds of cases.
  Cavovarus or calcaneocavus deformities are common as a result
  fo muscle imbalance and usually present at a younger age. Causes
  include Charcot–Marie–Tooth disease (hereditary sensory motor
  neurone disease), spinal dysraphism, benign spinal cord tumours,
  polio, degenerative disorders of central and peripheral nervous
  system, muscular dystrophy, and CP.
  - Trauma: after compartment syndrome and injury to sciatic nerve.
  - Associated with residual deformity of CETV.
- Clinical presentation include pain limiting mobility, inflamed callouses
in pressure areas (first and fifth metatarsal heads), and inversion ankle
injuries.
- Conservative treatment with orthosis and footwear modifications,
exercise, and casting
- Surgery depends on severity of deformity present, and involves multiple
incisions of foot and lower leg:
  - Plantar fasciotomy: singularly may correct mild to moderate
  deformity. Performed through small incision on medial side of foot
  over the plantar fascia.
  - Achilles tendon lengthening.
  - Tendon transfers: anterior tibial, posterior tibial, and peroneus longus
  tendon transfers, and transfer of toe extensors to metatarsal heads.

- Osteotomies:
  —Metatarsal dorsal closing wedge osteotomy: commonly first metatarsal to dorsiflex the head, through a dorsal incision over first metatarsal bone.
  —Calcaneal osteotomy: includes valgus and lateral wedge osteotomies.
  —Midfoot wedge osteotomy proximal to the cavus deformity.
- Triple arthrodesis.

Anaesthetic considerations

- The principles for anaesthetic perioperative management are the same as for hip surgery. However, most can be done on LMA with SV, but an ETT may be necessary if patient is positioned prone or for other clinical reasons.
- Tourniquet is routine, bleeding is not a concern, and therefore arterial line and tranexamic acid are generally not required.
- Type of LA blocks depends on the procedure. A single-shot sciatic nerve block in the popliteal region and a saphenous nerve block at the level of the adductor canal provide good pain relief for most procedures. Indwelling catheters are required for extensive surgery, redo procedures, chronic pain in foot, where muscle spasms are problematic, and where intensive physiotherapy is required postoperatively.

Leg length discrepancy (LLD)

- Due to either hemiatrophy or hemihypertrophy.
- Presentation: limp, scoliosis, low back ache, arthritis, and plantar fasciitis.
- Classified as functional or anatomical.
- Causes include congenital (femoral, fibular, or tibial deficiency, DDH) or secondary to trauma, infection (osteomyelitis, septic arthritis), inflammation, neuromuscular (CP, neural tube defects), or tumours (osteochondroma, Wilms').
- Treatment required if >2 cm LLD.
- Surgical options include:
  - Epiphysiodesis: interruption of growth in longer leg.
    —Permanent: percutaneous drilling resulting in permanent physeal growth arrest or removal of block of bone with physis plate.
    —Reversible: eight plates or staples, on removal of which physeal growth resumes.
  - Altering leg length: usually patients will have achieved skeletal maturity.
    —Altering length of femur is more common than tibia. Femoral osteotomy is usually performed just distal to lesser trochanter; and in the case of the tibia is usually performed just distal to tibial tuberosity between tibial metaphysis and diaphysis.
    —Osteotomies with external fixators (e.g. Ilizarov frame) are commonly used with intramedullary nail.
- Ilizarov frame is used for LLD and correction of angular deformity. It involves:
  - Percutaneously inserted trans-osseous wires and pins either side of fracture or osteotomy site
  - Fixation to an external circular fixator frame to achieve stability, using principle of distraction osteogenesis.
- Compartment syndrome is a risk. Avoid high-concentration LA since this may mask symptoms.

Preoperative assessment

- Focus on associated medical conditions.
- Eight-plate insertion is usually a day case.
- Patients may have undergone previous GA before and be very anxious; may require premedication.
- With Ilizarov frame, avoid NSAID owing to small risk of delayed bone healing (not confirmed).

Anaesthesia

- Induction as preferred.

Eight-plate insertion

- LMA and SV commonly used.
- Maintenance as preferred.

- Analgesia:
  - Preoperative or intraoperative paracetamol and NSAID.
  - Femoral and sciatic nerve blocks (preferred, since this is a very painful operation).
  - IV morphine and LA infiltration is an alternative.
  - Dexamethasone.

Ilizarov frame
- Often ETT and IPPV because of either comorbidities or prolonged duration of case.
- GA maintenance as preferred.
- Avoid muscle relaxants. Surgeons usually rely on muscle twitching secondary to motor nerve irritation during insertion of IO wires.
- Measure temperature and actively warm.
- IV maintenance fluids.
- Haemodynamic stability not a concern.
- Antibiotics as per local protocol.
- Analgesia (a major problem postoperatively):
  - Preoperative or intraoperative paracetamol
  - Sciatic and/or femoral nerve catheter (preferred for unilateral surgery) or epidural catheter with plain LA ± clonidine
  - PRN PO morphine
  - Dexamethasone
  - Consider magnesium.

Postoperative care
- PRN PO diazepam for muscle spasms.
- Regular IV paracetamol.
- Continue LA technique for 3 days. May need LA bolus prior to dressing changes or cleaning of pin sites.

Scoliosis surgery

- Scoliosis is defined as lateral curvature of spine >10° on an erect AP CXR. But clinically refers to a complex 3D spinal deformity including:
  - Increased lateral curvature
  - Rotation of vertebrae
  - Rib cage deformity.
- Classification:
  - Idiopathic: commonest (80%). Classified by age:
    —Infantile 0–3 years: <1% incidence, commoner in boys, more commonly left-sided, usually resolves spontaneously.
    —Juvenile 3–10 years: up to 20% incidence. Can progress to significant deformity and usually responds poorly to non-surgical treatment.
    —Adolescent >10 years: commonest type, predominantly girls. Curves may be thoracic, lumbar, thoracolumbar, or double-major curves, with right main thoracic curves being commonest type
  - Congenital (anomaly of vertebrae, increased risk of association with other congenital defects, including cardiac, renal, and VACTERL).
    —Failure of formation: hemivertebrae.
    —Failure of segmentation: vertebral bar.
  - Neuromuscular:
    —Neuropathy: upper motor neurone lesion, e.g. CP, or lower motor neurone lesion, e.g. polio, spinal muscular atrophy.
    —Myopathy: muscular dystrophy, arthrogryposis.
  - Miscellaneous:
    —Neurofibromatosis
    —Connective tissue disorders: Marfan syndrome
    —Trauma.
- Clinical implications depend on severity and location of curve at presentation, age and skeletal maturity of child, and associated comorbidities.
  - Severity of curvature assessed by measuring Cobb's angle—the angle between the intersecting lines drawn perpendicular to the top of the uppermost tilted vertebrae and the bottom of the lowermost tilted vertebra.
  - Curvatures <30° at skeletal maturity will remain stable and need no intervention, while curvatures >30° progress.
  - A double curve pattern involving thoracic and lumbar curves is more likely to progress than a single curve.
  - Curvature can result in reduced volume of chest cavity and restrict lung function:
    —<65° has no clinical effect.
    —>100° causes severe restriction of lung function with VQ mismatch, hypoxia, pulmonary hypertension leading to heart failure.
    —Surgery does not reverse lung dysfunction, but prevents further deterioration.
- Associated conditions:
  - May aggravate scoliotic effects on cardiorespiratory function.

- Idiopathic scoliosis is associated with asymptomatic mitral valve prolapse in up to 25% of otherwise-healthy cases.
- Management:
  - Curvatures < 5° need no intervention.
  - Curves between 25° and 40° require conservative treatment: brace.

Surgery
- Aim is to prevent progression of curvature, correct the deformity, and provide stability.
- Indications:
  - Idiopathic: skeletal immaturity and curve >45°, and adolescents with curve >50°.
  - Congenital: depends on underlying vertebral anomaly and effects on respiratory function.
  - Neuromuscular: depends on progress of underlying disease and effect of scoliosis on the already-compromised respiratory function. In DMD, if curvature >20°, surgery can be considered. Surgery may slow, but does not stop, decline in respiratory function; it aids posture and nursing care.

Adolescent idiopathic scoliosis
- Posterior instrumentation and fusion:
  - Commonest technique, used mainly for flexible thoracic curves.
  - Skin and supraspinous ligaments are incised and paraspinalis muscles retracted to expose the spine. The spinous processes and laminae are removed and facet joints destroyed. Pedicle screws or laminar hooks are inserted at multiple levels and Harrington rods fixed to these to distract and stabilize the spine. Bone graft is performed, then vancomycin powder is applied to site
- Anterior approach:
  - For major curves with reduced flexibility.
  - Retroperitoneal approach via thoracoabdominal flank incision to expose vertebral bodies and remove the intervertebral discs from the convex side. This improves flexibility and aids posterior instrumentation.
  - May need OLV in difficult cases.
- Combined anterior and posterior procedures are now commonly performed during the same admission.

Early-onset scoliosis
- Treatment options make allowance for normal development of thoracic cavity, lungs, and spine to ↓ risk of thoracic insufficiency syndrome.
- Posterior instrumentation and fusion impedes normal development and has been replaced by posterior insertion of spinal growing rods.
- Two rods are fixed by anchors placed either side of the curves, and serial distraction performed at regular intervals (6 months) to allow growth in the unfused spinal segments.

Neuromuscular scoliosis
- Treatment is influenced by underlying pathology: the main aim of limiting curve progression is to avoid cardiopulmonary deterioration. In

wheelchair-dependent children, it also improves posture, comfort, and nursing care.

Preoperative assessment

- Routine assessment with additional attention to cardiorespiratory function and optimization.
- ECHO and ECG:
  - Neuromuscular scoliosis patients may have reduced cardiac function and a higher risk of cardiomyopathy and rhythm abnormality.
  - Often their mobility is limited; a normal ECHO may be insufficient to predict perioperative cardiac complications
- Lung function test:
  - FVC <30% may predict need for postoperative IPPV.
  - Neuromuscular scoliosis patients may be unable to perform test.
- FBC, U+E. Anaemia: treat with iron and erythropoietin therapy.
- Cross-match.
- Review radiological investigations.
- Appropriate counselling is important. Risks vs benefits should be considered in children with significant comorbidities, especially neuromuscular diseases. Although perioperative outcomes have improved in children with significant reduction in lung function tests, a FVC <25% of predicted value and an ejection fraction <50% is considered a contraindication in children with progressive weakness, e.g. DMD.
- The anaesthetic plan, including pain management options, is explained in detail. Stress the importance of assessing lower limb movement at the end of surgery (as soon as patient is woken up before transfer from theatre) to confirm absence of neurological deficit.

Anaesthesia

- Premedication as preferred.
- Prepare all infusions before patient arrives in anaesthetic room.
- Induction as preferred.
- Volatile agents and neuromuscular blocking agents are avoided because of their effects on neurophysiological monitoring, but can be utilized at induction. TIVA with remifentanil is recommended.
- Various techniques of intubation without muscle relaxants are described with a combination of TCI induction dose of propofol and remifentanil bolus (1–2 mcg/kg) being common.
- Minimum of two large-bore IV cannulas sited in forearms for easy access.
- Arterial line (preferably radial).
- CVP line unnecessary for idiopathic spines, but indicated for difficult IV access, increased risk of bleeding, or need of inotropes (especially in non-idiopathic scoliosis).
- Urinary catheter.
- Hypothermia can affect spinal cord monitoring and coagulation. Start forced air warming in anaesthetic room; warm fluids intraoperatively.

- Technician sites electrodes for neurophysiological monitoring before positioning.
- Cefuroxime 50 mg/kg < 1 h before surgical incision and repeated every 3 h.

Maintenance
- TIVA with TCI propofol and a remifentanil infusion 0.05–0.25 mcg/kg/min. Guided by BIS monitoring, aim for BIS score <60.
- IV fluid is restricted until instrumentation. In idiopathic scoliosis, cell-salvaged blood is normally sufficient. The need for transfusion of allogeneic blood is higher with neuromuscular patients. Aim for haemoglobin >100 g/dL.

Positioning
- Prone for posterior instrumentation—may be difficult owing to fixed posture deformities.
- Procedure-specific frames and mattresses are used.
- Shoulders should not be abducted >90°; ensure adequate padding to minimize nerve injury.
- Check respiration is unrestricted.
- Check abdomen is free: if abdominal pressure is high, this elevates venous pressure and consequently increases risk of bleeding.
- Avoid pressure on eyes by using appropriate head rests. Loss of vision is thought to occur owing to ischemia of the optic nerve with prone position. Prolonged surgery, hypotension, and anaemia are risk factors.
- All monitoring is reinstated after turning prone.

Bleeding and coagulopathy
- Significant blood loss is common, the amount depending on duration of surgery, number of vertebrae fused, and presence of comorbidities.
- Blood conservation strategies to ↓ transfusion and their associated risks and costs include:
  - Avoid excessive IV fluid until instrumentation is complete.
  - Routine cell salvage.
  - Acute normovolaemic haemodilution to achieve target haemoglobin of 70 g/dL has been used to ↓ allogeneic blood transfusion.
  - Tranexamic acid (no consensus on dosing, higher doses associated with seizures) bolus 20 mg/kg followed by infusion 10–20 mg/kg/h intraoperatively.
  - Some surgeons infiltrate the tissues with dilute adrenaline (epinephrine) solution.
  - Controlled hypotension is a risk factor for spinal cord injury and should be avoided.
  - Anaemia is a risk factor for spinal cord injury.
- Remember to have a high suspicion of venous air embolism if there is a sudden loss of CO.

Risk of spinal cord injury
- Incidence 0.3–0.6%.
- Motor pathway is most commonly affected.
- Secondary to direct injury from instrumentation, or ischaemia from external pressure or disruption of radicular vessels.
- Intraoperative spinal cord monitoring is routine:
  - Somatosensory evoked potential (SSEP):
    —Stimulation of peripheral nerve (posterior tibial and or median nerve) and detection of spinal response from epidural electrodes or cortical response from scalp electrodes.
    —Tests ascending sensory pathways in dorsal column and not descending motor pathways in the anterior and lateral spinal tracts, which are most vulnerable.
    —Waveform is monitored: an ↑ >10% in latency or ↓ <50% amplitude is significant.
  - Motor evoked potential (MEP):
    —Stimulation of motor cortex with electrical impulse and detection of resulting signal at spinal level with epidural electrodes or generation of compound action potential from muscles.
  - SSEP and MEP are usually used in combination, being reliable and sensitive even in children with neuromuscular problems.
  - Both SSEP and MEP are affected by anaesthetic drugs:
    —Volatile anaesthetics and N_2O have a dose-dependent inhibitory effect on SSEP and MEP.
  - Complete neuromuscular blockade abolishes MEP.
  - IV drugs and opioids have no effect.
- Wake-up test:
  - Patient is woken in the middle of the operation and asked to obey simple commands (move feet or squeeze arm) to assess neurological pathway at that point in time.
  - Has largely been replaced by SSEP and MEP. If there are significant concerns raised by these tests, then a wake-up test may be used to confirm injury.
  - A gauze roll is placed between the teeth to prevent soft tissue injury and clamping down on the ETT (may compromise ventilation).
- If significant results are seen:
  - Surgery: remove instrumentation, ↓ distraction, abandon procedure.
  - Anaesthetic: normalize or ↑ BP, correct hypothermia, hypoxia or hyperCO$_2$, and anaemia.
  - Methylprednisolone 30 mg/kg followed by infusion 5.4 mg/kg/h if injury suspected.

Analgesia:
- Gabapentin may ↓ postoperative opioid requirements. Current practice in our institution (Alder Hey) is 10 mg/kg (maximum 300 mg per dose) the night before surgery. On morning of surgery, the same dose is given, with a second dose in the evening. This is continued 8-hourly for the next 3 days then stopped.
- IV paracetamol and PR diclofenac.

- Remifentanil at 0.05–0.25 mcg/kg/h.
  - Higher doses are not recommended, owing to risk of acute tolerance and opioid-induced hyperalgesia if used for prolonged periods, thereby resulting in higher pain scores postoperatively and increased opioid requirement
- Fentanyl 0.25–1 mcg/kg bolus at induction, then repeated every 2 h. May also ↓ hyperalgesic effects of remifentanil. Fentanyl infusion of 0.25–0.5 mcg/kg/h.
- Ketamine infusion:
  - Analgesic properties at sub-anaesthetic dose of 0.15–0.5 mg/kg, improving postoperative pain relief and reducing opioid consumption. May prevent hyperalgesia.
  - Followed by intraoperative infusion of 0.1–0.2 mg/kg/h.
- Magnesium infusion:
  - Shown to ↓ opioid consumption postoperatively. May prevent hyperalgesia.
  - Large doses may lead to hypotension and bradycardia, and potentiate the effect of sedatives and muscle relaxants.
  - Bolus and/or infusion described with huge variance in practice. Author's preference is 30 mg/kg bolus followed by 10 mg/kg/h until end of surgery
- Other described routes for opioids:
  - Intrathecal or caudal morphine has been shown to provide better postoperative analgesia when compared with systemic morphine. There is an increased risk of postoperative nausea and apnoea. If PCA is to be used, then a lower-dose demand bolus is used in the first 24 h, after which the bolus dose is increased to normal and a background infusion added.
- Epidural and PVB catheters sited surgically and LA infusion run postoperatively have been described. Response is variable owing to disrupted anatomy. Avoided in many institutions owing to fears of masking neurological signs.

Postoperative care

- Idiopathic cases cared for on designated wards with appropriate expertise.
- HDU or PICU for elective ventilation as warranted by comorbidities.
- Regular IV paracetamol and an NSAID.
- Gabapentin as discussed.
- PCA/NCA fentanyl +/- ketamine infusion if required.
- Laxatives as constipation a common problem.
- Early mobilisation encouraged (reduces complications).

Considerations in children with DMD/Becker muscular dystrophy

- Scoliosis develops as the child becomes wheelchair-dependent, usually by the end of the first decade of life. Increasing truncal muscle weakness and immobility and poor posture are thought to be causative; as these progress, positioning in the wheelchair and nursing become more difficult.

- Steroids are used to ↑ muscle strength and cardiorespiratory function, delay wheelchair need, and delay the onset, development, and progress of scoliosis.
- Conservative treatments, e.g. braces and orthoses, are usually ineffective and surgery is required in the majority. Surgery is indicated if curvature >20°; it is usually extensive, with fusion performed from T2 to the pelvis.
- The effect of changes in curvature and reduction in thoracic cavity with displacement and compression of intrathoracic organs, on top of pre-existing muscle weakness, can have a significant impact on pulmonary reserve. Note:
  - 6 weeks of preoperative physiotherapy and breathing exercises are needed to improve lung function and ↓ postoperative pulmonary deterioration.
  - Forced vital capacity <35% indicates a need for increased respiratory support postoperatively. If postoperative IPPV is necessary, non-invasive methods (CPAP and BiPAP) are often preferred.
- In addition, patients have significant cardiac impairment, with dilated cardiomyopathy (the commonest cause of death) common by adolescence and ECHO evidence of poor function present from an earlier age. Note:
  - Cardiology assessment should be performed (close to time of surgery) by a cardiologist with an interest in DMD. ECG may show ventricular hypertrophy from a young age. An ECHO with an ejection fraction <55% or a fractional shortening <28% indicate significant cardiac dysfunction. These changes may be late and not reflect a true picture of cardiac function—a dobutamine stress ECHO test or cardiac MRI may provide better evidence regarding cardiac reserve.
  - Children >10 years old may be on heart failure medications, e.g. ACE inhibitors and beta-blockers: a clear plan when to stop and restart these medications is required.
- Intraoperatively, these patients do not tolerate hypovolaemia and fluid overload. Effects of anaesthetic agents, positioning, blood loss, and procedure will add a significant stress to their compromised CO. Invasive monitoring is essential, oesophageal Doppler or TOE may prove useful to assess cardiac function. Have a low threshold for inotropes to maintain CO. Milrinone and/or dopamine are commonly used perioperatively.
- The risk of bleeding perioperatively is higher compared with idiopathic cases.
- For other significant anaesthetic considerations for DMD, ➲ Chapter 26.
- PICU postoperatively because of ↑ risk of complications and greater physiological dependency.
- Pain management is difficult, and routine postoperative measures for early mobilization or improving respiratory function may be impossible.

Forearm fractures

- Commonest non-elective orthopaedic case.
- 70% of fractures involve upper limb and 50% forearm and hand.
- Mostly independent children >5 years old; the result of falls during play or sport.
- Greenstick fractures commoner in younger children,
- Usually heal rapidly with active remodelling and little or no overgrowth. These factors allow conservative management with casting alone or manipulation under anaesthesia (MUA) followed by casting.
- Some require fixation with a percutaneous wire(s), while a minority require formal open reduction and plating.

Preoperative assessment

- Most deferred until fasted and listed on next trauma list. Usually treated as elective cases.
- In some cases, the child may be technically fasted but is pale and frightened. They may be in pain and have received opioid analgesia. Under these circumstances, the stomach is unlikely to have emptied and the child is regarded as a regurgitation risk.
- Some fractures require urgent surgery, irrespective of fasting status.
- Brachial plexus block rather than GA is poorly tolerated and not usually considered.

Anaesthesia

- Induction as preferred if fasted.
- RSI if regurgitation risk.
- For an MUA, an LMA with SV is suitable. For long cases or very young children ETT ± IPPV may be preferable—often depends on anaesthetist's experience.
- Laryngospasm may occur owing to surgical stimulation during manipulation of the fracture. Therefore, ensure an adequate depth of GA.
- All but MUAs require temperature monitoring, active warming, and IV fluids.
- Tourniquet used for open reduction and internal fixation, so blood loss minimal.
- Analgesia:
  - Preoperative or intraoperative paracetamol and NSAID.
  - Supraclavicular brachial plexus block with 0.125–0.25% levobupivacaine to minimize motor block and allow better neurological monitoring postoperatively.
  - If no block: IV morphine 50–100 mcg/kg ±IV ketamine 0.2–0.3 mg/kg plus LA infiltration to incision if an open reduction and internal fixation is performed.
  - Dexamethasone for PONV and analgesia

Postoperative care

- Regular PO paracetamol and NSAID.
- PRN PO morphine. PRN antiemetic.
- MUA can be discharged as day cases.

Supracondylar fracture

- Commonest elbow fracture; accounts for 75% of fractures in this area.
- Caused by trauma to elbow in hyperextension (95%) or hyperflexion (5%).
- Surgical options include closed reduction and casting, closed reduction and internal fixation with K-wires, or, commonly, open reduction and internal fixation.
- Significant incidence of neurological and vascular complications.
- Neurological injury is most commonly to the anterior interosseous branch of the median nerve, followed by radial and ulnar nerves. Usually neuropraxia, resolving spontaneously over 6–18 months; very rarely lacerated.
- Ischaemia distal to the fracture is relatively common, evidenced by weak radial pulse or slow capillary refill. Due to impingement of brachial artery on or between fragments of the fracture. Usually resolves with fracture reduction.
- Rarely, an arterial laceration occurs that requires exploration and repair.
- Risk of iatrogenic damage is uncommon. Commonest scenario is damage to ulnar nerve during percutaneous pinning of fracture. Usually resolves spontaneously. LA block is often discouraged since it prevents nerve assessment postoperatively. However, it could be avoided by identifying the nerve with US or PNS prior to pinning.

Preoperative assessment

- Urgent if there are concerns regarding neurological and vascular damage.
- Extremely painful and IV morphine is often administered in Emergency Department.
- Considerable force involved—exclude other injuries.
- Note any nerve damage.
- A regurgitation risk.

Anaesthetic technique

- RSI preferably IV.
- ETT and IPPV.
- Maintenance as preferred.
- Patient supine. Occasionally lateral position for a posterior approach to elbow.
- Tourniquet used and blood loss is usually minor.
- Require temperature monitoring, active warming, and IV fluids.
- Analgesia is not withheld because of compartment syndrome risk—consider pressure monitor:
  - Preoperative or intraoperative paracetamol and NSAID.
  - Supraclavicular nerve block: use 0.125–0.25% levobupivacaine. Use of regional nerve blockade is controversial owing to risk of compartment syndrome. There is no evidence that LA techniques delay diagnosis. Ischaemic pain does break through an LA block.
  - If LA block not performed: LA infiltration, IV morphine 50–150 mcg/kg IV, and ketamine IV 0.2–0.3 mg/kg.
- Extubate awake.

Postoperative care
- Regular PO paracetamol and NSAID.
- PRN PO morphine.
- IV fluids until drinking.
- Affected arm elevated in sling to help reduce swelling and allow observation of neurological function and vascular sufficiency distal to operation site.
- Breakthrough pain: consider compartment syndrome.

Femoral shaft fractures

- 1.6% of paediatric fractures. M2:1F.
- Bimodal distribution: 4–7-year-olds and adolescents.
- In young children, relatively weak bone may fracture with little force. In older children, when bone is mature, high velocity trauma is needed to fracture the femur. Resuscitation and treatment of other injuries takes priority over the femoral fracture.
- Age-dependent treatment:
  - <4 years old: traction or hip spica plaster cast.
  - Older children: traction, external fixation (compound fractures), intramedullary nailing or plating.
  - >10 years old: external fixation, intramedullary nailing or plating.
- Acute pain management at presentation and later to allow traction:
  - IV paracetamol
  - IV morphine; if no IV access, intranasal diamorphine.
  - Femoral nerve or fascia iliaca (single-shot or catheter)

Preoperative assessment

- Assess other injuries, volume status, fasting status, and analgesia administered.
- Usually surgery is planned for 1–2 days after injury. Fasted and treated as an elective case.
- Group and save blood.

Anaesthetic technique

- Induction as preferred.
- RSI if aspiration risk (even if technically fasted).
- LMA if treated electively.
- GA maintenance as preferred.
- Antibiotic cover if to be fixed.
- Require temperature monitoring, active warming, and IV fluids.
- Analgesia:
  - Preoperative or intraoperative paracetamol and NSAID.
  - SBYB, perform a femoral and lateral cutaneous nerve blocks
  - If no nerve block, then IV morphine (↓ dose if given recently)
  - ± IV ketamine 0.2–0.3 mg/kg.

Postoperative care

- Regular PO/IV paracetamol and PO/PR NSAID.
- PRN PO morphine if femoral nerve block.
- 24 h PCA/NCA if no femoral nerve block.
- IV fluids until oral intake established.

Septic arthritis

- Infection of a joint by pyogenic bacteria. Requires urgent surgery.
- Incidence 5–10:10,000.
- >50% are <2 years old.
- Hip, knee, shoulder, and elbow most commonly affected. Usually only one joint affected.
- Infection is usually haematogenous, but direct infection from trauma or surgery and local spread from infected tissues also occur.
- In infants the hip is most commonly affected, while in older children it is the knee.
- A febrile illness may precede symptoms and signs localized to the infected joint.
- Diagnosis may be difficult because of the subtle and non-specific presentation of a child who is generally unwell before localizing signs are identified. The child may appear septicaemic. Signs include abnormal posture, pain on passive movement, and a reduction in spontaneous movement of the joint.
- Differential diagnosis includes osteomyelitis, acute arthritis, post-traumatic joint effusion, Perthes' disease, and cellulitis.
- The commonest organisms are *Staphylococcus aureus, Staphylococcus epidermidis,* and *Streptococcus pyogenes.*
- Anaesthetic involvement may start with a request for IV access in a septic infant.
- Treatment requires rapid evacuation of the pus and antibiotics. Articular cartilage is particularly susceptible to the lytic effects of pus, and a delay in treatment may damage the joint and result in long-term deformity and disability.
- Joint aspiration may be performed, but in most cases, arthrotomy and generous irrigation of the joint are preferred. An arthroscope is usually used for the knee.

Preoperative assessment

- Older children may be systemically well, with symptoms and signs limited to the infected joint. Infants may be systemically unwell, febrile, tachycardic, and dehydrated.
- Some anaesthetists are prepared to anaesthetize the child as soon as possible, irrespective of fasting status, to ↓ chances of joint damage.
- GA can be delayed until the child is fasted, but in a septic infant oral intake will often have been poor for some time. Preoperative IV fluids may be needed.
- Respiratory symptoms are common in this situation.
- Recent paracetamol or NSAID should be noted to prevent intraoperative administration.

Anaesthesia

- Induction as preferred; note that IV access may already be present.
- RSI if regurgitation risk.

- In a fasted older child who is systemically well, an LMA and SV is a suitable technique. In infants and children who are 'toxic' or systemically unwell, ETT and IPPV are preferable.
- GA maintenance as preferred.
- Arthrotomy and irrigation is usually a short procedure, but large volumes of irrigation fluid are used, some of which soaks into the drapes and sheets. Temperature monitoring is required, particularly in infants, since the patient can cool rapidly in this environment. Actively warm patients, but this may not be necessary if they are febrile.
- Blood loss is minimal.
- IV fluids to replace fasting deficit and maintenance needs. Pyrexia ↑ insensible losses—therefore, ↑ maintenance fluids by 10% per 1°C temperature.
- Ensure secure IV access for long-term antibiotics: insert a long line or PICC line.
- Analgesia:
  - Preoperative or intraoperative paracetamol and NSAID
  - IV morphine 50–100mcg/kg (↓ dose if given recently)
  - ± IV ketamine 0.2–0.3 mg/kg.

Postoperative care
- Regular PO/IV paracetamol and PO/PR NSAID.
- PRN PO morphine.
- IV fluids until drinking.

Ophthalmology surgery

Anne Hunt

General principles

- Mainly day-case surgery
- Commonly include GA for procedures normally carried out in the outpatient clinic or under LA for adults and the more cooperative child.
- Age range: neonate to adulthood
- Mostly ASA 1, but may involve syndromic and autistic spectrum disorder patients.
- Multiple procedures leading to anxiety—may require sedative premedication, play specialists, and other psychological support.
- Surgery is in the vicinity of the airway, thus restricting access and in the case of nasolacrimal surgery a risk of aspiration of blood and injectates. Problems for the surgeon involve encroaching anaesthetic equipment, especially on a small face. Flexible LMAs (available in sizes 2 and above only) and south-polar tubes are therefore advised.
- PONV can occur, especially with extraocular muscle manipulation, e.g. strabismus surgery. Traction here sensitizes the vomiting centre via ciliary ganglion afferents (a trigemino-vagal reflex).
- Analgesia: usually only require paracetamol ± NSAID. Exceptions include strabismus surgery and some laser, glaucoma, and vitreoretinal work—these may be problematic.

Oculocardiac reflex (OCR)

- A trigemino-vagal reflex mediated by the ciliary ganglion, the ophthalmic division of the trigeminal nerve, and the vagus nerve.
- Most commonly seen with traction on the extraocular muscles (especially the medial rectus) and pressure on the globe, but may be seen with ocular manipulation and pain.
- Most frequent arrhythmia is sinus bradycardia, sometimes leading to sinus arrest. Others include junctional rhythms, atrial ectopics, ventricular dysrhythmias, rarely AV block, VT, or VF.
- Incidence 14–90%, depending on study and age of patient.
- Far commoner in children owing to dominance of parasympathetic nervous system causing heightened vagal tone. Incidence therefore decreases with age.
- Severity increases with hypoxia, hyperCO_2, acidosis, and light GA.
- Treatment:
  - Immediate cessation of surgical stimulus, i.e. tell surgeon to stop traction with squint hook.
  - If unresponsive, administer IV atropine 20 mcg/kg or glycopyrronium bromide 10 mcg/kg.
  - Optimize GA, i.e. depth and ventilation parameters
- Prevention:
  - Atropine 10 mcg/kg with induction. Glycopyrronium bromide may be used but it has a much longer $t_{1/2}$ and is likelier to cause a prolonged dry mouth.
  - Prevent light GA.
  - TIVA with propofol does not ↓ the risk; indeed, remifentanil increases incidence and severity.
- If OCR occurs, the risk of PONV is increased; consider prophylactic atropine to ↓ PONV risk.

Perioperative eye drops

- Analgesia: topical LA and diclofenac.
- Antibiotic and steroid drops may be used in initial postoperative period. Systemic effects are rare but possible.
- Cyclopentolate (0.5% or 1.0%): an anticholinergic that blocks muscarinic receptors in eye muscles. Onset 20–30 min (peaks at 30–45 min) to provide useful dilation. Duration 6–8 h, but can last up to 24 h. Systemic side effects are rare, but similar to atropine, i.e. tachycardia, dry mouth, etc. It often produces flushing of the cheeks postoperatively. Parental reassurance is required. Usually combined with phenylephrine preoperatively.
- Atropine (1%): rarely used, because of its slower onset (3 h), duration up to 14 days, and more common occurrence of side effects in infants. Mostly used in treatment of inflammatory eye conditions. Avoid in raised IOP.
- Phenylephrine (2.5%): α_1-adrenergic agonist that causes contraction of the dilator pupillary muscle and constriction of the arterioles in the conjunctiva. Peak effect 20–90 min and duration 3–8 h. Again systemic side effects are rare, but can be severe, including tachycardia, ventricular arrhythmias, hypertension, and myocardial infarction. Usually seen with the 10% solution—not routinely used in paediatrics.

Intraocular pressure (IOP)

- Adult range 11–21 mmHg; slightly lower in children.
- Mainly regulated by volume of aqueous humour, but also by tone of extraocular muscles, external pressure, choroidal blood volume, and vitreous volume.
- Aqueous humour is produced by ciliary body and is dependent on carbonic anhydrase, which is suppressed by acetazolamide. Production unaffected by IOP and is secreted at a constant rate.
- ↑ IOP/glaucoma in children is separated into two groups (both can be associated with other medical disorders, e.g. Sturge–Weber syndrome, neurofibromatosis 1, aniridia, and Lowe syndrome):
  - Primary: congenital or developmental. Congenital glaucoma results from abnormal development of the aqueous drainage system (1:10,000 births): 10% present at birth and 80% before 1 year of age. It is often inherited.
  - Secondary: caused by certain pathologies, e.g. uveitis, congenital cataract surgery
- Effects of GA on IOP:
  - Mechanical: ↑ with coughing, airway obstruction, pressure on eye from a poorly fitting face mask, and instrumentation of the airway (Guedel, LMA, and intubation may ↑ IOP by 30–40 mmHg).
  - Drugs:
    —Propofol and most IV induction agents ↓ IOP.
    —Ketamine slightly unpredictable. Probably causes an initial short-lived mild ↑ IOP, although some animal studies show a ↓ IOP.
    —All inhalational agents cause dose-related ↓ IOP.
    —Opioids and non-depolarizing muscle relaxants cause no effect or a slight ↓ IOP.
    —Suxamethonium ↑ IOP by up to 8 mmHg for about 7 min.
    —Steady-state maintenance with sevoflurane or propofol leads to same 50–60% ↓ IOP compared with awake values.
  - Miscellaneous: hypoxia and hyperCO$_2$ cause ↑ IOP; hypothermia causes ↓ IOP.

Examination under anaesthesia (EUA)

- Performed when not tolerated in outpatient clinic, e.g. babies, toddlers, learning difficulties, autism, and other uncooperative children. IOP is increased markedly in a screaming child.
- Often multiple GAs.
- Includes tests for IOP measurements, follow-up checks for retinoblastoma (during and post treatment, or a family history of the tumour), electrodiagnostic tests, post-cataract-surgery follow-up, retinal photography, refraction, fundoscopy, US, and multiple other investigations.
- Mydriasis and paralysis of the focusing ciliary muscles (cycloplegia) is usually required. This necessitates topical eye drops preoperatively, which sting and, in extremely uncooperative children, are impossible to administer awake, in which case they are applied immediately post induction and mydriasis is awaited.

EUA without IOP measurement

- Simple GA.
- Induction as preferred.
- Maintenance as preferred with LMA and SV (unless contraindicated by other patient factors).
- Use sufficient maintenance to avoid eye movements and rolling.
- Be aware that this may involve numerous tests and may be time consuming.

EUA with IOP measurement

- All induction agents affect IOP—the choice is debatable
- Two popular options:
  - IV ketamine 1–2 mg/kg, IOP measured before airway placement. If IV access is difficult, e.g. a chubby toddler, IM ketamine 5–10 mg/kg is possible, but sedative results are unpredictable and IM injections are usually avoided in children. Problems may occur with unpleasant side effects
  - Sevoflurane induction (with ophthalmologist on standby). IOP is measured immediately after induction before placement of IV cannula and airway (if safe).
- Some ophthalmologists are happy to measure IOP after propofol induction as long as it is measured immediately.
- IOP measurements usually take place in the anaesthetic room; the EUA is continued there or usually moved into theatre after LMA insertion.

EUA with other investigations

- Electrodiagnostic tests: performed by medical neurophysiologists, test function of visual pathway. They involve complex machinery and computers, in the dark, and there may be problems with interference from other electrical sources—e.g. electrical warming mattresses should be switched off (standard anaesthetic monitoring should not interfere). Duration 15–20 min. A simple GA with a flexible LMA is satisfactory. Avoid ketamine if possible, since it interferes with baseline readings.

- Fundus fluorescein angiography: uncommon test, used to investigate retinal disease, e.g. retinopathy of prematurity, Coats' disease, and familial exudative vitreoretinopathy. IV fluorescein is administered and retinal images taken. Simple GA is sufficient. Be aware fluorescein is allergenic and may cause urticaria or rarely an anaphylactic reaction.
- Children having EUA eyes under GA often present similar problems for other specialities, and other procedures may be 'tagged on', e.g. dental extractions, ENT procedures, and blood tests. This helps reduce the stress of multiple GAs for them and their parents, and within reason should be encouraged.

Squint/strabismus surgery

- Squint/strabismus is a condition where the visual axes are misaligned.
- Incidence 2–3%.
- Treatments include conservative (glasses, patching, exercises), surgery, or botulinum toxin injections.

Surgical technique

- Commonest paediatric eye operation.
- In young children may restore binocular vision, but in most cases is performed for cosmesis.
- The six extraocular muscles are innervated by the IIIrd, IVth, and VIth cranial nerves: the medial (III) and lateral (VI) recti; the superior (IV) and inferior (III) obliques; and the superior (III) and inferior (III) recti. The upper eyelid is supplied by the IIIrd cranial nerve.
- Surgical correction is achieved by recession (lengthening) or resection (shortening) one or more muscles. Occasionally, transposition (switching) of the muscles is performed and in older children an adjustable suture may be used (with adjustment in the outpatient clinic the day after the procedure using LA eye drops).

Preoperative assessment

- Usually ASA 1 with idiopathic aetiology.
- Occasionally associated with a family history, prematurity, Trisomy 21, Down syndrome, other circumstances causing the eye to have poor vision (e.g. cataract, retinal damage, ptosis), CNS disorders (e.g. cerebral palsy), intracranial disorders (e.g. tumours, infection, trauma), and other conditions leading to nerve/muscle palsies.
- Sedative premedication often required.

Anaesthesia

- The type of GA does not affect surgical success. However, some surgeons prefer to operate on paralysed muscles, and some require the use of a 'forced duction test' immediately prior to surgery. This involves the application of passive movement to the eye using forceps applied to the sclera to identify fixed restriction of movement rather than muscle imbalance. Again, some surgeons prefer muscle paralysis for this whilst others do not.
- Induction as preferred
- Flexible LMA or south-polar ETT.
- SV or IPPV as indicated (± paralysis with non-depolarizing muscle relaxant)
- O_2/air plus volatile or TIVA (avoid N_2O), which may be better for PONV.
- Atropine 10 mcg/kg prophylactically or have atropine 20 mcg/kg available.
- Ondansetron and dexamethasone.
- IV fluids may also help reduce PONV.

Analgesia

- Preoperative PO paracetamol and ibuprofen/diclofenac, or intraoperatively if preferred.
- Local anaesthetic block with 0.25% levobupivacaine.
- Topical LA eyedrops at end.
- Diclofenac eyedrops at end; 1 h onset, safe in combination with systemic NSAID.
- Consider IV fentanyl 1 mcg/kg (↑ PONV) or clonidine 1–2 mcg/kg; may help postoperative pain and distress.
- Lubricating gel drops.
- Eye patch reduces movement and prevents blinking of the eye—but obviously only one eye may be treated in this way, and some children find the patch adds to their distress.

Postoperative care

- Recover in a quiet, dark room.
- Pain management is difficult: patients often refuse to open their eyes and constantly try to rub them. The sutures in the conjunctiva cause the sensation of a FB; blinking and eye movements exacerbate the pain.
- Regular PO paracetamol.
- PRN PO morphine.
- 2nd dose of diclofenac eye drops (despite initial sting it has a cooling effect)
- PONV:
  - Incidence 50–75% without prophylaxis.
  - Incidence increased with opiates, adolescents, history of motion sickness (or previous PONV), medial rectus surgery, and the intraoperative occurrence of the OCR.
  - PRN antiemetic, also consider cyclizine and droperidol as third-line treatment.

Botulinum toxin for squint

- Used for short-term relief of diplopia, children with small to moderate esotropia, evolving or unstable conditions, unsuccessful surgery, and patients with binocular vision
- The effects wears off in 3–4 months, but the improved alignment may be long-lasting.
- Procedure is done awake using LA drops in compliant teenagers.
- Generally needs a GA, but the extraocular muscle to be injected is identified with a needle electrode and EMG. Muscle contraction is required—and a GA abolishes this.
- Ketamine sedation is used instead.
- Quick procedure in anaesthetic room.
- Possibly more PONV than formal squint surgery.
- Alternative option is to inject the muscle under direct vision, but this involves a short surgical procedure involving opening of the conjunctiva and sutures. Obviously a GA is employed here.

Sedation technique

- Preoperative explanation for parents and child: IV ketamine takes slightly longer to act than propofol; child's eyes may not close, but will cease to interact, and they will not recall anything.
- IV ketamine 1 mg/kg plus 0.5 mg/kg increments if child starts to move.
- Aim to sedate them enough for the procedure but leave some muscle tone; ideally, they blink a little to stimulation. Too sedated, and the EMG will be ineffective.
- If IV access cannot be established, then an inhalational induction is performed to site the cannula. Ketamine is administered once they start to wake.
- IV midazolam 1–2 mg (greater dose may interfere with muscle location) for older children to prevent hallucinations.
- Ondansetron and dexamethasone.
- Secretions due to ketamine are rarely a problem—atropine is seldom required.
- LA drops prior to procedure.
- Monitor with SpO_2 only with volume turned off (so muscle contraction may be heard via EMG).
- Rarely an occasional 'waft' of O_2 may be required via a facemask.
- Recover in a quiet, dark room. Ask parents to allow them to wake slowly to avoid 'nightmares'.
- PRN PO paracetamol.

Cataract surgery

- Cataracts are a major cause of blindness, especially in the developing world.
- Classified by numerous methods, including:
  - Age of onset: congenital, infantile (< 2 years), and juvenile (>2 years).
  - Aetiology:
    —Genetic (75%): non-syndromic (mainly autosomal-dominant) or, rarely, part of a syndrome, e.g. Trisomy 21, Rothmund–Thomson, Smith-Lemli-Opitz, myotonic dystrophy, Edwards, cri du chat, galactosaemia
    —Traumatic
    —Intrauterine infection, e.g. rubella, toxoplasmosis, varicella, CMV
    —Uveitis, e.g. juvenile idiopathic arthritis
    —Metabolic, e.g. hypoCa^{2+} and hypoglycaemia in infancy
    —Iatrogenic, e.g. radiation therapy, systemic steroids, post vitrectomy, post laser for retinopathy of prematurity.
  - Morphology: e.g. diffuse/total, anterior, cortical lamellar, persistent hyperplastic primary vitreous, traumatic disruption of lens.
- The neonate requires visual stimulation for maturation of neural pathways and the retina; hence dense cataracts need early intervention (before 2–3 months of age).

Surgical technique

- Bilateral cataracts are extracted 1–2 weeks apart to ↓ infection risk.
- An intraocular lens (IOL) is often inserted post extraction. Uncommon for patients <1 year old, who often have optic rehabilitation with contact lenses or glasses, with an IOL inserted later.
- Not all cataracts require surgery, e.g. if small, partial, paracentral. These are observed and operated on later if required when the eye has grown and is more amenable to IOL implantation.
- Postoperative complications include secondary opacification (requiring posterior capsulotomy—up to 90%), glaucoma (especially if baby at initial procedure), uveitis, endophthalmitis, and retinal detachment.

Preoperative assessment

- Often multiple visits and GAs previously.
- Associated comorbidities.
- Assessment of neonate/baby.

Anaesthesia

- Requires a motionless eye and avoidance of ↑ IOP.
- Note that procedure usually includes a EUA too.
- Induction as preferred (note that surgeon may wish to measure IOP).
- Usually ETT and IPPV to avoid hyperCO$_2$.
- Maintenance as preferred.
- If neuromuscular blockers used, monitor with a PNS (but difficult to use on neonates/babies).
- Ondansetron and dexamethasone.

- Infants will require IV fluids, active warming, and temperature monitoring.
- Analgesia:
  - Paracetamol ± NSAID
  - LA drops.

Postoperative care
- PO paracetamol ± NSAID.
- PRN PO morphine (PR codeine in neonates).

Glaucoma surgery

- Glaucoma causes blindness owing to reduction of capillary blood flow to the optic nerve. The first sign on fundoscopy is optic nerve 'cupping'.
- Conservative treatment with medication is challenging in children, and many drugs are unlicensed in paediatrics. Drugs are mainly used as an adjunct to surgery.
- Primary congenital glaucoma is caused by abnormal membrane obstructing normal outflow of aqueous via the trabecular network into Schlemm's canal and the venous system. It presents as a clinical triad: epiphora, blepharospasm, and photophobia. The cornea becomes cloudy at late presentation; 75% are bilateral. Diagnosis is often missed. 80–90% of babies with prompt surgical treatment will do well.

Surgical technique

- Two main operations:
  - Goniotomy: incision across trabecular network via the anterior chamber.
  - Trabeculotomy: incision via an external approach through Schlemm's canal. Drainage is from anterior chamber to sub-Tenon space. Antifibrotic agents, e.g. fluorouracil, may be applied.
- If these fail, possibilities include:
  - Tube implant surgery (aqueous shunts).
  - Trabeculectomy.
  - Cryoablation or laser surgery. Cryoablation causes less inflammation and is preferred. Used to ablate the aqueous-producing ciliary body. Used in management of refractory glaucoma. This is a painful procedure.

Anaesthesia

- As for cataract surgery. Note that opioids may be required, particularly in cryoablation or laser surgery.

Nasolacrimal surgery

- Indication: blocked tear ducts. Uni- or bilateral.
- Presentation: watering eyes and infections.
- Most ASA 1, but a minority have comorbidities, in particular craniofacial syndromes.
- Day case; simple PO analgesics suffice.

Syringe and probing

- Commonest form of surgery. Minor day-case procedure.
- Involves probing the nasolacrimal duct and syringing through a dose of diluted fluorescein. A suction catheter is place in the nostril and the oro/nasopharynx is suctioned to check for patency and presence of the dye.
- A simple GA with an LMA is required, as long as the fluorescein is suctioned well.

Nasolacrimal duct intubation

- After failure of syringe and probing.
- Entails the use of a nasal endoscope to insert a silicone tube through the duct, and may involve ENT surgeon. Adrenaline (epinephrine) pledgets used to ↓ bleeding.
- Simple GA with an LMA.
- Second GA required to remove the tube.

Dacryocystorhinostomy

- Creation of new low-resistance pathway bypassing the blocked nasolacrimal duct. Involves removal of bone adjacent to the nasolacrimal sac and incorporating the sac within the lateral nasal mucosa. Again a silicone tube is placed.
- There are two forms of surgery: endoscopic (more usual in paediatrics) and external.
- Both involve vasoconstrictors applied to nasal mucosa, ETT and a throat pack to avoid aspiration, a head-up tilt, and mildly hypotensive GA.
- Second GA 1–2 months later to remove tube.

Oculoplastic surgery

Ptosis repair
- Usually ASA 1; occasionally part of a syndrome or a manifestation of a neuromuscular disease.
- 70% are unilateral.
- If unilateral surgery, the eye should be marked preoperatively, since once the patient is asleep there is no way to tell which is the affected eye.
- Two main forms of surgery: using some form of sling (suture or tendon material) or muscle /tendon resection and advancement.
- It is superficial surgery and requires a simple GA with an LMA. LA infiltrated or block performed plus PO analgesia is adequate.
- The eye remains open after surgery and ointment is placed on the eye to avoid it drying out.
- Avoid trauma in recovery.

Entropion repair
- The eyelid (usually the lower) folds inwards and the eyelashes rub against the cornea, causing irritation.
- The causes are congenital, associated with facial nerve palsy, or due to lid scarring, e.g. trachoma. The GA is the same as for a ptosis repair.

Incision and curettage (I&C) of chalazion

- Cyst on eyelid (may be multiple) due to a blocked/chronically inflamed Meibomian gland.
- Initial treatment is medical with warm compresses and good lid hygiene. Chloramphenicol ointment is prescribed if acutely inflamed.
- If this fails, surgical treatment is incision of the tarsal gland (the eyelid is everted and a chalazion clamp is placed), with curettage of the retained secretions.
- Quick procedure requiring a simple GA.
- There may be profuse bleeding after removal of the clamp, so a patch is usually required.
- Simple PO analgesics.

Dermoid cyst

- A congenital choristoma of the eye.
- A benign tumour: 46% of orbital neoplasms in children. Slow-growing, usually superficial, near the lateral eyebrow (occasionally form deep in the orbit).
- Superficial ones require a simple GA, LA infiltration, and oral analgesia. Note that the surgery is delicate and operating time may be up to 45 min.

Retinopathy of prematurity

- Occurs in infants <32 weeks gestation. It is affected by degree of prematurity, birth weight, and supplemental O_2 concentrations.
- It is treated by laser or cryotherapy while on neonatal unit and usually while still on a ventilator; often does not involve an anaesthetist. These therapies destroy the peripheral area of the retina, slowing or reversing the abnormal growth of blood vessels.
- It is painful and requires an opiate.

Ophthalmology emergencies

- Very uncommon and almost all related to trauma. General principles as discussed with the addition of a possible full stomach.

Penetrating eye injury

- Commoner in boys. Ratio of 2.6:1 M:F in >3-year-olds.
- May be associated with a FB.
- Risk of visual loss and endophthalmitis.
- Often lead to further GAs for EUA and cataract extraction for example.
- Require wound closure (and removal of FB).
- Urgent operation, but surgeons are usually happy to wait until the child is fasted.
- If risk of a full stomach, then a RSI is performed. In the past, the use of suxamethonium was thought to be a grave danger here since it is known to increase IOP, possibly leading to expulsion of globe contents on induction. However, the rise in IOP is thought to be relatively minor (~7 mmHg) and there has never been a case reported of a patient losing the contents of their eye after the use of suxamethonium—so it should not be avoided if required. However, nowadays, the use of suxamethonium is thought by many to be relatively obsolete in these circumstances with the introduction of rocuronium and sugammadex.

Anaesthesia

- Avoid ↑ IOP: avoid crying, struggling, vomiting, and coughing. A sedative may be helpful.
- Induction as preferred, but beware of pressure from the facemask (ketamine is not indicated).
- Intubation and coughing may ↑ IOP markedly, so ensure response to laryngoscopy and intubation is attenuated by full paralysis and a dose of opiate or beta-blocker.
- Maintenance as preferred.
- Paralysis (PNS monitoring) and IPPV to avoid hyperCO$_2$.
- Avoid N$_2$O in case of air in the eye.
- Active warming, temperature monitoring, and IV fluids advisable.
- Ondansetron and dexamethasone.
- Often a painful procedure, Analgesia:
  - IV paracetamol and PR diclofenac
  - Topical LA drops
  - IV opiate usually required.
- Smooth extubation, attempting to minimize coughing and straining.

Postoperative care

- Regular simple analgesics.
- PRN PO morphine and antiemetics.
- A patch/clear plastic shield to avoid further trauma.

Retinal detachment

- Paediatrics account for <10% of all cases.
- Up to 30% are bilateral.

- Main disposing factors:
  - Trauma (40%)
  - Comorbidities (Stickler syndrome, Marfan syndrome, coloboma, cataract surgery, uveitis, Coats' disease)
  - Myopia
  - Retinopathy of prematurity.
- Rarely presents as an emergency, because progress is slower than in adults, visual loss is less acute, children are less likely to recognize it (only 40–70% report symptoms on diagnosis); in trauma, detachment develops late owing to the support of a well-formed vitreous.
- GA technique is that of intraocular surgery, although it may be painful, so opiates are often required.

Eyelid trauma

- Not uncommon.
- Always fasted; therefore, require a simple GA with an LMA/ETT and LA infiltration.
- Operate on within 24 h.
- There are two injuries of note:
  - Lacerations involving lid margin. If not closed early, the child may suffer intractable watering and ingrowing of lashes.
  - Lacerations involving the lacrimal canaliculi within the medial aspect of the lower eyelid. Require early surgical intervention involving some form of stent. Late treatment leads to risks of scarring, infection, corneal exposure, and poor drainage.

Radiology

Laura Bowes

Overview

- Most adults undergo radiological investigations awake. However, the requirement to remain still for long periods of time within enclosed and often noisy spaces, e.g. for MRI, mean a large proportion of children will require GA.
- An increasing range of investigations and procedures are performed in the radiology department, thereby increasing the demand for GA provision.
- Radiology departments are increasingly designed to enable GA, providing designated areas for induction and recovery. Planning for these involves piped gases, integrated monitors, and anaesthetic machines suitable for use in all settings, e.g. MR conditional.
- Many children manage these scans awake owing to the skill of the radiographers in guiding them and their carers through the process. Other patients will have sedation prescribed and administered by non-anaesthetists to facilitate their scan as per local policy.
- Where the infrastructure does not allow for the routine provision of GA, or where staff are unfamiliar with working with anaesthetized children, the combined challenges of working in a remote site and with a complex patient population mean good communication and planning are essential.

General considerations

The patient

- Standard preoperative assessment with special attention to syndromes and concomitant illnesses.
- Patients for investigation of CNS pathology are common and frequently have associated CVS, respiratory, or endocrine conditions. Assess the airway with care.

Staffing and facilities

- Staffing levels are as for any GA. Appropriately trained radiology staff may be required to assist transferring children on and off the scan table (especially when logrolling).
- Appropriate standards should be met for induction, maintenance, and recovery. All staff should be familiar with the equipment used. Equipment used within the MRI should be either MR safe or MR conditional and invasive monitoring may need to be discontinued for the duration of the scan. Where TIVA is required, MR-conditional pumps are required or longer infusion lines must be used so the pumps can be outside the Faraday cage.
- O_2 is often supplied from a cylinder—have a spare.
- Dedicated anaesthetic suction.
- Resuscitation trolley and defibrillator present.
- Planned and known drill for extricating a child in an emergency.
- In the event of a cardiac arrest, removing the patient to the induction room is usually preferable—be familiar with the protocol. Do not let the resuscitation team enter the MRI room.

The procedure

- There are multiple factors to consider when planning the anaesthetic:

General
- Duration
- Will the patient be anaesthetized in one location then transferred to another room?
- Patient position: supine/prone/lateral?
- Head or feet first into scanner?
- Will the patient be moved during the procedure?
- Patient access is often difficult owing to limited space, immovable tables and equipment, dark rooms, and numerous staff. This can make it impossible to position anaesthetic equipment close to the patient.
- Will the airway and IV cannula be accessible?
- Long ventilation tubing and IV lines are easily caught or dislodged.
- Ask the radiographer to do a trial run with the table into the scanner so that the extra 'slack' required can be ascertained.
- What is being done first? Risks and complications? Stimulating or non-invasive? Will contrast or heparin be used? Will you be asked to administer drugs?
- What are the likely sequelae of the procedure: PONV, pain, bleeding from puncture or biopsy site, CVS or respiratory complications, anaphylactoid or anaphylactic reactions to contrast solutions?

Temperature
- Radiology suites often contain superconductors (for MRI), which require cooling. Measure patient temperature for all but the briefest scans.
- Warming blankets and underbody warmers can interfere with the quality of imaging.

Radiation
- Modern equipment (shielded and coned) causes negligible radiation exposure >2 m from the source.
- However, all personnel should take precautions to minimize total exposure, wearing a lead apron, thyroid shield, and an exposure badge if exposure is frequent. Take advice from radiographers.
- If possible (and the patient is appropriately monitored), leave the immediate vicinity and observe from behind leaded-glass screen. Protect the patient from unnecessary exposure (testes, ovaries, thyroid, and eyes).

Contrast media
- Iodinated contrast media are frequently administered during a scan to enhance the images obtained. Occasional side effects:
  - Dose-dependent reactions due to the physiochemical properties of the agent include heat, pain, vasodilation, cardiac depression, and hypotension.
  - Dose-independent reactions:
    —Nausea and vomiting.
    —Hypersensitivity reactions: minor (flushing, nausea and vomiting, pruritis, urticarial, arm pain); moderate (severe urticarial, facial oedema, hypotension, bronchospasm); severe (shock, laryngeal oedema, convulsions, cardiac arrest). Most reactions are anaphylactoid and true anaphylaxis with contrast media is rare. Mortality rate is 1:75,000.
    —Adverse reactions are uncommon with low-osmolarity media, which should be used in all intra-arterial injections (less painful).
  - Contrast-induced nephropathy is a concern with pre-existing renal impairment and may influence the use of contrast.
- Gadolinium is the standard MRI contrast medium; ➔ section on MRI.

Computed tomography (CT)

- A rotating X-ray emitter and detector provide images taken at numerous different angles such that a 2D image of a thin cross-sectional slice of the body is produced.
- Structures of differing densities (bone and muscle) within the body are clearly separated, while those of similar densities are less well differentiated.
- Quick: head scans are often produced in <30 s, meaning that GA is usually avoidable.
- Modern 'spiral' CT machines are very quick, but so is the table movement. Check the full extent of movement that the patient will experience during the scan and ensure that the anaesthetic circuit and IV extensions are long enough with no potential for catching.
- No restriction on type of anaesthetic and monitoring equipment.
- Relatively large doses of radiation are used. If possible, monitor from the control room.
- Discuss positioning and use of contrast before scan, so that the dose can be decided and the method of administration; note allergies to iodine and pre-existing renal impairment.
- Patients range from well infants with a CCAM who are fasted and scanned electively to trauma patients who are undergoing resuscitation during the scan. Where CT scans are performed before surgical intervention, e.g. stereotactic guided neurosurgery, subsequent access to the airway may be limited. Use a standard ETT, since the metallic coils of a reinforced ETT interfere with the CT images.
- Limited access to the head and airway, especially for head scans. Ensure airway is secure prior to scanning.
- Keep IV sites visible and accessible.
- Keep metallic leads, e.g. ECG cables, away from the scan site, since they cause interference
- Ensure enough trained staff for a controlled transfer from trolley to scan table, especially if log-rolling.

Anaesthetic technique

- Induction as preferred.
- An LMA is sometimes appropriate for airway management. In many cases, an ETT is preferable, either because the child is small and access is limited or because they are undergoing a CT of the thorax and the radiographers will request a 'breath hold' in inspiration. This is easier with an ETT and either a muscle relaxant or a bolus of remifentanil. Expertise may allow this to be facilitated with an LMA.
- Where cases are planned for stereotactic guided neurosurgery, consideration should be made of suitability for induction within the CT suite prior to transfer to theatre and accessibility to airway after the frame has been applied.
- Maintenance as preferred. Syringe pumps are small and lightweight, and can usually be placed on the scan table with the patient and the monitor if required.
- Emergency head injury cases with a reduced LOC require an IV RSI.

Postoperative care
- Elective cases where the scan is the sole procedure usually recover rapidly, feed, and are discharged within 1–2 h. Emergency cases go to theatre, ICU, or HDU, depending on the result of the scan and the clinical situation.

Magnetic resonance imaging (MRI)

- Increasingly the imaging modality of choice, since there is no ionizing radiation. It produces high-quality images giving clear differentiation between soft tissues and is used in conjunction with CT when bony images are also required, e.g. internal auditory meati for preoperative assessment for cochlear implants.
- A static magnetic field is generated that causes protons within hydrogen atoms to align and precess on their axes at an angle related to the strength of the magnetic field. Radiofrequency radiation applied at the resonance of these protons causes a transfer of energy, increasing the angle of spin until it is at 90° to the magnetic field. When the radiofrequency is turned off, the hydrogen atoms give off energy as they 'relax' back to align with the magnetic field; this is detected by the coil. The entire process is repeated, with the coil receiving multiple signals. These signals are assembled to create a digital image. Different tissues relax at different rates and so appear different on the resulting image.
- In order to generate the large magnetic field (static—always on), a superconductor is used (a wire is cooled by liquid helium to −269°C so that its electrical resistance vanishes and it can carry a massive current).
- Field strength: 0.5–3 tesla (T) (1 tesla = 10,000 gauss).
  - Earth's magnetic field: 0.3–0.7 gauss, i.e. the magnet is 10,000 times stronger.
  - Any ferromagnetic material is influenced
  - <0.5 mT (5 gauss) has minimal influence. This boundary should be marked within the scan room.
  - No magnetic material (including syringe pumps) should be closer than the 0.5 mT line.

Equipment

- All equipment must be 'MR safe' or 'MR conditional' and labelled as such. This includes patient trolleys, O_2 cylinders for transfer to wards, and laryngoscopes.
- MR safe: not hazardous in any MRI environment, i.e. non-conducting, non-metallic, non-magnetic items.
- MR conditional: no known hazard when subjected to a specified environment with specified conditions of use, e.g. anaesthetic machines located beyond the 5 gauss contour. Equipment that is conditional in a 1.5 T scanner may be MR unsafe in a 3 T scanner.
- MR unsafe: hazardous in all MRI environments, e.g. ferromagnetic scissors.

Monitoring

- Minimum standards of monitoring as for any GA.
- Cables should be padded or directed away from the skin and should not be coiled (may burn skin).
- MR-compatible fibreoptic pulse oximeter cables, temperature probes, and carbon fibre ECG electrodes are available.

- Capnography tubing is long, increasing the interval between sampling and recording.
- ECG may be inaccurate—currents generated in the large vessels and heart by the magnetic field may be displayed as artefact.
- Audible alarms may be unnoticed above the MR noise, especially if ear defenders are worn. Many anaesthetists prefer to remain outside the scanning room with a slave monitor and observe the patient through a window.
- All patients wear ear defenders or ear plugs, since the noise levels can reach 130 decibels in a 3 T scan. Staff present in the scanning room should also wear ear defenders.
- The superconducting magnet coils in an MRI require liquid helium to keep them cool and allow them to function. This means the environment in the scan room is cool and patients should be kept warm during the scan.
- Gadolinium is the standard contrast used, it shortens the relaxation time, thereby enhancing T1-weighted images. Mild side effects: nausea, vomiting, pain on injection.
- Anaphylactoid reactions are possible. The contrast is metabolized entirely in the renal system, so care should be taken in renal failure since it can cause nephrogenic systemic fibrosis. Incidence is also increased in concurrent liver disease. Check preoperative renal function.

Preoperative assessment
- Standard preoperative assessment.
- GA has more risks than MRI. Many children attending for MRI come regularly as part of surveillance for the treatment of cancer. However, increasingly, scans are performed as part of the 'work-up' for developmental delay and informed consent must be obtained for the GA.
- Consent is required—follow local policy regarding whose responsibility this is.
- A safety questionnaire must be completed and checked prior to induction.

Anaesthetic technique
- Induction as preferred. Many patients have permanent lines, which can be used for induction. However, many radiology departments have a policy of avoiding their use for contrast administration, in which case a temporary cannula should be sited.
- Maintenance as preferred.
- Increasingly, patients present directly to the radiology department, have their scan, and are discharged directly from radiology recovery. Minimizing GA side effects is therefore very important.
- Many institutions use propofol sedation with supplementary O_2 via a nasal cannula with capnography monitoring attached. Induction can still be with volatile gas, but following IV access the volatile is discontinued, a bolus of 2–4 mg/kg propofol administered, and a propofol infusion commenced (usually 100 mcg/kg/min). During the administration of contrast and for diffusion scans, the maintenance dose may need to be

increased, since these are stimulating, but for the remainder of the scan the only requirement is for the patient to stay still and the dose can be reduced to facilitate a rapid discharge.
- Head nodding is relatively common with sedation and can cause artefacts; for head scans this can be countered by scanning the child in the recovery position. This is not possible for scans of other parts of the body, in which case a small shoulder roll or the careful placement of a Guedel airway helps (deepen sedation for insertion). Rarely, a change to GA technique with either an LMA or ETT is required; the latter requires the patient to return to the anaesthetic room.

Nuclear medicine

- This requires the administration of a radioactive substance, which is then detected by a gamma camera pinpointing where the tracer substance has preferentially accumulated, providing information about the organ and its function. Beyond the administration of the radioactive substance, this is a non-invasive test; however, the cameras move in close proximity to the body and whole body scans can take >1 h so are poorly tolerated in young children.
- Single photon emission computed tomography (SPECT) relies on multiple gamma cameras rotating around the body to create a more detailed 3D image.
- A positron emission tomography (PET) scanner has multiple rings of detectors and looks similar to a CT or MRI scanner. It can give detailed 3D images, which can be combined with CT or MRI to provide further information.

Anaesthetic technique

- Most children requiring GA are 0–24 months old.
- Access to the airway and IV lines may be challenging—secure them well. Use an extension line to aid drug administration.
- Maintenance as preferred.
- Temperature monitoring and active warming should be used from the start of the scan to minimize interruptions.

Interventional radiology

- Paediatric interventional radiology is a rapidly expanding speciality, covering a range of minimally invasive procedures that rely on image guidance to assist in the diagnosis or treatment of many conditions.
- Techniques performed include central venous access, aspiration or drainage of collections (nephrostomy, ascites, abscesses), angiography and venography for embolization and stenting, sclerotherapy, lymphangiography, image-guided biopsies, and targeted administration of chemotherapy.
- Unlike in adult practice, access to interventional radiology out of hours is still in its infancy and it may be unavailable even in major centres in an emergency. Adult interventional radiologists with an interest in paediatrics may form part of an out-of-hours provision.

Angiography/venography

- Elective angiography and venography is performed to assess arteriovenous malformations (AVMs), tumour blood supply, and vessel mapping for IV access, and in transplant surgery to assess the portal venous system. Cardiac angiography is mentioned in Chapter 15. It also has a role in the assessment of brain function when planning epilepsy surgery by enabling one hemisphere to be electively anaesthetized so that cognitive tests can be performed.
- The majority of angiography and venography is performed under GA. LA is used at the site of catheterization and minimal analgesia is required. Cerebral angiography can cause a post-procedural headache and it is useful to administer paracetamol and encourage fluid intake post procedure.

Embolization

- Multidisciplinary teams discuss angiography and venography results to plan subsequent management. Many patients return to the interventional radiology department to undergo embolization. Embolization can be used in the treatment of AVMs and aneurysms and to ↓ tumour blood flow prior to surgery.
- Methods of embolization include the use of solid embolic agents (coils, balloons, PVA agents, absorbable gelatin sponge), and liquid embolic agents (onyx, alcohol).

Intra-arterial chemotherapy/transarterial chemotherapy embolization (TACE)

- Intra-arterial chemotherapy is used to deliver chemotherapy directly to the vessels supplying a tumour, thereby reducing the effects on surrounding healthy tissues.
- TACE is used to target the hepatic blood supply of solid liver tumours, thereby causing necrosis.
- Intra-arterial chemotherapy has an increasing role in retinoblastoma treatment.
- Infants undergoing intra-arterial chemotherapy require GA in order to stay still and provide optimal conditions for catheter placement.

- Close monitoring of $ETCO_2$ and BP is maintained throughout, particularly during administration of chemotherapy, which has been known to cause a ↓ in $ETCO_2$ and SpO_2 with subsequent hypotension and even cardiac arrest. While this chain of events is documented to occur more during the second dose of chemotherapy, it can occur at any time; consider using invasive arterial monitoring.

Sclerotherapy

- Used to ↓ the size of lymphatic malformations by causing irritation or inflammation followed by scarring. The antibiotic bleomycin is used, since it causes less pain and swelling, and is the best agent for reducing the size of microcystic lymphatic malformations. However, it can cause lung scarring in high doses, and preoperative lung function tests are performed. Rarely, it causes skin and nail discoloration; this may be precipitated by scratching or the placement of monitoring leads, plasters, and cannulas.

Anaesthetic considerations

- Restricted access—ensure airway and IV access are secured and extensions available.
- Consider arterial access. If this is impossible and vessels are large enough, a side port on the femoral introducer sheath can be used; however, this may be impossible in small infants.
- IR suites are cold. Monitor temperature and consider active warming.
- Crucial to IR procedures: immobility, maintenance of physiological stability, and, for neurological cases, the means to manage cerebral blood flow.
- Contrast media are associated with nephropathy and rarely anaphylactic reactions.
- Contrast media can cause PONV—keep hydrated and give an antiemetic.

Plastic surgery

Doug Johnson

Lumps and bumps

- These include lipomas, haemangiomas, lymph nodes, naevi, dermoid cysts, calcified hair follicles, and rarely skin cancers, e.g. malignant melanoma.
- 99% of superficial lumps excised are benign.
- Approximately 80% of malignant lesions are recognized by:
  - Presentation as a neonate
  - A history of rapid or progressive growth
  - Skin ulceration
  - Fixation
  - Presence of a firm mass >3 cm in diameter.
- 5–10% of benign lumps regress spontaneously; the remainder persist or slowly enlarge. The latter are excised for cosmetic reasons, to prevent infection or inflammation, or to avoid missing a malignancy.

Preoperative assessment

- Usually unremarkable. Occasional parental anxiety about possible malignancy.

Anaesthetic technique

- Simple analgesics preoperatively.
- Inhalational or IV induction.
- Usually LMA with SV.
- Anaesthetic maintenance as preferred.
- A tourniquet may be used.
- In most cases, the surgeon infiltrates LA with adrenaline (epinephrine) to provide analgesia and aid haemostasis.
- Opiates are usually not required.

Postoperative care

- Most will be discharged 1–2 h postoperatively.
- PONV is rare.
- Low-dose PO morphine for rescue analgesia.
- Paracetamol and a NSAID for discharge.

Otoplasty

- Indications: prominent ears and microtia (both may be unilateral or bilateral).
- Prominent ears are not usually associated with other malformations. Surgery aims to correct the specific area of prominence by reshaping the antihelical fold through a post-auricular elliptical incision.
- Microtia can be part of hemifacial microsomia with associated malformations, e.g. an asymmetric mandible. Surgery is reconstructive and often involves harvesting costal cartilage.
- Age: >6 years.
- M:F ratio 2:1.

Preoperative assessment

- Mostly ASA 1.
- A minority of microtia patients are difficult intubations, though they usually have an easy airway (❯ Chapter 9).

Anaesthetic technique

- In these older children, an IV induction is usual unless airway problems are anticipated.
- Airway management with an armoured LMA or south-facing preformed (RAE) ETT. An ETT is indicated if costal cartilage is to be harvested for ear reconstruction.
- IPPV or SV as preferred.
- Maintenance as preferred, avoid N_2O.
- High risk of PONV. Administer ondansetron and dexamethasone, and a 20 mL/kg bolus of maintenance fluid. Consider TIVA.
- Analgesia:
  - Paracetamol and an NSAID.
  - Greater auricular nerve block. 2 mL 0.25% bupivacaine ± adrenaline is injected superficially at the junction of the posterior body of the sternocleidomastoid and a line drawn laterally from the superior border of the cricoid cartilage. The nerve (from superficial cervical plexus C3) becomes superficial at this point before running up to supply the external ear and mastoid.
  - US-guided superficial cervical plexus block.
  - Or infiltration with LA and adrenaline
  - Options for managing postoperative pain from costal cartilage harvest site include LA infiltration, intercoastal block, LA wound catheter or paravertebral block.
  - Opioids are usually unnecessary.

Postoperative care

- Otoplasty is a day case.
- If PONV occurs despite prophylaxis, administer an antiemetic from another class.
- Regular paracetamol and NSAID, plus PRN PO morphine.
- CXR after costal cartilage harvest to exclude pneumothorax.
- There is a low incidence of postoperative haemorrhage requiring exploration.

Syndactyly

- Congenital failure of fingers or toes to separate. Can involve two or more digits.
- It is 'complete' if fusion extends to the fingertips.
- It is 'complex if there is fusion of phalanges, 'simple' if not.
- Incidence 1:2,500.
- M:F ratio 2:1.

Aetiology

- Failure of differentiation during first trimester.
- Family history in up to 50%.
- Isolated malformation or part of a syndrome e.g. Apert (most commonly).
- Epidermolysis bullosa (EB).
- Polydactyly.
- Poland syndrome (unilateral absence or underdevelopment of pectoralis muscle plus syndactyly of the ipsilateral hand).

Treatment

- Early repair around 12 months of age gives the best aesthetic and functional results.
- Complex syndactyly usually require several staged procedures.
- A full-thickness graft is often necessary to cover defects and may be taken from the thigh or antecubital fossa.
- Fixation of digits with K-wires may be required to prevent contractures.
- Morbidity—scarring and contractures requiring revision, infection.

Specifics in preoperative assessment

- Presence of a syndrome e.g. Apert, that may present airway difficulties.
- Consider sedative premedication (unless there are airway problems), since children usually undergo a number of procedures for this and associated conditions.
- Syndactyly secondary to EB is managed in a specialist centre.

Anaesthetic technique

- Inhalational induction is common. Patients are usually toddlers, venous access may be difficult, and in Apert syndrome there may be a difficult airway.
- LMA or ETT. An ETT is preferable for longer complex cases.
- SV or IPPV as preferred.
- Maintenance as preferred.
- A tourniquet is usually required.
- Analgesia is provided by:
  - Paracetamol and NSAID.
  - LA infiltration for minor cases.
  - Forearm nerve blocks.
  - Brachial plexus block for complex procedures.
  - LA infiltration or nerve block to donor site.
  - IV opioid is not usually required with a working LA block.

Postoperative care

- Regular paracetamol and NSAID, plus PRN PO morphine.
- A further procedure will probably be required about a week later for removal of sutures and change of dressing. This is usually quick and can often be done in the anaesthetic room under GA.

Reconstructive free flap surgery

- Used for large wounds unsuitable for linear (primary) closure.
- Uncommon in children.
- The defect is usually caused by trauma or tumour excision.
- It involves the transfer of a free tissue flap (usually musculocutaneous, possibly with bone) to a site of tissue loss, where its circulation is restored with microvascular anastomoses.
- A muscle flap produces a better appearance and defence against infection than a skin graft.
- Flap success rate is better than in adults (better vessels, increased blood flow).
- The principles of GA for flap reconstruction apply to reimplantation surgery.

Surgery involves

- Elevation of the flap and clamping of vessels.
- Primary ischaemia as blood flow ceases and intracellular metabolism becomes anaerobic.
- Reperfusion as the arterial and venous anastomoses are completed and the clamps released. Ideally, re-establishment of blood flow reverses the transient physiological derangement produced by primary ischaemia.
- Secondary ischaemia occurs after a free flap has been transplanted and reperfused. This period of ischaemia is more damaging to the flap than primary ischaemia. Flaps affected by secondary ischaemia have intravascular thrombosis and interstitial oedema. Local fibrinogen and platelet concentrations ↑. Skin flaps can tolerate 10–12 h of ischaemia, but irreversible changes in muscle occur after 4 h.
- Surgery is prolonged (6–12 h), with several incisions. There may be significant blood and fluid losses as well as heat loss. Hypovolaemia, vasoconstriction and hypothermia ↓ blood flow to the flap and contribute to flap failure.
- Causes of flap failure:
  - The arterial anastomosis may be inadequate, in spasm, or thrombosed.
  - The venous anastomosis may be defective, in spasm, thrombosed, or compressed.
  - Oedema reduces flow to the flap and may be a result of excessive crystalloids, extreme haemodilution, trauma from handling, or a prolonged ischaemia time. Flap tissue has no lymphatic drainage and is therefore susceptible to oedema.

Specifics of preoperative assessment

- Background to the surgical condition.
- The child is likely to have had several related procedures; therefore, it is important to assess need for premedication, and assess previous GA and analgesia experiences.
- FBC, U+E, cross-match.

Anaesthetic technique

- Induction as preferred.
- ETT and IPPV. Avoid hypocapnia, which causes vasoconstriction.
- Anaesthetic maintenance of choice, bearing in mind the need to provide safe, prolonged anaesthesia and to provide optimal conditions for the free flap.
- Standard monitoring plus arterial and central lines, UO, and core and peripheral temperature.
- ↑ ambient theatre temperature, use a warming mattress/blanket and fluid warmer.
- Measure ABG and haematocrit throughout the case.
- Take great care to protect pressure areas and the corneas.
- Aim to provide the flap or reimplanted tissue with the best environment to re-establish blood supply. Optimum blood flow to and from the flap requires:
  - Vasodilation. Vessel radius is the most important determinant of flow. Adequate vasodilation requires:
    - —Maintenance of normothermia. It is essential to avoid hypothermia as it causes vasoconstriction and a ↑ in haematocrit and plasma viscosity. Monitor central and peripheral temperatures, aiming for a difference of <1°C (indicating a warm, well-filled, and vasodilated patient).
    - —Normovolaemia or mild hypervolaemia. Strict attention to fluid input is required. Maintenance fluids, replacement of insensible losses, and replacement of bleeding (from both donor and recipient site) should be considered. Provided CO is maintained, a haematocrit of 30% is ideal. Modest hypervolaemia increases CO, and decreases sympathetic vascular tone; however, excessive fluid (especially crystalloid) will accumulate in the flap, causing swelling and obstruction to venous drainage. Hypovolaemia can cause vasoconstriction.
    - —Spasm of the transplanted vessels may occur after surgical handling; the surgeon may apply a local vasodilator, e.g. papaverine.
    - —Sympathetic blockade. The ideal block is an epidural followed by a postoperative epidural infusion. Other advantages of epidural analgesia may include a ↓ in intraoperative bleeding and rapid postoperative recovery. Alternatively, a combination of PNB ± catheters may be appropriate, depending on the donor/recipient sites. Good analgesia reduces the level of circulating catecholamines and the vasoconstrictor response to pain.
  - Perfusion pressure:
    - —Usually attained by adequate depth of GA and fluid administration.
  - Viscosity:
    - —Haemodilution to a haematocrit of 30% improves flow by reducing viscosity.
    - —If the haematocrit falls further, the marginally improved flow characteristics may be offset by a ↓ in O_2 delivery.

- As the flap is mobilized, moderate hypotension provides good operating conditions and ↓ blood loss. Titrated volatile agent is ideal since it provides direct vasodilatation.
- By the time the flap is reperfused, the patient should be normothermic, vasodilated, and slightly hypervolaemic ('*warm and wet*') with a CO higher than normal.
- Vasodilators or inotropes are rarely required.
- Smooth emergence prevents sympathetic stimulation and vasoconstriction.

Postoperative care

- It is essential that the techniques employed to maintain tissue perfusion intraoperatively are continued postoperatively.
- HDU.
- Maintenance fluids. Boluses of crystalloid/colloid, if required, to maintain CVP and UO. Maintain haematocrit around 30%.
- Maintain normothermia and avoid shivering.
- Analgesia is managed with an opioid-based technique, and/or a continuous regional block. Epidural infusion analgesia (➲ Chapter 10) is ideal for lower limb flap surgery. A combination of an epidural infusion of LA to provide analgesia and vasodilation for the recipient site and an IV opiate infusion or PCA for the donor site may be required, depending on the exact procedures performed.
- Maintain normovolaemia in patients with epidural, since sympathetic blockade-mediated vasodilation may precipitate a 'steal phenomenon' in the flap if the patient is hypovolaemic.
- Prescribe regular paracetamol, NSAID, and an antiemetic PRN.
- Regular checks are performed on the flap: if ischaemia or congestion are identified early, then the flap may be salvageable.

Laser treatment for pigmented lesions and scars

- Used for cosmetic and functional management of scars, pigmented and vascular lesions, and depilation.
- Usually requires a course of treatments several months apart.
- Majority are suitable for day case.
- Older children can tolerate treatment under LA (EMLA/Ametop) ± Entonox.
- Different lasers are indicated for different pathologies, but common issues of fire safety and eye protection apply to all.
- May be isolated-site surgery.
- Laser safety for patient and staff:
  - Dedicated 'laser-safe room' with locking door, external warning light, and blackout blinds.
  - Experienced surgeon.
  - Patient protection: laser-specific external eye shield unless laser work is on the face or close to the eyes, in which case an internal eye shield is mandatory.
  - All staff must wear laser-specific external eye shields.

Preoperative assessment

- Patients have multiple treatments, so good early experiences help ↓ anxiety for future sessions.
- Commonly 'frequent fliers' with experience of GA.
- Usually well children, but may have associated comorbidities from underlying pathology (e.g. neurological aspects of Sturge–Weber syndrome).

Anaesthetic technique

- Most small lesions take minutes to laser.
- Induction and maintenance as preferred.
- Airway management:
  - Due care is required in patients with neck or facial scarring that may limit neck extension or mouth opening.
  - Intubation is rarely necessary and spontaneous ventilation with mask or LMA is usual. Some centres continue to wrap/cover ETT or LMA to minimize risk of fire. Ensure adequate scavenging of anaesthetic gases. There is a risk of fire with a high concentration of O_2 in the laser field.
- Analgesia:
  - Preoperative paracetamol and NSAID.
  - For CO_2 or erbium:YAG laser treatment, consider surgically administered LA and/or an opiate, e.g. fentanyl.
  - Cool/ice packs or gel (e.g. Aloe vera) to treated area to improve comfort.

Minor non-elective surgery

- The majority are peripheral lacerations or finger injuries.
- Emergency procedures are rare; the majority can wait until fasted and listed semi-electively for the following day.

Lacerations

- Lacerations to the head and peripheries, and fingertip injuries, are very common.
- Surgery involves exploration to exclude damage to underlying structures, debridement of dead and dirty tissue, and cleaning and suturing of the wound.
- Many procedures can be performed under LA only, but this is often poorly tolerated, especially in younger children.

Preoperative assessment
- Most are ASA 1 or 2.

Anaesthetic management
- Induction and maintenance as preferred.
- Usually LMA with SV.
- Paracetamol and NSAID.
- PNB or LA infiltration.
- A tourniquet is often required and blood loss is usually minimal.
- Antibiotics, if required, are given prior to inflating tourniquet.
- The procedure may become prolonged if damage is found during exploration.

Postoperative care
- Prescribe regular paracetamol and NSAID, plus PRN PO morphine.
- Day case unless surgically complex or requiring continued IV antibiotics.

Bite injury

- Child protection considerations may be necessary.
- Classically dog bites to extremity or face (infrequently human bite).
- High risk of underlying structural injury through crush or rotational force, and a high degree of suspicion is required.
- High infection risk; all but the most minor injuries need thorough washout and repair.
- GA management as for lacerations.
- Patients and families may be particularly psychologically traumatized.

Nerve, tendon, and digital vessel repairs

- Classically a broken-glass injury to the hand.

Preoperative assessment
- Usually ASA 1 or 2. Surgery is delayed until fasted unless perfusion is compromised.
- If opioid analgesia has been given in the emergency department, consider the regurgitation risk.

Anaesthetic technique
- An RSI is performed if indicated.
- IPPV may be preferable to SV for prolonged procedures and in younger children.
- Surgery may be prolonged; consider pressure-area care, temperature monitoring, and maintenance IV fluids.
- A tourniquet is usually used and blood loss is minimal.
- Paracetamol and NSAID.
- Nerve blocks are a relative contraindication in nerve repair procedures since they can make postoperative assessment of neurological function difficult. Weak solutions of LA may minimize motor block.
- LA wound infiltration.
- An opioid, e.g. morphine or fentanyl, may be required.

Postoperative care
- Prescribe regular paracetamol and NSAID, plus PRN PO morphine.
- Frequent assessment of neurological function required.
- IV fluids until oral intake resumes.

Burns and scalds

- Burns and scalds require anaesthetic involvement in initial resuscitation, ICU, surgical procedures, and acute and chronic pain management.
- They account for 6% of paediatric injuries. In the UK, approximately 40,000 children attend hospital yearly with a burn or scald and between 6,000 and 7,000 require admission.
- The majority involve preschool children, most commonly between 1 and 2 years.
- The most common injuries are scald burns from hot beverages, followed by contact burns.
- House fires are the cause of most fatal burns (approximately 80%), with smoke inhalation being the immediate cause of death in many cases.
- Non-fatal flame burns generally involve flammable clothing and liquids.
- Children have nearly three times the BSA:mass ratio of adults. Fluid losses are proportionally higher and consequently they require relatively greater fluid resuscitation.
- Children <2 years old have thinner skin and insulating subcutaneous tissue than older children and adults. Because of this, a burn that may initially appear to be partial thickness may instead be full thickness in depth.
- Severity is related to the temperature and the duration of contact. At 44°C, contact with a heat source would require 6 h for tissue damage to occur; at 70°C, epidermal injury occurs in 1 s.
- The extent of a burn is categorized by the %BSA involved and the depth of the burn. There are several age-related assessment charts (Fig. 25.1), and for assessment of smaller areas, the child's hand is used as an indicator of approximately 1% BSA.
- Superficial burns (erythema):
  - Involve the outer epidermal tissues, are erythematous and painful, but cause minimal tissue damage.
  - The protective function of the skin remains intact.
- Partial thickness burns:
  - Involve entire epidermis and variable portions of the dermis. There is blistering of the skin and weeping transudates, and they are extremely painful.
  - Superficial partial thickness burns heal quickly with re-epithelialization from hair follicles and sweat glands and minimal scarring.
  - In deep partial thickness burns, there are few viable epithelial cells. Re-epithelialization is very slow and scarring occurs if skin grafting is not performed.
- Full thickness burns:
  - Destroy the dermis and epidermis.
  - The surface has a dry leathery firm consistency with charring or pearly white discoloration.
  - Not painful.
  - This tissue is avascular and there is a zone of ischaemia between the dead tissue above and the live tissue below.
  - Skin grafting is always required.

% Total Body Surface Area Burn
Be clear and accurate, and do not include erythema
(Lund and Browder)

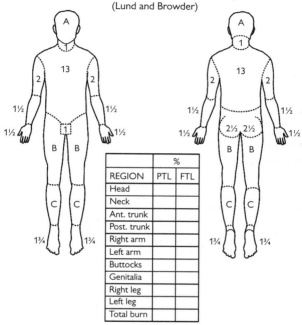

	%	
REGION	PTL	FTL
Head		
Neck		
Ant. trunk		
Post. trunk		
Right arm		
Left arm		
Buttocks		
Genitalia		
Right leg		
Left leg		
Total burn		

AREA	Age 0	1	5	10	15	Adult
A = ½ OF HEAD	9½	8½	6½	5½	4½	3½
B = ½ OF ONE THIGH	2¾	3¼	4	4½	4½	4¾
C = ½ OF ONE LOWER LEG	2½	2½	2¾	3	3¼	3½

Fig. 25.1 Lund and Browder burns chart.

Reproduced with permission from Hettiaratchy, S., et al. Initial management of a major burn: II—assessment and resuscitation. *British Medical Journal*. 2004, **329**: 101–103. Copyright © 2004 The BMJ Publishing Group Ltd

Reproduced with permission from Hettiaratchy, S., *et al. British Medical Journal* 2004, **329**: 101–103

- Major burns are defined in different ways:
  - Partial and full thickness with >10% BSA affected, <10 years old.
  - Partial and full thickness with >20% BSA affected, >10 years old.
  - Full thickness with >5% BSA affected.
  - Partial or full thickness involving face, hands, feet, perineum, or major joints.
  - Partial or full thickness involving an electrical or chemical burn.
  - Partial or full thickness involving an inhalational injury.
  - Partial or full thickness associated with a pre-existing comorbidity.
- Morbidity and mortality ↑ with the size and depth of the burn and with ↓ age.
- Commonest cause of death within the first hour is smoke inhalation.
- When assessing a severe burn, it is easy to become distracted and focus solely on the burn. The structured approach to major trauma is followed with burn assessment occurring during the secondary survey.
- It is important that the exact mechanism is sought—consider NAI.

Primary survey

- High-flow O_2 from a face mask with a reservoir bag.
- Consider fitting a cervical collar if there is potential injury to the spine from a fall or escape attempt and if no history is available.
- Seek information from witnesses, firefighters, and paramedics whilst the primary survey is taking place. A history of exposure to smoke in a confined space for any length of time indicates a potential inhalational injury.
- There could be airway compromise related to a thermal injury to the upper airway from inhalation of hot gases or smoke, because of burns to the face or neck, from chemical injury to the lung, and from asphyxia. Look for singeing of facial hair and carbonaceous deposits in the oropharynx. Listen for wheeze and stridor.
- Oedema of the airway and face can occur very rapidly following burn and/or significant smoke inhalation. If there is concern that the airway may deteriorate, the patient should be anaesthetized and the airway secured with an appropriately sized uncut ETT at an early stage in the assessment.
- A RSI is appropriate if respiratory function is inadequate and there are no concerns about the airway. If there are concerns that maintaining the airway or intubating the patient may be difficult, an inhalational induction and ETT without neuromuscular blockade should be considered.
- If the airway is adequate, breathing is assessed looking for abnormal chest movement, RR, wheeze, crepitations, and cyanosis. If there are signs of hypoventilation, and the patient is not already intubated and ventilated, this should be carried out.
- A full thickness circumferential chest burn (or abdominal burn in infants) can hinder respiratory movements of the chest; escharotomies should be performed. Although the full thickness burn is insensate (dermal nerve endings are destroyed), effective incisions must extend into innervated tissue and so GA is required.
- Large-bore IV access on two limbs is secured expediently (US may assist). Burnt areas should be avoided where possible. The IO route can be used for initial fluid resuscitation. Samples for FBC, U+E, and group and save are taken. An ABG is required to measure the percentage of carboxyhaemoglobin (can cause a deceptively high SpO_2 reading).

- Although major burns are associated with large volumes of fluid loss in the first 4–6 h, signs of hypovolaemia on initial presentation should be assumed to be due to other causes, e.g. fractures.

Secondary survey

- With a major burn, there is a rapid reduction in plasma volume owing to loss of the skin's barrier function and to oedema. Oedema is caused by an ↑ in microvascular permeability and tissue osmotic pressure that leads to interstitial fluid accumulation.
- Unburned tissue becomes oedematous owing to a transient endothelial injury related to a ↑ in the concentration of systemic inflammatory mediators and the presence of hypoproteinaemia.
- Cover burned areas to ↓ heat and fluid loss, protect against infection, and aid analgesia. Initially, cling film can be used, with specialized dressings being applied later.
- There are a number of formulas for *estimating* fluid requirements. The simplest is the Parkland formula:

  %BSA burnt × weight in kg × 4 = volume of crystalloid fluid (mL) required in the first 24 h *from the time of burn*

  - Usually given as Hartmann's solution.
  - 50% of calculated volume given in first 8 h, the remainder given over next 16 h.
  - Maintenance fluids are required in addition to resuscitation fluids.
  - It is essential that fluid balance be assessed regularly. UO should be 1 mL/kg/h and the fluid regimen adjusted as necessary to achieve this.
  - Other signs of adequate resuscitation are rapid capillary refill, a decline in a high haematocrit and a normal or normalizing pH. It is important to ↓ fluids as necessary, because over-resuscitation is a cause of significant morbidity.
- Opiate analgesia is usually required, e.g. intranasal diamorphine (effective, well tolerated, and a rapid onset) or IV morphine Bolus (100 mcg/kg bolus- may be repeated every 5 minutes to effect) followed by IV morphine infusion of 20–60 mcg/kg/hr. Many centres use NCA/PCA systems for IV opiate infusions.
- Urinary catheter.
- Cyanide is a product of combustion of common household materials. Suspect cyanide poisoning in a patient from a house fire with lactic acidosis unresponsive to fluid resuscitation, high SvO_2, and reduced LOC. There are specific antidotes, e.g. hydroxocobalamin.
- Once the child has been stabilized, a management plan is made by a senior plastic surgeon. This usually involves multiple visits to theatre for assessment, staged skin grafting, and dressing changes.
- In the UK, there are regional burns networks giving clear guidelines for the transfer and management of increasingly severe and complex paediatric burns. Regional burns centres concentrate the necessary resources and expertise needed to manage these complex patients.

Anaesthesia for patients with burns and scalds

- Patients range from toddlers with small contact burns or small chest wall scalds caused by pulling a cup of hot liquid on to themselves who

are well, feeding normally, and playing on the ward to children with extensive burns and smoke inhalation being ventilated on ICU.
- GA is usually required for the initial cleaning and dressing of burns or scalds, subsequent skin grafts, and extensive changes of dressings.
- Minor dressing changes are performed on the ward with a combination of PO sedation and analgesia, e.g. midazolam and morphine, intranasal diamorphine, ketamine IV/IM, or Entonox® (➔ Chapter 12).

Preoperative assessment
- Patients may be on ICU, intubated and ventilated with arterial and central venous access.
- Assess the history related to the burn, extent of burn, adequacy of resuscitation, and comorbidities. Correct electrolyte imbalances preoperatively.
- Anticipate significant blood loss during extensive grafting. Group and save or cross-match blood.
- Patients usually undergo a series of operations. Family members may have died in the fire. Minimize the psychological and physiological disruption: quiet environment preoperatively and at induction, sedative premedication if necessary, minimize fasting time.
- Nasogastric or nasojejunal feeds are continued in intubated patients. Minimizing starvation times and maximizing essential nutrition is an important consideration. There is a general move towards establishing NJ feeding and, if tolerated, not stopping feeds even if unintubated.
- Chest symptoms are common secondary to infection, significant opioid consumption with cough suppression, and restriction of chest movement and coughing by circumferential dressings around the trunk.
- Wounds are frequently colonized/infected and patients may be febrile and tachycardic from sepsis or simply in a hypermetabolic state.
- Parents are usually devastated and require sensitive communication. Following a house fire, it is not uncommon for the parents to be patients in an adult hospital and unavailable to give a history or to comfort the child.

Anaesthetic technique
- ICU patients are transferred to theatre with sedative and analgesic infusions continued. Additional volatile anaesthetic is usually given.
- Given that most patients are preschool, an inhalational induction is easier in most cases without IV access.
- Facial burns may present a challenge with regard to airway management. Mask ventilation may be problematic with difficulty achieving a seal owing to dressings and NG/NJ tubes.
- Venous access is obtained once anaesthetized. This is often difficult if limbs are burnt. Do not place IV access where grafts are to be harvested from.
- Central venous access may be required owing to a lack of cannulation sites. A femoral vein is often used (➔ Chapter 10), since the groin skin creases are often unburnt. Avoid cut-downs, because they ↑ infection risk.
- LMA with SV can be used for minor scalds and burns.

- ETT and IPPV are usually indicated.
- Securing the ETT in the presence of facial burns requires some consideration. Nasal ETT may be considered less mobile. Simple ties are often employed. Securing to a nasal sling or oral fixation to teeth are also well-described techniques.
- Although suxamethonium can be used safely during the initial treatment of a burn (<24–48 h), it is later contraindicated for up to 18 months because of the danger of hyperK$^+$. There is often a relative resistance to non-depolarizing neuromuscular blockers for several weeks after a major burn.
- Application of monitoring equipment, e.g. ECG, SpO$_2$, and NIBP cuffs, may be difficult. Consider invasive monitoring for major cases.
- Maintenance as preferred.
- There is risk of hypothermia. Increase the ambient theatre temperature, use a warming mattress, and warm IV fluids. A warming blanket is often unfeasible, given the extent of access to the patient required by the surgical team. Vigilance from all staff to heat conservation and minimizing heat loss is necessary.
- The application of circumferential dressings around the trunk requires a team of people to lift and hold the child off the operating table, and for this reason, if no other, in many cases a secure ETT is chosen. Ensure that these dressings allow adequate ventilation.
- Skin grafts are often taken from a thigh if this is unburnt. If the thighs are unavailable or the burn is very extensive, skin may be harvested from the back. This requires the child to be positioned lateral or prone.
- ↓ infection risk: minimal theatre personnel; use aseptic techniques where possible.
- Major haemorrhage can occur during grafting of extensive burns. Adequate-gauge IV access is required and equipment for a rapid transfusion prepared. Blood loss can be reduced by staging the necessary procedures and infiltrating the burn sites generously with a very dilute solution of 1:500,000 adrenaline.
- Analgesia:
  - IV paracetamol
  - Morphine sulfate 100–150 mcg/kg IV or fentanyl citrate 2–4 mcg/kg IV. Many children have been receiving regular opioids and other sedatives during admission and may be resistant to normal doses of opioid.
  - Consider co-analgesics, e.g. ketamine and clonidine.
  - Regional anaesthesia can be a useful adjunct.
  - Harvest sites can be covered with swabs soaked in a dilute solution of LA.
- A GA presents the opportunity to perform additional procedures, e.g. change of NGT, peripheral or central venous access, or urinary catheter that would distress the child if performed when awake.

Postoperative care
- The patient may be returned to ITU anaesthetized and ventilated. Otherwise, the child is extubated awake and observed closely to ensure circumferential dressings around the chest do not impede ventilation.

- Maintenance fluids are given until feeding resumes. FBC and U+E are checked after extensive grafting. Blood is transfused if necessary.
- Burn pain can be very severe, and the pain threshold is decreased because of the local inflammatory response. The patient will have background pain and procedural pain. Use a multimodal approach to pain management.
- Analgesia requirements are very variable and depend on the extent of the burn and grafting and previous analgesia administration. For minor procedures a combination of paracetamol PO 6-hourly and morphine sulfate 200–300 mcg/kg oral 4-hourly is adequate.
- In many cases, an NCA/PCA (➲ Chapter 12) will be appropriate.
- NSAIDs are a relative contraindication, particularly in the resuscitation phase.
- Major or complex burns require input from paediatric pain services, e.g. ketamine and/or clonidine infusions, opioid rotation, and gabapentin 10 mg/kg oral 8-hourly (started gradually over 3 days).
- Pruritus can be a significant issue for patients with healing burns. Initially, moisturizing and cooling may be of benefit, but frequently pharmacological intervention is necessary. Gabapentin 5 mg/kg oral 8-hourly, chlorphenamine, and cetirizine can all be used in isolation or combination. Laser treatment is sometimes beneficial.

Long term
- If symptoms of neuropathic pain occur, refer to chronic pain specialist. The patient may need low-dose tricyclic antidepressants or long-term gabapentin.
- Consider TENS machine and relaxation techniques in older children.
- Anxiety and post-traumatic stress disorder require expert psychological input for both the patient and their family.

Section 6

Syndromes and diseases

Comorbidities and syndromes

Anthony Moores

Arthrogryposis multiplex congenital

- A descriptive term for the occurrence of multiple non-progressive congenital joint contractures within a syndrome or symptoms complex. Can affect joints of all four limbs, the spine, and the jaw with varying degrees of severity. May be associated with other congenital malformations.

Aetiology

- Incidence 1:3,000–1:10,000 live births.
- Unknown aetiology; however, the effect of early fetal akinesia on joint and muscle development is thought to play a role.
- Causes of this can be classified into external mechanical factors (oligohydramnios, twin pregnancy, amniotic bands, fibroids), neuropathic, myopathic (central core disease, myotonic dystrophy, congenital myasthenia), and abnormal connective tissue. Maternal disease, e.g. myasthenia gravis or drug consumption during pregnancy, can be causal.
- The commonest diagnostic subgroup is associated with hypoplastic muscle (amyoplasia congenita), probably arising from a developmental defect in fetal muscle. Amyoplasia tends to occur sporadically. Those affected have fatty and fibrous tissue replacement of their limb muscles. In these cases, all four limbs are involved in a symmetrical pattern.
- The 'neuropathic' forms show denervation atrophy of muscles and reduced number and size of anterior horn cells in the spinal cord. Demyelination may be seen in the pyramidal tracts and motor roots.
- >200 other syndromes and conditions are associated with congenital contractures, e.g. CP, and rarely ARC syndrome (arthrogryposis, renal dysfunction, and cholestasis).

Clinical features

- Usually normal intelligence.
- The upper limbs have internally rotated shoulders, extension contractures of the elbows, deformities of flexion, and ulnar deviation of the wrists and flexed fingers.
- The lower limb abnormalities may include equinovarus deformities of the feet, the hips are flexed and dislocated, and the knees hyper-extended and dislocated.
- Distal muscles are usually small and wasted with absent reflexes, and there may be webbing of soft tissues.
- The skin is often thickened and tense with dimples over the affected joints and lack normal skin creases.
- Other abnormalities may be present, e.g. micrognathia, CHD, scoliosis, cleft palate, hypoplastic lungs, and genitourinary abnormalities.
- Patients commonly present for diagnostic muscle biopsies, MRI, and correction of orthopaedic abnormalities.

Anaesthetic management

- Potential airway difficulties in up to 25%. Typical reasons for this include micrognathia, temporomandibular joint involvement, trismus, cleft palate, Pierre Robin sequence, high-arched palate, small mouth, cervical spine involvement (scoliosis, short neck, Klippel–Feil syndrome), large facial haemangiomas, and limited tongue protrusion.

- Potential for chronic lung disease from recurrent aspiration and restrictive lung function owing to scoliosis.
- Difficult IV access owing to extensive contractures, tense skin, and minimal subcutaneous tissues and muscle mass.
- Careful positioning and padding of pressure point areas.
- Association with hypermetabolic responses to GA, although this is more likely to be due to an underlying primary neuromuscular disorder. In cases where hyperthermia occurred, active cooling has been sufficient in treating the patient. A link with MH remains unproven. However, patients with an associated myopathy may be at risk of MH.
- More susceptible to the depressant effects of GA agents and possibly opiates.
- Avoid suxamethonium in patients with a recognized underlying myopathic cause of their AMC due to the risk of an exaggerated hyperK$^+$ response.
- A small increased sensitivity to non-depolarizing muscle relaxants due to lower muscle mass and underlying neurogenic and myopathic changes. Use lower doses and use neuromuscular function monitoring.
- Regional techniques may be difficult or impossible owing to problems positioning the patient and to associated spinal anomalies.

Asthma

- Presents as recurrent episodes of wheezing, coughing, breathlessness, chest tightness, airway oedema, and reversible airflow obstruction within the lungs. A nocturnal cough may be the only symptom.
- Increased risk for perioperative respiratory complications. Overall morbidity and mortality have decreased as a result of improved prevention.
- Drug classes include inhaled short and long-acting β_2-adrenergic agonists, inhaled or oral corticosteroids, inhaled anticholinergics, and leukotriene-receptor antagonists. Methylxanthines have benefit as rescue medication in severe cases.
- In most cases, asthma is well controlled and there is no need to modify standard GA practice. Most suggested modifications only required in a severe asthmatic or in a symptomatic child anaesthetized for emergency surgery.

Preoperative assessment

- Is the diagnosis of asthma correct? Some children aged <3 years will get occasional symptoms of cough and wheeze following a respiratory viral illness for which they may be prescribed inhalers but not necessarily develop asthma. Gastro-oesophageal reflux may also give rise to a nocturnal cough.
- Establish severity of disease and level of control. Patients on a single inhaler, e.g. salbutamol, are likely to have mild disease, whereas children on several different classes of medications are likely to have more severe disease.
- Enquire about any recent changes in their medication regime. Nocturnal cough can be a sign of poor control. Exercise tolerance is an indicator of severity.
- History of recent exacerbations requiring an ↑ in inhaler use, PO corticosteroids, and visits/admissions to hospital/ICU (requiring IPPV or IV infusions) all suggest severe disease.
- The use of >2 weeks of systemic corticosteroids in the past 6 months requires consideration of perioperative steroid supplementation to avoid an adrenal crisis.
- Determine triggers for asthma: cold, exercise, pollen, RTI, exposure to allergens.
- Passive smoking may also ↑ the risk of perioperative respiratory adverse events.
- Children may have a history of atopy or allergies to agents, including latex.
- Children with an RTI or current wheeze should have elective surgery postponed until their symptoms are better controlled, ideally for 4–6 weeks.
- Continue all current medication.
- β_2-agonists are often given pre induction to ↓ airway irritability.
- Poorly controlled asthmatics may have been started on inhaled steroids (in severe cases PO steroids) the week before surgery.

Intraoperative management

Induction

- Inhalational or IV.
- Compared with thiopental and etomidate, propofol attenuates the bronchospastic response to intubation in asthmatics and non-asthmatics.
- Ketamine is the agent of choice for haemodynamically unstable asthmatic patients owing to its ability to produce direct smooth muscle relaxation without any negative cardiovascular effects. An anticholinergic is often given also to ↓ airway secretions.
- Consider supplemental dose of IV corticosteroid.
- ETT increases airway resistance. This is not observed with LMA or facemasks, but their use must be balanced with the risks of an unsecured airway.
- An inadequate depth of GA is a common cause of bronchospasm.
- IV lidocaine 1.0–1.5 mg/kg 1–3 min prior to tracheal intubation has been shown to ↓ reflex airway bronchoconstriction. Topical administration to the larynx may provoke bronchospasm.

Maintenance

- Sevoflurane is first choice—bronchodilator.
- Avoid desflurane—increases airway resistance.
- Humidify inspiratory gases.
- Non-histamine-releasing neuromuscular blocking drugs, e.g. rocuronium, are safe.
- Ventilation strategies to avoid air-trapping and auto-PEEP include limiting the peak inspiratory pressures and V_T, and increasing the I:E ratio assist.
- If required, tracheal suctioning should only be performed at deep levels of GA.
- Have a high index of suspicion for complications, e.g. bronchospasm and anaphylaxis.

Emergence

- Muscarinic side effects of acetylcholinesterase inhibitors may provoke bronchospasm.
- There is a small incidence of sugammadex causing bronchospasm in adult studies.
- The decision to extubate "deep" or awake depends on the experience of the anaesthetist and the clinical situation. Deep extubation avoids mechanical stimulation from the ETT, while awake extubation ensures a secure airway immediately after extubation.

Analgesia

- NSAIDs are contraindicated if there is a history of adverse reaction or nasal polyps.

Attention deficit hyperactivity disorder (ADHD)

- ADHD is a heterogeneous neurobehavioural syndrome characterized by a combination of the core symptoms of hyperactivity, poor impulse control, and inattention.
- Increasing prevalence; 3–9% of school-age children and young people are affected.
- 3M:1F
- Commoner in lower socio-economic groups.
- Multifactorial aetiology; approximately 50% have coexisting disorders of mood, conduct, learning, motor control, communication, and anxiety disorders.
- Inadequate dopamine and noradrenaline (norepinephrine) in the fronto–subcortical–cerebellar regions may cause under-stimulation of inhibitory pathways. The effectiveness of stimulants in treatment supports this theory.
- The main issues are management of perioperative anxiety, agitation at induction and emergence, and postoperative behavioural changes.
- Drug treatment is reserved for severe symptoms or patients who have refused or not responded to non-drug interventions. There is concern over the possibility of drug interactions between their current medication and GA agents.

Stimulants
- Methylphenidate. Mechanism of action is to block dopamine and noradrenaline reuptake.
- Dextroamphetamines block dopamine and noradrenaline reuptake and inhibit the enzyme monoamine oxidase.
- Lisdexamfetamine is a prodrug of dextroamphetamine (dexamfetamine) with a longer duration of action and less potential for abuse.
- Consequences are potentially an ↑ in the MAC of volatile agents and an increased dose for sedative medications, including propofol and dexmedetomidine.
- Pro-seizure activity and cardiovascular effects may be exacerbated by a number of drugs, including tramadol, pethidine and ephedrine.

Non-stimulants
- Atomoxetine is a selective noradrenaline reuptake inhibitor, especially in the prefrontal cortex. It also is a NMDA receptor antagonist. Glutaminergic dysfunction has been implicated in the pathophysiology and aetiology of ADHD.
- Side effects are much milder than those of stimulants. Potentiates CVS effects of salbutamol. Use sympathomimetics with caution.
- Clonidine has been used alone and in combination with stimulants.

Perioperative management
- Children with ADHD are intolerant of long waiting times, becoming agitated and disruptive. Schedule to be first on the list.

- Provide a quiet, calm environment with age-appropriate toys or activities to help minimize anxiety and disruptive behaviour.
- Distraction techniques provided by play specialists may minimize distress preoperatively and at induction of GA.
- Premedication may prove beneficial. The effects may be difficult to predict and less effective if the child is on stimulants.
- Medications modify noradrenergic and dopaminergic function in the CNS. They may ↓ the seizure threshold and predispose to PONV.

Autistic spectrum disorder (ASD)

- ASD is a neurodevelopmental disorder characterized by functional impairments in social communication, and restricted or stereotyped patterns of behaviour. There may be touch, visual, taste, or sound hypersensitivity.
- About 1% incidence. Usually diagnosed before 3 years of age. The male-to-female ratio varies with intellectual impairment. 4M:1F in the higher-IQ group, dropping to approximately 2M:1F in the lower-IQ group.
- Associated with IQ <70 in about 55% of patients, although up to 3% have a higher than average IQ.
- Unknown aetiology.
- The recent diagnostic classification systems are based on observation and assessment of behaviour and cognition: the Diagnostic and Statistical Manual of Mental Disorders 5 and the International Classification of Diseases 10.

Clinical features

- Social communication and interaction:
  - Speech delayed or absent. May have difficulty initiating or maintaining a conversation. Language may be repetitive, stereotyped, or idiosyncratic. They may not understand synonyms in context, humour, or metaphors.
  - Possible difficulties with non-verbal communication, e.g. facial expressions.
  - May have difficulty with social/emotional reciprocity, affecting interactive flow of conversation with others, reduced sharing of interests and emotions, or an inability to respond to social interactions.
  - Possible difficulty developing and understanding relationships amongst their developmental peers; may show no interest at all in interacting with others.
- Behaviour and interests:
  - May have ritualistic and repetitive behaviour. This may include inflexible routines or patterns of behaviour, e.g. eating the same food each day, or having a particular cup that they use.
  - There can be extreme distress if their routine is altered, e.g. hospital admission.
  - They often develop a special and often abnormal fixated interest in unusual objects. The presence of these can often help with cooperation and reduction of anxiety in stressful situations.
  - They may also have stereotypical or repetitive motor movements.
- Sensory input:
  - There may be an exaggerated or reduced response to sensory input and unusual fascination with sensations, e.g. lights.
  - May get upset with tactile sensation during a medical intervention/examination, or the strange feeling of being made to wear an unusual item of clothing of a different texture to their clothes, e.g. a theatre gown.

- Certain noises may upset them, e.g. a vacuum cleaner or even a stranger speaking.
- May not appear to sense/react normally to pain or extremes of temperature.
- May have other associated psychiatric problems: social anxiety disorders (29%), ADHD (28%), conduct disorder (30%), and major depressive disorder (1%). Self-harm and aggressive or challenging behaviour may be common, especially in response to stressful situations.
- Epilepsy is common: 18% of males and 30% of females.
- Sleep problems are common.

Perioperative management
- Advance warning and preparation prior to admission allows time to assess the child's needs and to put measures in place to meet them.
- Where possible, surgical specialties should coordinate multiple interventions under the same GA.
- The pre-assessment nursing staff should contact the parent/carer by telephone to ask questions about the child's routines, special interests, likes, and dislikes. They can establish their level of intelligence and what level of information the child may benefit from receiving. Social stories and videos can be used (at home and in school) to prepare them for admission.
- It may be possible for height, weight, and baseline observations to be carried out in the community.
- Encourage parents to bring in comforters, e.g. a favourite toy.
- It is important to be flexible with the admission process; ensure all staff are aware of and accommodate the needs of the child.
- Place first on morning list to minimize fasting and upset from altered routines.
- There should be a quiet waiting area away from other children, and equally one for the recovery period.
- It may be sensible to leave the child in their own clothes rather than changing them into an unfamiliar hospital gown.
- May get upset with the application of ID bracelet or LA cream to their hands: accommodate their wishes.
- It is important to recognize that the child may not want to interact with you during your visit.
- The parents may have had previous experience of their child undergoing GA; this information is invaluable in forming a plan. It is important to speak quietly and calmly, giving clear explanations of what is going to happen and what will happen if things do not go to plan.
- May be on antipsychotic medication, e.g. risperidone and clozapine, which may interact with GA agents. Discuss their perioperative use with psychiatrist and consider alternative agents. Psychostimulants, e.g. methylphenidate, may alter the response to sedatives and GA agents, and ↑ the risk of sudden hypertension.
- Premedication is often required where parental presence and non-pharmacological calming methods are not enough to achieve a smooth induction. It may be a challenge to persuade the child to take

premedication, and often it must be disguised in cordial—consider using their favourite drinking cup.
- If there have been difficulties with premedication on previous visits it may be necessary to give it to the child at home, e.g. lorazepam.
- For very difficult, children consider ketamine 5–10 mg/kg PO. This can be mixed with midazolam 0.5 mg/kg; use a lower ketamine dose of 3 mg/kg. If PO premedication is refused and it is not possible to perform a gas induction, IM ketamine 5 mg/kg may be required.
- Avoid restraint where possible. If it is considered the only option and surgery is essential, then this should be discussed with the parents to explain what to expect. The parents or carers may be skilled in restraining their child, and together with the help of trained staff this will facilitate induction.
- Some parents prefer restraint to the side effects of premedication, which can be very distressing and delay discharge to the safe environment of home.
- Document the pre-induction events to inform future admissions.
- The anaesthetic room should be quiet (perhaps with low-level lighting), with only necessary staff present. Generally it is best to have both parents present.
- If the child is still uncooperative despite premedication, a discussion about whether to proceed should take place with all concerned.
- Multimodal analgesia as per normal. Antiemetics and a fluid bolus of crystalloid solution to ↓ PONV. It may be difficult to get the child to take any analgesic medicines postoperatively.
- For day surgery, a rapid smooth recovery with early removal of the IV cannula and discharge home can help ↓ distress.
- Pain assessment can be difficult; a non-verbal tool may be required, e.g. FLACC scale.
- For major surgery, NCA may be required. Secure all forms of lines to avoid them being pulled out.

Branchial (pharyngeal) arch syndromes

- Structures of the mandible, ear, and neck develop from six pharyngeal (branchial) arches. The 1st, 2nd, and 3rd give rise to supralaryngeal structures, the 4th and 6th become the larynx and trachea, and the 5th arch regresses.

Goldenhar syndrome

- A congenital defect of the 1st and 2nd branchial arch derivatives resulting in asymmetric craniofacial abnormalities.
- It is a variant of the oculo-auriculo-vertebral spectrum. It consists of hemifacial microsomia, epibulbar dermoids, and vertebral abnormalities.
- Cardiac and limb abnormalities and renal, lung, and CNS defects may occur.
- Cases occur sporadically, but rarely are inherited in an autosomal dominant manner.
- 3M:2F.

Clinical features

- Patients present with unilateral hypoplasia of the mandible, zygoma (malar), and maxilla accompanied by epibulbar dermoids.
- Facial asymmetry may worsen with age.
- The ear on the affected side may be absent or abnormal in shape or size. There may be atresia of the external auditory canal, preauricular skin tags, pretragal fistulae, and a high incidence of unilateral deafness.
- Coloboma of the upper eyelid is common. There may be defects of the extraocular muscles, cataracts, or atrophy of the iris.
- Associated CHD (VSD, TGA, or tetralogy of Fallot) and vertebral abnormalities: cervical spine instability, spinal fusions, scoliosis (40%).
- May have a cleft lip and/or palate.
- Pulmonary hypoplasia/agenesis, tracheoesophageal fistula, oesophageal atresia, and laryngomalacia may be present.
- Often have a low IQ.
- Patients tend to present for reconstructive ear surgery, ophthalmic surgery, or mandibular advancement surgery.

Perioperative management

- Airway management may become more difficult with age, with the facial asymmetry becoming more pronounced. Previous GA charts may give a reassuring false impression of laryngoscopy grade to expect.
- Facial asymmetry may result in difficulty in achieving a facemask seal.
- Laryngoscopy and intubation can be difficult, especially if the right side is affected; fibreoptic intubation, tracheostomy, and video laryngoscopy may assist.
- CHD and craniovertebral anomalies require assessment.
- OSA is common and may be exacerbated by GA and perioperative opioids.
- Awake extubation recommended.

Treacher Collins syndrome (mandibulofacial dysostosis)

- Autosomal dominant disorder of craniofacial development resulting from developmental anomalies of the 1st and 2nd branchial arches. It results in symmetrical malformations of the head and neck.
- Nager syndrome presents similar GA problems. In addition to mandibulofacial dysostosis, there are preaxial limb anomalies (hypoplastic or absent thumbs, radial aplasia/hypoplasia).

Clinical features

- Hypoplasia of the facial bones (mandible and zygomatic complex), downslanting palpebral fissures, colobomata of the lower eyelids, and absent eyelashes medial to the defect.
- Abnormalities of the external pinnae, auditory canals, and middle ear ossicles resulting in a high incidence of conductive deafness.
- There may be a high-arched or cleft palate (35%), macroglossia, and malocclusion of the teeth.
- Associated with CHD, skeletal defects, chronic upper airway obstruction, OSA, and sudden death.
- Usually normal intelligence.

Perioperative management

- Difficult facemask ventilation in up to one-third of patients.
- Inhalational induction can be difficult: get an assistant to pull the mandible and tongue forward.
- An antisialogogue reduces secretions during induction.
- Difficult laryngoscopy should be anticipated. Even if previous laryngoscopies were not difficult, they may become so with increasing age.
- Fibreoptic endotracheal intubation or a videolaryngoscope are often necessary.
- The risks of apnoea and upper airway obstruction mean that sedative drugs are relatively contraindicated. Even after awake extubation, residual GA agents and opioids may result in airway compromise. Use opioid-sparing techniques, e.g. LA.
- Extubate awake.
- Monitor postoperatively on HDU or PICU owing to high incidence of respiratory complications. Occasionally, postoperative CPAP is required.

Pierre Robin sequence (PRS)

- A triad of micrognathia, glossoptosis (backward, downward displacement of the tongue) and airway obstruction.
- Commonly associated with cleft palate.
- Aetiology unknown.
- Occasionally associated with certain syndromes, specifically Treacher Collins, Stickler, fetal alcohol, and velocardiofacial (22q, 11.2 deletion).
- Incidence 1:5,000–1:85,000.
- Presentation: variable degree of airway obstruction and respiratory distress. The extent is judged clinically and/or with a formal sleep study. The severity determines the neonate's ability to feed and thrive and influences treatment options.

- Mild airway obstruction is usually improved by proning the patient.
- Airway obstruction, swallowing difficulties, gastro-oesophageal reflux, and the presence of a cleft palate can result in feeding difficulties, risks of aspiration, and laryngeal oedema (worsening airway obstruction). Active assessment and management of feeding in the neonate is essential to encourage growth and ↓ morbidity.
- Airway obstruction is thought to improve with age, although there is evidence to suggest that catch-up growth of the mandible does not occur before 22 months of age.
- Therapeutic options for more severe obstruction include insertion of a NPA, tongue–lip adhesion, mandibular distraction osteogenesis, and occasionally tracheostomy.
- GA may be required for microlaryngobronchoscopy to assess levels of airway obstruction, tracheostomy, mandibular distraction, cleft palate repair, gastrostomy insertion, radiological investigations, or Nissen fundoplication.

Perioperative management
- Plan for difficult airway. If significant difficulties are anticipated, discuss with ENT colleagues.
- High incidence of OSA. They may be more sensitive to the effects of opioids postoperatively and at risk of respiratory complications. Therefore ↓ opiate doses, use LA techniques where possible, regular NSAIDs and paracetamol.
- Consider inserting a NPA before emergence.
- Awake extubation.
- Consider PICU or HDU postoperatively.

Stickler syndrome
- Autosomal dominant disorder of connective tissue
- Incidence 1:1,000.
- Often diagnosed following prenatal polyhydramnios, micrognathia, and a positive family history.
- Characterized by ocular/orofacial/musculoskeletal changes, and deafness. There is a great variation owing to the genetic heterogenicity of the syndrome.
- Most serious features are ocular with risk of retinal tears or detachment, high myopia, and vitreoretinal degeneration eventually resulting in blindness.
- Patients have a flat midface, depressed nasal bridge, short nose with anteverted nares, and micrognathia. These features become less pronounced with age. Midline facial clefting may be present, ranging in severity from a full PRS to clefting of the hard and/or soft palate, or a bifid uvula. There may be a high-arched hard palate.
- There may be joint hypermobility, arthritis from the third to fourth decade of life, and progressive conductive or sensorineural deafness.
- Patients present for cleft surgery, ENT procedures, ophthalmic surgery, and orthopaedic procedures in adult life.
- GA challenges are often similar to those for PRS.

Velocardiofacial syndrome (VCFS)

- A genetic abnormality caused by a microdeletion on chromosome 22. It may occur as a new mutation or occasionally there is autosomal dominant inheritance.
- Abnormal 3rd and 4th pharyngeal arch development affects the parathyroid glands, thymus, and conotruncal region of the heart.
- There are genetic and phenotypic similarities to DiGeorge syndrome (22q.11.2 deletion): cardiac abnormality, hypoparathyroidism (hypoCa^{2+}), and thymic aplasia.
- VCFS is the most common syndrome associated with cleft palates, representing approximately 8% of this group. These may be isolated cleft palates or submucous clefts, which may cause velopharyngeal incompetence and hypernasal speech.
- 15–20% have PRS.
- Approximately 75% have CHD: interrupted aortic arch type B (50%), truncus arteriosus (35%), tetralogy of Fallot (16%), pulmonary atresia, and VSD.
- Parathyroid dysfunction in up to 50% of patients. HypoCa^{2+} and tetany can be fatal.
- An absent or hypoplastic thymus gland results in an impaired T-cell immune response, thereby predisposing to infection. All blood products must be irradiated.
- Developmental delay and/or behavioural problems are common.
- Ophthalmological, musculoskeletal, and renal abnormalities may occur.

Cerebral palsy (CP)

- A spectrum of non-progressive neurological disorders of motor, sensory, and intellectual function that present early in life. They are the result of lesions or anomalies that occur in the early stages of brain development.
- There is a wide range in clinical severity, from a mild monoplegia to severe spastic quadriplegia. Commonest cause of childhood motor disability.
- The motor deficits are often accompanied by intellectual impairment, developmental delay, speech difficulties, and epilepsy.
- Incidence is 1–2.5:1,000 live births among babies of normal birth weight.
- Multifactorial aetiology. It may be prenatal (congenital infection, e.g. rubella, toxoplasmosis, CMV, herpes, or cerebral malformation), perinatal (asphyxia), or postnatal (IVH, cerebral ischaemia, trauma, NAI, or meningitis). There may be a genetic origin to pure ataxic or dyskinetic CP.
- Often associated with low birth weight and prematurity.

Clinical features

- Classified according to the predominant type of motor defect, i.e. spasticity (70%), ataxia (10%), dyskinesia (10%), or mixed (10%).
- Intellectual function is impaired in about two-thirds of patients; however, communication disorders and sensory deficits may mask normal intelligence.
- Spasticity may present as hemiplegia, diplegia, or quadriplegia.
- Ataxic patients have poor balance, tremor, and hypotonia, and may have uncoordinated movements.
- Dyskinesia may present with involuntary movements (athetosis or dystonia), poor postural tone, or fluctuating muscle tone.
- Epilepsy is common (30%).
- GOR and poor swallowing result in recurrent chest infections.
- May develop a progressive scoliosis that impinges on respiratory function or makes sitting difficult.
- A multidisciplinary approach is adopted, aiming to preserve motor function and mobility in those who can walk, but also to improve ease of care in those more severely affected. This is achieved by regular physiotherapy, limb splints, and antispasticity drugs.
- Antispasticity drugs include:
  - Centrally acting: baclofen (PO or intrathecal), diazepam, vigabatrin, and tizanidine. The main side effects are sedative
  - Peripherally acting: dantrolene and botulinum toxin type A. The latter is injected IM, thereby inhibiting the release of acetylcholine at the motor end-plate; the aim is to improve range of movement and reduce pain from contractures (lasts 3 months)
- Patients often present for orthopaedic surgery for muscle or tendon releases/ transfers, botulinum toxin type A injections, and osteotomies of the feet or femurs to maintain mobility and range of movement.
- Patients in wheelchairs are at risk of recurrent hip dislocations, causing problems with sitting and often chronic hip pain. Femoral and pelvic osteotomies and scoliosis surgery may be necessary to improve their position in the wheelchair.
- Patients may require GA for PEG, fundoplication, imaging, and dental work.

Perioperative management

- Usually multiple previous hospital admissions.
- Good communication and early involvement of a multidisciplinary team are important.
- The main ongoing problems are associated with recurrent chest infections, poor nutritional status, and seizure control. Continue anticonvulsant and antispasticity medications.
- Establish the child's level of communication and understanding to potentially enable provision of information and reassurance. Establish the carer's ability to assist communication, alleviate anxiety, and assess pain/distress.
- Review GA records.
- Screening questions should enquire about latex allergy.
- Use sedative premedication with caution in hypotonic patients with poor upper airway tone.
- Have the patient's carer present during induction to help alleviate the child's distress.
- GOR is common: consider an RSI.
- Induction may be challenging. IV access may be difficult owing to previous scarring and limb contractures. Gas induction may be difficult owing to excessive drooling, GOR, and an anxious, uncooperative patient. A second pair of hands is often useful.
- Position carefully on the operating table; pad pressure areas to prevent nerve, soft tissue, and bone injury.
- Patients may be especially susceptible to hypothermia if they are poorly nourished or have hypothalamic dysfunction; consider actively warming them on the ward for transfer and in the anaesthetic room during procedures, e.g. epidural insertion.
- May be resistant to suxamethonium and vecuronium.
- Intraoperative MAC values for volatiles are about 20% lower, and more so for those on anticonvulsant medications.
- Postoperative pain and muscle spasms can be difficult to manage:
  - Pain assessment can be difficult: ➔ Paediatric Pain Profile, Chapter 12.
  - 'Continuous' rather than 'on demand' multimodal analgesia regimens should be used: regular simple analgesics, nerve blocks, and opioid infusions.
  - Epidurals can be difficult to site in scoliosis patients.
  - Combinations of LA with clonidine in epidurals are beneficial in controlling spasms and pain after major orthopaedic surgery.
  - Regular PO/PR diazepam can be given prophylactically for spasms; in resistant cases, a midazolam infusion may be required.
- Restart postoperative feeding and medications as soon as possible. Adequate hydration, chest physiotherapy, care with positioning, and ensuring that plaster casts are not too tight are important to minimize morbidity.

Diabetes mellitus

- Commonest metabolic disease of childhood.
- 90% of cases are type 1 IDDM.
- Usual onset is late childhood or early adolescence.
- Unknown aetiology (partly autoimmune). There are also genetic and environmental components. Children with a family history of IDDM have an increased incidence.
- Associated with other autoimmune diseases.
- Rare forms of IDDM are due to mitochondrial disorders, steroids or chemotherapy, Prader–Willi syndrome, and CF.

Clinical features

- There may be a short history of a few weeks of polydipsia, polyuria, fatigue, anorexia, and weight loss.
- Some present acutely with ketoacidosis and coma.
- Diagnosis is confirmed in symptomatic patients with:
  - A random venous plasma glucose >11.1 mmol/L, or
  - A fasting plasma glucose >7.1 mmol/L, or
  - Plasma glucose >11.1 mmol/L 2 h after a 75 g glucose load.
- Diagnosis in asymptomatic patients: a plasma glucose >11.1 mmol/L repeated on another day (fasting, random or 2 h post 75 g glucose load).
- Impaired glucose tolerance is when fasting plasma glucose is <7.0 mmol/L and plasma glucose 2 h post 75 g glucose load is 7.8–11.1 mmol/L.

Treatment

- Three types of insulin preparations: short-, intermediate-, and long-acting.
- Treatment regimen is personalized, usually combining an intermediate/long-acting with a short-acting insulin.
- Increasing use of insulin pumps, which deliver a rapid-acting insulin SC at a basal rate supplemented by bolus doses before meal times. Potentially provide better control.
- Aiming for blood glucose level of 4–9 mmol/L, while avoiding hypoglycaemia.
- Glycosylated haemoglobin gives a better measure of glycaemic control over the preceding 6–8 weeks. A level of 6.5% or lower is ideal, although achieving this can run the risk of hypoglycaemia.
- Optimal glycaemic control helps to avoid long-term complications. Retinopathy, neuropathy, and nephropathy are rare in children, but are screened for 5 years after first being diagnosed or annually from 12 years of age.
- Diet, exercise, and avoidance of obesity are important for long-term management.

Type 2

- Due to a combination of relative insulin deficiency and peripheral insulin resistance.
- Rare in children, but incidence is increasing as obesity becomes more prevalent.

- Maturity-onset diabetes in the young (MODY) is characterized by impaired glucose tolerance; treatment focuses on dietary management.
- Oral hypoglycaemic agents (metformin) may be used, and occasionally insulin is required in symptomatic or hyperglycaemic patients. MODY represents a common phenotypic manifestation of several genetic abnormalities.

Perioperative management

- A multidisciplinary approach is essential, ensuring good communication between the surgeon, anaesthetist, and diabetic team.
- Use hospital's protocols, which can then be fine-tuned to the individual patient under the guidance of the diabetic team.
- Surgical stress response is characterized by increased catabolism, increased metabolic rate and protein and fat breakdown, periods of starvation, and glucose intolerance. Insulin secretion is suppressed at the same time that cortisol, glucagon, and catecholamine secretion are increased. This results in hyperglycaemia from an ↑ in glycogenolysis and gluconeogenesis by the liver, increased lipolysis and ketogenesis, and reduced uptake and use of glucose by muscle and fat.
- In IDDM, the stress response is exaggerated and can result in ketogenesis, hyperglycaemia, ketosis, or ketoacidosis. The type and duration of surgery, and presence of infection, can influence this response.
- The aim is normoglycaemia (target range 5–10 mmol/L), avoidance of electrolyte abnormalities (↓ K^+, ↓ Mg^{2+}, ↓ phosphate), and getting the patient eating/drinking as soon as possible postoperatively.
- Management depends on type and duration of surgery.
- Minor procedures: lasting <30 min, where patients are expected to eat within 4 h postoperatively. Often managed as day cases.
- Poorly controlled IDDM and those undergoing emergency or major surgery are managed with infusions of glucose, insulin, and K^+.
- Non-day cases are admitted the day before surgery. First on morning list.
- A common approach is outlined below.

Minor procedure
- First on morning list.
- Aim for blood glucose 5–10 mmol/L during and after surgery.
- If preoperative glucose >15 mmol/L, check urine for ketones. If negative or a small trace, continue but monitor. If positive for ketones, surgery may need to be postponed: seek advice from diabetic team.

Morning list
- Normal insulin on day before surgery.
- Fast 6 h for solids and milk, with clear fluids up to 1 h before surgery.
- Monitor capillary blood glucose hourly from time insulin given.

Afternoon list
- Must be first on list.
- Light breakfast on morning of surgery, then fast.
- 20% of insulin TDD as slow-acting analogue insulin by SC injection immediately before breakfast.

- 10% of insulin TDD as rapid-acting analogue immediately before breakfast.
- IV fluids (NaCl 0.45% with glucose 5%) at maintenance rate from time insulin given.
- Monitor capillary blood glucose hourly from time insulin given.

Postoperative
- If patient eat or drink within 2 hours:
  - Give 10% of insulin TDD as rapid-acting insulin analogue after food to ensure uptake established and PONV not a problem.
  - Monitor blood capillary glucose 2–4-hourly once stable.
- If patient is not going to eat within 2 h:
  - Slow-acting analogue insulin should prevent ketosis and maintain blood glucose control for several hours postoperatively.
  - If unable to eat, either a combined infusion of glucose, insulin, and K+ or separate infusions of glucose and insulin (as for major surgery) is required.
- If patient is using an insulin pump, seek advice from the diabetic team.

Major or emergency surgery
- Best managed with a continuous infusion of insulin separate to the IV fluids.
- Insulin: 50 units of soluble insulin dissolved in 50 mL NaCl. Infusion rate = 0.01 units (mL)/kg/h if blood glucose <4 mmol/L; 0.02 units (mL)/kg/h if glucose 4–7.9 mmol/L; 0.04 units (mL)/kg/h for glucose 8–13.9 mmol/L; 0.07 units (mL)/kg/h if glucose 14–22 mmol/L; and 0.1 units (mL)/kg/h if glucose >22 mmol/L.
- This should maintain blood glucose between 5 and 12 mmol/L.
- IV fluids 0.45% NaCl/5% glucose + 10 mmol KCl/500 mL. Infusion rate 2.5 mL/kg/h.
- If insulin and IV fluids are attached to the same cannula, an anti-syphon/anti-reflux valve must be used to separate the infusions.
- Blood glucose measured hourly perioperatively. U+E measured preoperatively and daily while on IV fluids.
- IV insulin has a $t_{1/2}$ of 3–4 min and should not be stopped unless hypoglycaemia occurs (blood glucose <3 mmol/L). Ketosis will develop if insulin is omitted. If hypoglycaemia continues, change to 10% glucose solution.
- Continue IV regimen until eating and drinking again.
- The usual SC dose of insulin is given after first meal and infusion is stopped 1 h later.
- Insulin requirements may initially be higher than normal in the postoperative period.
- The diabetic team will regularly review perioperative management.

Hypoglycaemia
- The commonest acute complication of IDDM. Secondary to missed meals (excessive fasting), unexpected exercise, or errors of insulin administration.
- Awake patients tend to get symptoms of feelings of hunger, sweating, tremor, tachycardia, anxiety, weakness, change in affect, slurred speech,

and confusion. This can progress to convulsions and coma if left untreated.
- If patient is conscious and able to eat, then give PO carbohydrate. If unconscious, give 2 mL/kg of 10% glucose solution followed by IV infusion of 5% or 10% glucose.
- If unconscious or fitting, give glucagon SC or IM:
  - <20 kg: 0.5 mg (0.5 unit) or a dose equivalent to 20–30 mcg/kg
  - >20 kg: 1 mg (1 unit).

Down syndrome (DS)

- Commonest chromosomal abnormality; incidence 1:700 live births. The incidence for mothers aged 25 years is 1:1,400; increasing to 1:46 for mothers aged 45 years.
- 95% have trisomy 21 caused by meiotic non-disjunction. The remainder arise from chromosomal translocations (2–3%) or mosaic trisomy 21 (2–3%).
- Life expectancy has improved owing to proactive management of life-threatening congenital abnormalities. About 20% die in the first year and 45% survive to 60 years of age (86% of the general population survive to 60 years), in contrast to a generation ago, when approximately two-thirds died in early childhood.

Clinical features

General appearance
- Small head circumference, brachycephaly, often a third fontanelle, short thick neck, upwardly sloping palpebral fissures, epicanthic folds, Brushfield spots (small white spots on the periphery of the iris), flat nasal bridge, large protruding tongue, and small mouth and ears.
- Usually low birth weight, but tend towards obesity in childhood.
- Often small in stature.
- A single transverse palmar (simian) crease in both hands (50%).

CHD
- Occurs in 40–60%.
- Most common abnormalities are atrioventricular canal defects, ASD, VSD, PDA, and tetralogy of Fallot.
- Pulmonary hypertension is more severe and earlier in onset with left-to-right shunts.

Respiratory tract
- OSA in 50%.
- Subglottic stenosis (2–3%).
- Chronic lower respiratory tract infections are relatively common, often secondary to reduced immunity and GOR.

Gastrointestinal anomalies
- Occur in 7%.
- 33% of patients with duodenal atresia have DS.
- GOR, oesophageal atresia, Hirschsprung's disease, and coeliac disease are commoner.

Neurological
- Neonates may be hypotonic.
- Intellectual function is limited. A steady decline in IQ with age in adults has been attributed to a presenile (Alzheimer's) dementia.
- Up to 10% have epilepsy.

Haematological
- Leukaemias have a 10–18-fold higher incidence than in the general population.

- 5% of DS neonates show a transient leukaemoid reaction that resolves spontaneously by 3 months of age, but may be associated with leukaemia in later life.
- In the first year of life, acute non-lymphoblastic leukaemia predominates and has an excellent prognosis.
- In older children, acute lymphoblastic leukaemia predominates and is associated with higher relapse rate and increased treatment-related mortality.
- Lymphomas may be commoner.

Immune system
- Infections are commoner, secondary to defects in cell-mediated immunity, granulocyte abnormalities, and a decreased adrenal response.
- Higher incidence of hepatitis B.

Endocrine
- Hypothyroidism without antibodies occurs commonly in childhood.
- In adults with DS, thyroid antibodies may result in hypothyroidism or hyperthyroidism.

Skeletal
- Asymptomatic atlanto-axial instability (20% incidence) due to lax transverse ligament and/or malformation of the odontoid peg. Subluxation or dislocation may result in cord compression.

Perioperative management
- Higher incidence of perioperative morbidity and so thresholds for referral to HDU or PICU for postoperative care should be lower.
- Often have a low IQ and poor understanding of clinical situations. The induction process may come across as being scary and intimidating, and normally pleasant cooperative children may become uncooperative, disruptive, and aggressive towards theatre staff, possibly causing harm to themselves or others.
- Have a supportive parent or carer present at induction to alleviate their fears. Sedative medication may be required; use with caution and appropriate monitoring owing to incidence of OSA.
- Several airway issues exist:
  - Difficult intubation is rare.
  - Slightly higher incidence of subglottic stenosis should prompt the anaesthetist to choose an ETT 0.5–1.0 mm smaller than that predicted by age.
  - Atlanto-axial instability. Lateral cervical spine X-rays only if there is a history of neurological symptoms of spinal cord compression, e.g. ataxia, abnormal gait, exaggerated reflexes, clonus, quadriplegia. New symptoms require investigation before elective surgery. Avoid excessive neck movement during laryngoscopy and positioning on the table.
- Cardiac anomalies should be assessed. Cardiac conduction defects may be present as a result of cardiac surgery. Sometimes these have been treated with medication or a pacemaker may have been fitted. Consider antibiotic prophylaxis.

- Chronic chest infections are common, as is postoperative atelectasis and respiratory tract infection. Postoperative chest physiotherapy may be prescribed to minimize chest complications.
- OSA may result in airway obstruction during GA or recovery. Avoid sedative premedication.
- Pain assessment and management is not always simple. Regional techniques may avoid the respiratory depressant effects of opioids and improve compliance with chest physiotherapy. Some patients are able to use PCA.
- Postoperative agitation may be a problem: facilitate the early presence of their carer in the recovery room; rarely, sedation is required.

Epidermolysis bullosa (EB)

- A heterogenous group of rare genetic diseases characterized by blistering of the skin and mucosa following minimal mechanical trauma. The severity and course range from minor disability to death in infancy.
- Secondary to a deficiency of structural proteins of the dermo-epidermal junction. Classification depends on the skin level at which the blistering occurs.
- Common operations used to manage the disease include plastic surgical procedures (syndactyly release and dressing changes), excision of squamous cell carcinoma with split skin grafts, dental surgery, and oesophageal dilation.

Clinical features

- There are three major types:

Epidermolysis bullosa simplex

- Autosomal dominant inheritance
- Commonest type, has three major subtypes:
  - *Weber–Cockayne type*: Onset in early childhood. Mild variant localized to hands and feet, not involving the nails and rarely affecting the mouth.
  - *Koebner type*: Onset in perinatal or postnatal period (often improves with age). Nails and mouth rarely affected.
  - *Dowling–Meara type*: Onset in early infancy. Severity ranges from mild to extremely severe resulting in death in the neonatal period. Blisters are often haemorrhagic, involving hands, feet, face, trunk, and limbs. There may be oral involvement (affecting feeding) and occasionally laryngeal involvement (hoarse cry). Keratoderma of the palms and soles is characteristic.

Epidermolysis bullosa letalis (junctional EB)

- Severe form.
- Autosomal recessive inheritance.
- Blisters in the lamina lucida.
- All parts of the skin are affected. There is often blistering of the respiratory tract (hoarse cry, stridor, acute airway obstruction) and GIT (pain, feeding difficulties, and failure to thrive).
- Lifespan rarely beyond 2 years of age, with death usually due to septicaemia or acute airway obstruction.

Dystrophic epidermolysis bullosa

- Two types, secondary to mutations in the *COL7A1* gene responsible for type VII collagen synthesis. The collagen anchors the lamina densa within the superficial dermis.
- The autosomal dominant variant is less severe than the recessive form.
- The more severe autosomal recessive form can present at birth or in infancy and includes widespread atrophic scarring blisters resulting in limb contractures, fusion of digits (mitten deformity), and mouth contractures. Blistering of the mucosal membranes of the oesophagus results in strictures, problems with oral feeding, malnutrition, and

iron-deficiency anaemia. Oesophageal strictures ↑ risk of reflux, regurgitation, and pulmonary aspiration. Nails are dystrophic, teeth are malformed with chronic decay, hair is sparse, and corneal ulceration occurs. There is an increased incidence of squamous cell carcinoma, porphyria, and amyloidosis.

Perioperative management

- Manage in a specialist centre familiar with the complex aspects of patient care. An admission for surgery should be planned well in advance and all specialties concerned with care involved from the start.
- A protocol with a list of essential equipment and things to be avoided may help in the planning of anaesthetic management.
- The main aim is to prevent any new bullae or wound formation secondary to any physical action that results in a shearing or friction force.
- Admit ideally to a dermatology ward under joint care with the surgeons. Ensure the patient is scheduled first on the list to allow time to accommodate additional necessary precautions.
- History and examination with particular attention to identifying potential airway issues. Potential of GORD and renal and cardiac involvement. Rarely, muscle weakness may be associated with muscular dystrophy.
- Review GA records and discuss perioperative plan with patient and carers.
- Adrenal suppression from long-term steroids may require perioperative supplementation with hydrocortisone.
- Antacid prophylaxis if history of GOR or oesophageal stricture.
- Premedication with PO midazolam or clonidine can be beneficial for anxious patients, who may move excessively during induction.
- EMLA™ (lidocaine/prilocaine) or Ametop® (tetracaine) may be used with a non-adhesive dressing, e.g. clingfilm.
- Minimize transfers, in particular avoiding frictional forces associated with sliding the patient on and off trolleys or beds. If possible, allow them to position themselves before induction on the operating table in the anaesthetic room. Use Gamgee or a crease-free sheet with foam padding to protect their heels.
- Venous access can be difficult, owing to scarring or contractures.
  - Caution with application of pressure with hands to assist with cannula insertion.
  - Secure cannulas with a non-adhesive technique, e.g. paraffin gauze and wrapping with a crepe bandage or using silicone-based products.
  - A central line may be necessary; suture in place.
- Monitoring:
  - Pulse oximeter clip on probe applied to ear or digit.
  - Avoid self-adhesive ECG electrode pads. Instead, use paraffin gauze over the ECG leads in contact with the patient.
  - Place more gauze, cotton wool, or PVC film and padding between the BP cuff and the skin.
  - Avoid rectal or nasopharyngeal temperature probes.

- There is sensitivity and unpredictable response to non-depolarizing muscle relaxants owing to reduced muscle bulk and poor nutritional status with hypoalbuminaemia.
- Suxamethonium is safe, but there is some concern over movement secondary to muscle fasciculations, and potential for cardiac dysrhythmias due to hyperK⁺ (secondary to muscle atrophy).
- Airway management:
  - Be prepared for potentially difficult mask ventilation and laryngoscopy.
  - Paraffin gauze used to lubricate/pad facemasks and areas of skin where anaesthetic fingers support the airway. Lubricate gloves.
  - Intubation with a lubricated laryngoscope blade and a smaller than predicted size of ETT minimizes laryngeal trauma
  - Cricoid pressure is not contraindicated, but should be applied evenly. Protect the area over the cricoid cartilage and back of the neck with paraffin gauze.
  - Oropharyngeal suctioning and poorly placed oropharyngeal airways can result in life-threatening bullae formation.
  - LMA can be used, although lingual bullae have been reported. A smaller size should be used and the shaft wrapped with gauze to protect the lips. Remove under deep GA.
  - Avoid adhesive tapes; tie ETT and LMA in place
- Lubricating eye ointments should be used instead of tape.
- Bipolar diathermy is preferred, to avoid the use of an adhesive diathermy pad.
- Regional anaesthesia can avoid many potential problems.
- Postoperative analgesia:
  - IV and regional are acceptable. Suppositories given to an awake patient are relatively contraindicated because of potential trauma
  - PO is preferred, where appropriate using liquids or effervescent preparations because of swallowing difficulties.

Epilepsy

- Abnormal paroxysms of neuronal activity lead to seizure activity; seen clinically as altered consciousness, motor, sensory, or autonomic events.
- Diagnosed when there are at least two unprovoked seizures >24 h apart; can be considered after one unprovoked seizure in an individual who has other factors that give them a high recurrence risk (e.g. structural lesions, stroke, inborn error of metabolism, CNS infection, or trauma) or if they have an epilepsy syndrome.
- Incidence 4–9:1,000; 60% of all cases of epilepsy are diagnosed in childhood.

Clinical features

- Classified according to the clinically observed features. The two main groups are generalized seizures and partial seizures.
- Generalized seizures are associated with bilateral symmetrical electric brain activity and usually involve loss of consciousness. Patients may have a prodromal period with behavioural changes or an aura. Following the seizure, they may remain unconscious and sleepy for a period
- They are further subdivided into:
  - Absence seizures where there is transient impaired consciousness without evidence of abnormal motor activity. Sometimes accompanied by reduced tone and autonomic behaviour.
  - Seizures with abnormal muscle activity (atonic, myoclonic, tonic, clonic, or combination of tonic–clonic) and impaired consciousness
- Partial seizures have a localized onset in the brain, sometimes spreading to become generalized. May present with jerking of a limb, altered sensation involving a strange taste or smell, a hallucination, or paraesthesia. Activity may spread to involve other limbs or areas of the body.
- Complex partial seizures are localized seizures with an impaired conscious level typically lasting 30 s to 2 min and often preceded by an aura, which may be visual, auditory, somatosensory, gustatory, olfactory, autonomic, abdominal, and psychic (déjà vu). They may be accompanied by automatisms (non-purposeful, stereotyped, and repetitive behaviours) specific to the seizure site.
- 'Epilepsy syndromes' include:
  - Infantile spasms
  - Juvenile myoclonic epilepsy
  - Temporal lobe epilepsy
  - Childhood absence epilepsy
  - Benign rolandic epilepsy
- Febrile convulsions occur in 2–5% of children <5 years. Associated increased risk of developing epilepsy later (1% in general and up to 10% if there is a family history).
- Diagnosis is made from the history and by observation of a seizure. EEGs aid diagnosis and often localize epileptic foci in the brain. MRI, SPECT, and PET scans can locate abnormal brain lesions and look at cerebral blood flow during seizures. These may provide useful information for surgical resection of foci in patients with intractable seizures.
- Antiepileptic drugs (AEDs) have several modes of action:
  - Increasing inhibitory neurotransmitter activity (GABA): benzodiazepines, gabapentin, vigabatrin, barbiturates.

- Reduction of inward voltage-gated currents: phenytoin and carbamazepine (Na^+ channel), ethosuximide (Ca^{2+} channel).
- Decreasing excitatory neurotransmitter activity: topiramate (glutamate antagonist). Lamotrigine is a Na^+ channel blocker with effects on Ca^{2+} channels. Sodium valproate has several sites of action, including K^+ channels. Some patients may need multiple medications.
- Some patients with intractable epilepsy or intolerable side effects to AEDs respond to a ketogenic diet (high-fat low-carbohydrate). Glucose containing solutions and lactated Ringer's solution are avoided intraoperatively, since they can exacerbate the pre-existing metabolic acidosis. Careful monitoring of plasma glucose levels are necessary to detect and avoid hypoglycaemia in susceptible infants.
- Surgical management for intractable seizures is becoming more common (➔ Chapter 21). This may include lesionectomy, anterior temporal lobectomy, hemispherectomy, or division of the corpus callosum. Cervical vagus nerve stimulation devices can be effective in patients refractory to AEDs but unsuitable for resective surgery.

Perioperative management

- History of seizure type, frequency, last seizure, control, and AEDs.
- Continue AEDs up until the time of surgery and restart as soon as possible postoperatively. If oral intake is delayed, some medications can be given PR (carbamazepine), IM (phenobarbital), or IV (phenytoin or sodium valproate).
- Learning difficulties and behavioural problems are common. Sedative premedication with midazolam may help. Hyperventilation decreases the seizure threshold.
- GA drugs may alter seizure threshold.
  - Thiopental has powerful anticonvulsant properties
  - Propofol is associated with abnormal movements and epileptiform changes in the EEG at low doses; however, it suppresses EEG activity during GA.
  - Sevoflurane causes epileptiform EEG changes and there are case reports of seizures under GA, although it is accepted practice to use in epileptic children. Isoflurane and desflurane both have anticonvulsant properties
  - Methohexital and enflurane (especially with hyperventilation) are associated with causing seizures. Ketamine has anticonvulsant properties.
- AEDs may induce liver enzymes (cytochrome P450), so drugs metabolized in the liver may have a shorter duration of action, e.g. vecuronium.
- Regional techniques may allow a more rapid return to oral intake and medication.
- Status epilepticus has an 8% mortality. Defined as a seizure >30 min or when intermittent seizure activity occurs over a 30 min period without regaining consciousness. Prolonged convulsions result in hypoxia, cerebral oedema, metabolic acidosis, cardiac dysrhythmias, hypertension, pulmonary oedema, DIC, rhabdomyolysis, and multi-organ failure.

Haemophilia and von Willebrand's disease

- The three commonest hereditary bleeding disorders are haemophilia A (factor VIII deficiency), haemophilia B (factor IX deficiency), and von Willebrand's disease (vWD)—von Willebrand factor (vWF) deficiency.

Haemophilia A

- An X-linked recessive bleeding disorder affecting 1:5,000 males arising from a mutation in the long arm of chromosome X at the *F8* gene.
- Positive family history in 66% of cases. Females are gene carriers.
- Severity and frequency of bleeding correlates with the level of FVIII coagulation activity (FVIIIc) measured by clotting assay. Levels are commonly expressed as a percentage of the normal expected level and severity is inversely related to the amount of factor present. (<1% = severe; 1–5% = moderate; 6–30% = mild; 50–200% = normal). The proportions of patients who are severe, moderate, and mild are 50%, 10%, and 40% respectively.
- Age at presentation depends on the level of severity and the type of trauma.
- Patients commonly present with spontaneous bleeding into joints (ankles, knees, hips, and elbows; this results in painful swelling and eventually degenerative arthritis) and muscles (necrosis and contractures).
- More severely affected may suffer intracranial haemorrhage with mild head trauma.
- Haematuria is common.
- Even in mild disease, haemorrhage can be life-threatening, e.g. dental extraction.
- Preoperative blood tests elicit abnormalities of the intrinsic coagulation pathway, with a prolonged activated partial thromboplastin time (APTT) and normal thrombin time (TT), prothrombin time (PT), platelet count, and fibrinogen level. Bleeding time is normal except in the most severe cases. It is important to have a baseline FVIIIc assay.

Perioperative management

- Seek advice of consultant haematologist and haemophilia nurse specialist. Good communication is essential in coordinating perioperative management.
- Elective surgery should be scheduled early in the week. Preferably in the morning, although not first on the list, owing to the practicalities of giving the factors and measuring post-transfusion levels preoperatively.
- IV access may be difficult. Patients usually have a portacath for their treatment.
- Manufactured recombinant FVIII concentrate is the mainstay of treatment. It is useful to establish preoperatively how much, how often, and what response a dose has on FVIIIc assay levels. It is essential to know if there are any anti-FVIII antibodies. FVIII has a $t_{1/2}$ of 8–12 h and may have to be given two or three times daily. Generally maintenance

therapy is given three times/week from walking age to minimize long-term joint damage.

- The FVIIIc assay target level depends on the type and location of surgery. Major surgery, e.g. neurosurgery, requires an initial assay >100%, which may be required for up to 6 weeks postoperatively. The details of specific patient management will be closely monitored and managed by the haematology team.

- Each FVIII unit/kg body weight will ↑ the plasma FVIII level by approximately 2%. Usually about 50 IU/kg are given just before surgery, followed by 25 IU/kg that evening and twice daily thereafter for the first week. The peak level should be measured about 20 min post dose, with the aim of having a level >100% post infusion. FVIIIc assays are repeated daily during the first postoperative week to ensure the target is achieved.

- 10–15% of patients develop antibodies to FVIII that ↓ its effectiveness. Surgery in this group is only performed when essential. In the lower-risk groups (inhibitor level <5 Bethesda units/mL), a higher dose of factor is needed. In the higher-risk groups (inhibitor level >5 Bethesda units/mL) recombinant activated factor VII (rFVIIa) or factor eight inhibitor bypassing activity (FEIBA) may be used as an alternative.

- Tranexamic acid inhibits fibrinolysis through competitive inhibition of the conversion of plasminogen to plasmin (which degrades fibrin). Given PO or IV and continued for up to a week postoperatively.

- Desmopressin causes the release of vWF from endothelial cells and this forms a complex with FVIII, thereby preventing its breakdown. It is used mainly in patients with the milder forms of haemophilia A who are undergoing minor surgery (e.g. dental extractions) and results in a 2–5-fold ↑ in FVIII levels. IV/SC dose is 0.3 mcg/kg.

- Avoid IM injections, NSAIDs, and regional techniques.

- The incidence of transfusion-related hepatitis B and C and HIV has decreased with the use of recombinant FVIII concentrate.

Haemophilia B (Christmas disease)

- X-linked disorder (long arm of X chromosome at *F9*) due to FIX deficiency.

- Less common than haemophilia A.

- Clinically resembles haemophilia A; only distinguished by assay of FVIIIc and FIX. Other results include a long PTT, and normal PT, TT, fibrinogen, and bleeding time.

- Treatment: heat-treated or recombinant FIX concentrate. Each unit/kg body weight will ↑ the plasma FIX level by 1 IU/dL. Levels are recorded approximately 15 min after the infusion. The $t_{1/2}$ is 18–24 h, so given once daily.

- Desmopressin is ineffective.

Von Willebrand's disease

- Commonest inherited bleeding disorder; approximately 1% incidence.

- It is caused by deficiency or dysfunction of von Willebrand factor (vWF) due to a defect on chromosome 12 and occurs in both sexes.

- vWF has two main functions:
  - Promoting platelet aggregation and adherence at the sites of vascular injury.
  - Acts as a carrier protein for FVIII, protecting it from premature activation and degradation. This results in a secondary deficiency of FVIII.
- vWF deficiency produces a defect in platelet plug formation and fibrin formation.
- There are three main phenotypes:
  - Type I. The mildest and commonest variant (60–80%). It is characterized by moderate deficiencies of vWF and FVIII (5–30% of normal levels). Inheritance is autosomal dominant. Patients may present with bruising after trauma or surgery. They usually do not bleed spontaneously but may suffer epistaxis or menorrhagia. Symptoms are often so mild that it is never diagnosed.
  - Type II (10–30%). Inheritance is autosomal dominant or recessive and results in a qualitative abnormality of vWF. It has several subtypes: IIA, IIB, IIM, and IIN. Type IIB has a reduced vWF associated with decreased platelet survival and thrombocytopenia. Patients may present with spontaneous skin and mucosal bleeding, e.g. epistaxis.
  - Type III. The severest. Inheritance is autosomal recessive. Bleeding is more frequent and severe owing to an absence of both vWF and FVIII. This group suffer intra-articular and IM bleeds.
- Test results may vary in an individual and need to be repeated to make a diagnosis. Tests include:
  - The bleeding time tends to be grossly prolonged (normal in haemophilia A).
  - The PTT is ↑, while PT, TT, and fibrinogen are normal.
  - Platelet aggregation and adhesion are ↓.
  - FVIII and vWF antigen levels are ↓. The disease is considered mild if vWF antigen level is 20–40% normal and severe if <10%.
  - vWF activity is measured by ristocetin cofactor activity and ristocetin-induced platelet agglutination tests.
  - Analysis of the vWF multimers helps classify the type of vWD and has treatment implications
- Main treatments are desmopressin (administered IV, SC, or intranasally), which induces autologous secretion of FVIII and vWF into the plasma; plasma concentrates (cryoprecipitate); recombinant FVIII, or purified vWF concentrate. Fibrinolysis inhibitors, platelet concentrates, and the oral contraceptive pill may be useful adjuvant therapies.
- Desmopressin is ineffective in some type II and all type III patients. In type IIB, it can lead to platelet aggregation and thrombocytopenia.
- Patients with type III vWD require prophylaxis if they have recurrent bleeding into mucosa or joints.
- In types I and II, prophylactic treatment is only given before invasive procedures or if spontaneous bleeding occurs.

Perioperative management

- Good communication between haematologist, anaesthetist, and surgeon is essential.
- For surgery involving mucosal membranes, the bleeding time must be normalized.
- The pharmacological agents most commonly used are desmopressin and tranexamic acid.
- Desmopressin 0.3 mcg/kg IV diluted in 10 mL of normal saline and given over 10 min. Monitor for side effects (tachycardia, hypotension, facial flushing).
- For elective surgery, patients are often admitted for a trial of treatment to assess the efficacy of the desmopressin. Blood is taken 45–60 min post dose and it is hoped that FVIII and vWF levels exceed 50% of normal values following treatment.
- If desmopressin is administered for >2 days, monitor levels, since tachyphylaxis can occur.
- Desmopressin is not given to known 'non-responders', type IIB or III disease, and those <2 years of age.
- It has an antidiuretic effect; if several doses are given, then monitor fluid balance and electrolytes. Consider fluid restriction. Children <2 years are at increased risk of hypoNa⁺.
- A combination of desmopressin with a fibrinolytic inhibitor (tranexamic acid 15–25 mg/kg PO and as a mouthwash for up to 7 days) can be used for dental extractions.
- For desmopressin non-responders, give a single dose of recombinant FVIII or vWF.
- For major surgery, seek haematological advice on appropriate use of cryoprecipitate, vWF concentrate, pasteurized FVIII preparation (Humate-P) and platelet transfusion.
- Treatment continues as long as the haemostatic challenge from surgery persists, e.g. 1–5 days for minor surgery or up to 2 weeks for neurosurgery. Special care is needed with tonsillectomy patients when, at day 6–7 postoperatively, the scab falls off with inherent risk of further bleeding.
- Avoid IM injections, aspirin, and other NSAIDs.
- Universal precautions, as there is a higher incidence of hepatitis C and HIV from multiple blood product transfusions.

Human immunodeficiency virus (HIV)

- Paediatric acquired immune deficiency syndrome (AIDS) refers to those <13 years old who are infected with HIV, and represents 5% of worldwide cases. Approximately 90% of cases are found in developing countries in south and central Africa and southern Asia.
- HIV preferentially infects T-helper cells (CD4+ T cells) and destroys them. This has a direct effect on cell-mediated immunity and results in increased susceptibility to opportunistic infections and malignancies.
- Two distinct subtypes exist: HIV-1 and HIV-2. HIV-2 is found almost exclusively in West Africa; disease progression is slower and vertical transmission from mother to child is less common.
- 80% of paediatric HIV results from vertical transmission from an infected mother to the fetus. This may occur in utero, intrapartum, or postpartum through breast feeding. Transmission rates vary from 30% in Europe to 50% in developing countries.
- Transmission rates are higher for mothers who have more advanced disease, have prolonged rupture of membranes (>4 h), chorioamnionitis, or premature delivery. Perinatal antiretroviral therapy may ↓ transmission rates to 8%. The combination of an elective caesarean section and antiretrovirals can further ↓ the risk to about 2%.
- HIV transmission may result from sexually transmitted infection, sexual abuse from an infected individual, or from IV drug abuse using contaminated needles. It is less common now to be transmitted as a result of receiving infected blood products.
- Children born to HIV antibody-positive mothers acquire HIV antibodies by passive transfer across the placenta. These remain detectable for the first 12–18 months of life, making diagnosis difficult in the first 15 months. Virology assays, specifically HIV DNA polymerase chain reaction (PCR), can identify 30–50% of infected infants at birth and nearly 100% of infected infants by 3–6 months of age. Enzyme-linked immunoassays and western blot analysis are used to test for antibody activity, but are limited in their ability as reliable predictors of future infection.
- Although virtually all infants born to HIV mothers are antibody-positive at birth, only 15–30% go on to develop AIDS. However, if antibodies persist beyond 15 months, the child is assumed to be infected.

Clinical features

- CD4+ T-lymphocyte levels are used to classify severity of immunosuppression secondary to infection. HIV infection results in depleted levels and is responsible for many of the manifestations of the disease. Interpretation of levels is age-specific.
- Incubation period is 6 months to several years. Patients may present with non-specific signs and symptoms: failure to thrive, oral thrush, recurrent diarrhoea, respiratory infections, unexplained fever, anaemia, lymphadenopathy, dermatitis, hepatosplenomegaly, and thrombocytopenia.
- Vertically acquired infections are more aggressive than other forms. 15–30% develop profound immune deficiency and an AIDS-defining illness before 1 year of age. More commonly, the disease is slowly progressive, with 75% of infected infants surviving to 5 years of age.

Infection

- Respiratory sepsis, meningitis, osteomyelitis, cellulitis, and gastrointestinal and urinary tract infections all occur. Causative organisms include *Streptococcus pneumoniae, Haemophilus influenzae, Salmonella* spp., *Escherichia coli, Staphylococcus aureus*, and *Pseudomonas* spp.
- Commonest opportunistic infection is *Pneumocystis carinii* pneumonia, commonly diagnosed between 3 and 6 months of age and associated with a poorer prognosis than in adults (median survival time from infection is only 1–4 months).
- *Pneumocystis carinii* pneumonia is treated with high dose co-trimoxazole. Systemic prednisolone therapy (1 mg/kg/day) is advised for patients with a PaO_2 <9.3 kPa. Respiratory support and O_2 therapy may be required. Prophylaxis with co-trimoxazole or inhaled pentamidine is recommended for children who have had an episode of *Pneumocystis* pneumonia, for those born to infected mothers but not yet diagnosed HIV antibody-positive, and for infected children with low CD4$^+$ lymphocyte counts.
- Candidal, tubercular and viral pneumonias can occur with cytomegalovirus, respiratory syncytial virus, varicella-zoster virus, herpes simplex, *Candida albicans, Toxoplasma gondii*, and atypical mycobacteria.

Respiratory system

- The main cause of mortality and presents the biggest anaesthetic challenge. Opportunistic infections may progress to acute respiratory failure.
- Lymphoid interstitial pneumonitis presents with dyspnoea on exertion, a non-productive cough, diffuse reticulonodular shadowing on CXR, and finger clubbing. Onset is insidious, with an uncertain pathophysiology. Treatment is with steroids and bronchodilators. Opportunistic infection is less common in these children and the overall prognosis is improved. They can also get episodes of parotid gland enlargement, adenotonsillar enlargement, and mediastinal lymphadenopathy potentially causing airway obstruction.

Cardiovascular system

- Commonly affected, although the pathogenesis is not always clear. Myocarditis may result from infection with coxsackie B virus, CMV, *Cryptococcus*, aspergillosis, or HIV. This can result in a dilated cardiomyopathy.
- Infective endocarditis, pericardial effusions, and autonomic neuropathy may be present.

Central nervous system

- Most infected children have an encephalopathy that may be progressive, with developmental delay, symmetrical motor deficits (abnormal gait, tone, and reflexes), behavioural changes, and seizures.
- Abnormal brain growth results in microcephaly and cerebral atrophy, with early demyelination of cerebral white matter.
- *Cryptococcus neoformans, Candida*, aspergillus, HIV, and tuberculosis can cause meningitis.
- Patients have an increased susceptibility for primary CNS lymphomas and cerebrovascular accidents.

Gastrointestinal system
- With disease progression, patients may fail to thrive or lose weight. Adequate nutritional intake is made difficult by pain from oral and oesophageal candidiasis and by recurrent diarrhoea due to infection or HIV enteropathy. Medication side effects can also contribute to this and affect hepatic function.

Haematological system
- Microcytic anaemia, thrombocytopenia and leukopenia may occur secondary to the disease or drug therapy.

Other features
- Recurrent skin infections: bacterial (staphylococcal), fungal, viral (molluscum contagiosum).
- Kaposi sarcoma occurs in about 10%.
- Between 5% and 10% develop nephrotic syndrome secondary to a focal glomerulosclerosis affecting renal function and requiring a review of their medication.

Drug therapies and side effects
- Antiretrovirals slow disease progression but are toxic, and complicated regimens make compliance difficult. They suppress viral replication, reducing viral load, and are given as a combination therapy to ↓ drug resistance.
- Four categories of drug are available:
  - Nucleoside-analogue reverse transcriptase inhibitors (NRTIs), e.g. zidovudine (side effects include bone marrow suppression, gastrointestinal upset), lamivudine (anaemia), didanosine (peripheral neuropathy and pancreatitis). They act as false nucleotide and prevent reverse transcriptase from synthesizing DNA.
  - Non-nucleoside reverse transcriptase inhibitors (NNRTIs), e.g. nevirapine (rash, hepatitis) and efavirenz (rash). These bind to reverse transcriptase and inhibit enzyme activity. Lactic acidosis is a recognized complication (inhibition of mitochondrial DNA replication) with an associated high mortality.
  - Protease inhibitors, e.g. saquinavir (diarrhoea and elevated transaminases—can inhibit midazolam metabolism, prolonging action), ritonavir, and lopinavir (gastrointestinal upset, hyperlipidaemia, circumoral paraesthesia). They prevent the processing of viral proteins into their functional forms.
  - Fusion inhibitors, e.g. enfuvirtide, inhibit viral binding or fusion to target host cells.
- Patients may be taking other drugs that are nephrotoxic (amphotericin, aciclovir, or pentamidine) or cause thrombocytopenia (zidovudine, co-trimoxazole, or ketoconazole).

Perioperative management
- 20–25% need surgery during their illness. They may be asymptomatic at presentation for surgery or have multi-organ involvement with opportunistic infections.

- Commonly present for central line insertion, PEG, drainage of infected lesions, and diagnostic procedures (lung or liver biopsies). As survival improves, more children are presenting for other types of surgery, e.g. dental or ENT.
- A careful history and examination needs to focus on the current status of HIV infection. Low $CD4^+$ counts suggest more advanced disease and potentially more organ involvement.
- Assess respiratory function for the presence of infection. CXR if indicated.
- Cardiovascular investigations performed where indicated. Abnormal ECGs are common (>90%).
- Blood tests include FBC, U+Es, LFTs, and coagulation for evidence of abnormalities relating to HIV infection or side effects of drug therapy. Inform laboratory personnel of the high-risk specimen.
- Often have complex social backgrounds and may not present with their biological parents. It is important to ascertain (sensitively) who has legal guardianship in order to obtain informed consent.
- Central neural blockade is usually avoided in the presence of neurological signs or symptoms related to HIV infection. Other contraindications may be related to side effects of medications, e.g. thrombocytopenia. Regional anaesthesia in this immunocompromised group of patients may carry a higher risk of CNS infection.
- 20–60% are affected by pain. This may be complex and related to the disease process or to toxicities and side effects of medications.
- Postoperative mortality is not higher in this group.
- The incidence of postoperative fever, anaemia, and tachycardia is higher.

Risk of infection transmission

- Patient-to-anaesthetist. Universal precautions (gloves, gown, mask, eye protection) for high-risk patients. Avoid spillage of infected body fluids. Disposal of needles without re-sheathing into sharps containers is essential. The risk of HIV transmission from a significant needle-stick injury is approximately 0.31%.
- Post-exposure prophylaxis. A significant needle-stick injury from a high-risk patient should be immediately discussed with occupational health. Post-exposure prophylaxis is started within 1–2 h of exposure. Toxicity and compliance with treatment may be a problem.
- Patient-to-patient. HIV is destroyed by heat and chemicals (glutaraldehyde or sodium hypochlorite). Disposable airway devices, HME filters, and circuits are used. Other non-disposable anaesthetic equipment is routinely cleaned and decontaminated.

Klippel–Feil syndrome

- Congenital anomaly characterized by a failure of formation or segmentation of the cervical vertebrae. Incidence 1:42,000 newborns.
- Clinical triad: short neck, low posterior hairline, and a severe restriction in neck movement. <50% demonstrate all three clinical features. Usually present in early childhood.
- Associated abnormalities of other organ systems may be present.
- Most cases occur sporadically, although inheritance has been reported to be both autosomal dominant and recessive.

Clinical features

- Early classification systems recognized three morphological types of cervical fusion:
  - Type I:
    —Extensive fusions of cervical and upper thoracic vertebrae.
    —Most often associated with other severe syndromic abnormalities.
    —Autosomal dominant.
  - Type II:
    —Commonest form. Fusions occur at one or two cervical interspaces.
    —C2/3 is the commonest site.
    —Often associated with other skeletal deformities, e.g. Sprengel's deformity (congenital upward displacement of the scapula:30%), cervical rib, hemivertebrae, occipito-atlantal fusion.
    —Can be associated with Arnold–Chiari malformation and syringomyelia.
    —Autosomal recessive.
  - Type III:
    —Fusions at cervical and lower thoracic or lumbar spine.
    —Autosomal dominant.

Types I and III have greater risk of scoliosis (60%).

- May be associated with spina bifida (45%), profound deafness (30%), rib abnormalities, e.g. fused ribs (30%), cleft lip and/or palate (15%), renal aplasia or other genitourinary abnormalities, CHD (10%: commonly VSDs). Less commonly: cervical rib, micrognathia, syringomyelia, Moebius syndrome (congenital facial palsy with impairment of ocular abduction), webbing of soft tissues (neck and syndactyly), and flattening of the base of the skull (platybasia). Anomalies are present at birth but often undiagnosed until a later stage.
- Patients may present for surgery to resect fused or cervical ribs, lower elevated scapula, genitourinary procedures, and neurosurgical procedures for neck instability or cord compression. They may present for cleft palate repair, scoliosis correction, and eye surgery.

Perioperative management

- Undiagnosed Klippel–Feil can present as an unexpectedly difficult intubation.
- If already diagnosed, the areas of spinal fusion should be identified (C-spine AP and lateral X-rays) and cervical stability assessed. If

there are signs or symptoms of cord compression, an MRI should be
performed: discuss with neurosurgical and neurological colleagues.
• Cervical spine instability may result in spinal cord injury if the neck is
manipulated for intubation. Airway management may require fibreoptic
intubation or use of a videolaryngoscope blade. LMAs have been used
successfully with minimal neck movement. Consider a neck collar to
support the neck during GA.
• An unpredictable neuraxial block may occur where there is distortion of
the vertebral column or compression of the epidural space.

Acute liver failure

- Acute liver failure or fulminant hepatitis is a rare complex disease with mortality >70% without supportive treatment and/or liver transplantation.
- The adult disease is a clinical syndrome consisting of the acute onset of encephalopathy, coagulopathy, and evidence of acute liver necrosis with hepatic dysfunction starting within 8 weeks of the first signs of liver disease. This assumes the absence of any pre-existing liver disease.
- However, in infants and children, encephalopathy may be absent, late onset, or undiagnosed even in severe disease. Acute liver failure may also be the first presentation of an underlying metabolic (Wilson's disease) or autoimmune disease.
- Paediatric definitions emphasise the presence of a significant coagulopathy due to acute hepatic dysfunction unresponsive to parenteral vitamin (in the absence of sepsis or DIC). It may be defined as hyperacute (up to 10 days), acute (11–30 days), or subacute (>30 days) in onset, depending on the duration of liver dysfunction. Jaundice is more common in subacute-onset liver failure. Encephalopathy is associated with a poor prognosis and may be a pre-terminal event.

Aetiology

- Varies with the age of the child. 40–50% have no identifiable cause. Neonatal haemochromatosis is the commonest cause of acute liver failure in infants. Viral hepatitis accounts for 50% of cases of fulminant hepatic failure in children of all age groups. Hepatotoxic drugs account for approximately 20% of cases.

Neonates and infants

- Infection: septicaemia, HBV, adenovirus, parvovirus B19, echovirus, coxsackie, non-A–G hepatitis, EBV, HIV.
- Metabolic: neonatal haemochromatosis, tyrosinaemia type 1, mitochondrial disorders, fatty acid oxidation defects, α_1-antitrypsin deficiency.
- Drugs: paracetamol, iron, vitamin A, salicylates, anticonvulsants, isoniazid.
- Vascular: CHD, asphyxia, Budd–Chiari syndrome.
- Others: neuroblastoma, hepatoblastoma, leukaemia, familial erythrophagocytic syndrome.

Older children

- Infection: viral hepatitis A–G, EBV, CMV, HSV, leptospirosis, bacterial sepsis.
- Metabolic: Wilson's disease
- Drugs: paracetamol, isoniazid, salicylates, valproic acid, drugs of abuse in adolescents (glue sniffing, ecstasy), halothane hepatitis.
- Toxins: carbon tetrachloride, *Amanita phalloides* (death cap mushroom), iron poisoning.
- Neoplastic: lymphoma, leukaemia, hepatocellular carcinoma.
- Vascular: sequelae of cardiac surgery, CHD, shock, sickle cell anaemia.

Clinical features

- Usually affects previously healthy children with no risk factors.
- Jaundice is the commonest presenting symptom, often preceded by a prodromal flu-like illness. Anorexia, nausea, vomiting, and ascites are common.
- Encephalopathy is not always obvious, especially in neonates and infants, where jaundice and coagulopathy may be the presenting features. Encephalopathy in infants may present with irritability, poor feeding, and altered sleep patterns, while older children may present with confusion or aggressive behaviour.
- Hepatic encephalopathy is graded according to severity (West Haven Criteria) and this correlates with disease severity and worsening prognosis:
  - Grade 1: behavioural changes with minimal change in conscious level.
  - Grade 2: drowsy, disorientated, inappropriate, combative.
  - Grade 3: markedly confused, incoherent speech, sleeping most of the time but responds to vocal stimuli.
  - Grade 4: comatose, unresponsive to pain, decorticate and decerebrate posturing.
- Acute liver failure is a multisystem disorder associated with numerous complications: sepsis, acute renal failure, severe coagulopathy, GIT bleeding, ascites, cerebral oedema, high CO failure (with low SVR), hypoglycaemia, hypoK$^+$, and a metabolic acidosis. These patients are only anaesthetized for emergency procedures, since perioperative morbidity and mortality are high.

Chronic liver failure

- Incidence is 6:100,000 live births.
- Suspected in any infant with jaundice continuing beyond 14 days.

Aetiology

- Commonest cause is extrahepatic biliary atresia. Infants undergo hepatic portoenterostomy (Kasai procedure) within their first 8 weeks of life. If successful, the procedure achieves a 90% 10-year survival. Failure of this procedure represents the commonest indication for liver transplant worldwide.
- Other causes of chronic liver disease include:
  - Biliary obstruction: choledochal cyst, cystic fibrosis, sclerosing cholangitis.
  - Infective: acute viral hepatitis B, chronic active hepatitis, CMV.
  - Metabolic: Wilson's disease, α_1-antitrypsin deficiency, tyrosinaemia, haemochromatosis.
  - Autoimmune: chronic active hepatitis.

Clinical features

- Patients may be asymptomatic or may present with symptoms of acute liver failure, or there may be a more insidious onset of symptoms.
- Features suggesting chronicity are a small hard liver, splenomegaly, jaundice, cutaneous manifestations (spider naevi, palmar erythema, caput medusae), ascites, fluid retention, impaired renal function, growth failure, or muscle wasting.
- Encephalopathy can be precipitated by sedative medication, infection, GIT bleeds, high protein diets, hypoK$^+$, and surgery. A deteriorating conscious level may mark the onset of cerebral oedema, necessitating intubation and ICU management.

Perioperative management

- Patients represent a significant risk when presenting for surgery. The Child–Pugh classification is a scoring system that assesses the severity of chronic liver disease and is used to predict prognosis and the risk of major surgery.
- Serum bilirubin, serum albumin, and prothrombin time are accurate markers of disease progression. Rising bilirubin and prothrombin time with a falling albumin are poor prognostic signs.
- Assessment of encephalopathy, nutrition, and ascites, although subjective, are still useful.
- Standard liver function tests are poor markers of function and have no prognostic value. Alanine aminotransferase and aspartate aminotransferase serve as markers for liver damage, but may fall in the late stages of the disease. Alkaline phosphatase is elevated in cholestasis and biliary obstruction.
- Mortality in this group may result from sepsis, massive haemorrhage, renal failure, or deterioration in hepatic function with encephalopathy.

Haemorrhage

- The liver is responsible for the synthesis of all coagulation factors except vWF. PTT is usually prolonged and INR usually high, and these are good indicators of liver function.
- There is often a quantitative and qualitative ↓ in platelets, primarily from splenic sequestration.
- There is a risk of massive haemorrhage from oesophageal, gastric, or rectal varices secondary to portal hypertension. Screen regularly for varices. They may need treatment with prophylactic beta-blockers, sclerotherapy or banding of varices, or a portosystemic shunt.
- Patients tend to be anaemic, as a consequence of chronic disease, chronic bleeding, and malnutrition.
- Preoperatively, there should be a FBC, coagulation screen, cross-match, platelets, and clotting factors where required.
- These patients often handle fluid loads poorly owing to their inability to excrete excess fluid, and so infusion of large volumes of clotting factors and platelets to correct for surgery may result in circulatory overload.

Ascites

- Oedema and ascites indicates advanced liver dysfunction.
- Raised intra-abdominal pressure may cause diaphragmatic splinting, respiratory distress, and hypoxia. FRC is reduced.
- Patients may be on diuretics (spironolactone) or may have a peritoneovenous shunt.
- Intraoperative drainage of ascites may result in marked hypovolaemia and hypotension postoperatively as the ascites recollects. Extra fluid should be given to account for this loss.

Respiratory

- PaO$_2$ may be low because of intrapulmonary shunts, with resultant ventilation–perfusion mismatch (hepatopulmonary syndrome), pleural effusions, and ascites.
- Atelectasis and chest infections are more common perioperatively.

Cardiovascular

- Patients have a hyperdynamic circulation with a high CO and low SVR.
- A variety of shunts occur (cutaneous, portopulmonary) and portal hypertension resulting in ascites and varices.

Renal function

- Decreased renal function is common with liver failure and carries a poor prognosis.
- A ↓ SVR with low perfusion pressures activates the renin–angiotensin–aldosterone axis, causing a further ↓ in GFR. Antidiuretic hormone secretion is also increased in response to hypoperfusion and UO falls further.
- There is a risk of hepatorenal syndrome, producing pre-renal failure secondary to intense renal vasoconstriction in the presence of liver failure. It is characterized by a hyperosmolar urine and low urinary Na$^+$ (<10 mmol/L). Na$^+$ and water retention may occur. This is rare.
- Renal failure in liver disease may occur secondary to sepsis or acute tubular necrosis.

Metabolic
- Reduced glycogen stores and impaired gluconeogenesis mean there is a risk of hypoglycaemia. Monitor blood glucose closely: infants and children may need an IV solution containing glucose.
- Acid–base balance may be altered by renal dysfunction or diuretic therapy.

Infection
- Reduced immunological function increases the risk of sepsis.
- Procedures should be carried out aseptically.
- A high index of suspicion should exist for the presence of infection as a cause of cardiovascular instability or worsening encephalopathy.

Altered drug pharmacokinetics
- Liver disease reduces the hepatic clearance of certain drugs, e.g. opioids and benzodiazepines. The degree of impairment of the metabolic reactions can be variable, making appropriate dose adjustments difficult. It can, however, be predicted that drugs with sedative effects will likely have enhanced effect and prolonged action.
- Obstructive disorders may result in reduced biliary excretion and clearance of drugs or their metabolites in bile, e.g. pancuronium, resulting in prolonged neuromuscular blockade.
- Reduced plasma albumin will ↑ the free active portion of the drug in the plasma, resulting in a greater drug effect for a given dose, e.g. thiopental.
- The V_d for protein-bound drugs in hypoalbuminaemia is increased, since the free portion is more able to redistribute in the body compartments. Ascites, Na^+, and water retention also ↑ the V_d of drugs.
- Drugs that ↓ CO and hepatic blood flow during GA have a deleterious effect on hepatic metabolism. Avoid halothane

Preoperative investigations
- FBC, coagulation, U+Es, LFTs, plasma glucose, CXR, ABGs, hepatitis B serology.

Anaesthesia
- Manage in tertiary centre with experience of the disease.
- Midazolam and diazepam premedication should be used with caution since they may precipitate encephalopathy.
- Increased intra-abdominal pressure from ascites will ↑ the potential for reflux, regurgitation and aspiration. H_2 receptor antagonists or proton pump inhibitors should be given. Induction in a slight head-up position may ↓ this risk and diminish the effect of diaphragmatic splinting.
- Consider a RSI.
- Low threshold for invasive monitoring and booking ICU/HDU for postoperative care.
- The clearance of thiopental is unchanged (high fat solubility and rapid redistribution). However, patients may be sensitive to it and the induction dose should be reduced.
- Propofol similarly has unchanged clearance. With prolonged infusions, the $t_{1/2}$ is prolonged in liver failure. Induction doses should be reduced to avoid hypotension.

- Cisatracurium or atracurium are the muscle relaxants of choice. Rocuronium, vecuronium, and pancuronium all have extended duration of action. Decreased synthesis of plasma cholinesterase prolongs the effect of suxamethonium and mivacurium. Monitor neuromuscular blockade.
- Maintenance with isoflurane or sevoflurane (theoretical risk of compound A) may be used. Desflurane may be the safest choice owing to its low rate of metabolism implying a low risk from toxic metabolites. It also preserves hepatic blood flow.
- Patients have increased sensitivity to morphine, fentanyl, and alfentanil. The $t_{1/2}$ of morphine is prolonged and so the frequency of administration should be reduced. PCA lockout times should be increased. Metabolism of remifentanil is unaffected.
- Avoid NSAIDs perioperatively.
- Peripheral regional anaesthesia is safe. Neuraxial block is often contraindicated. Coagulation studies should be normal. LA doses should be reduced owing to their reliance on hepatic clearance.
- Detailed attention to fluid balance, replacing blood loss, insensible losses, and ascites is important to avoid the risk of circulatory instability or renal failure.
- Lactate solutions should be avoided and glucose solutions should be titrated to avoid hypoglycaemia. Losses are often best replaced with albumin solutions to maintain an adequate intravascular volume. Patients who have a coagulopathy may need fresh frozen plasma as their primary replacement fluid. Maintain UO at 1 mL/kg/h. Mannitol may be necessary.

Marfan syndrome

- An inherited multisystem disorder of fibrous connective tissue caused by a mutation in the fibrillin-1 gene (*FBN1*) on chromosome 15. This mutation reduces the tensile strength and elasticity of connective tissue.
- Incidence 1:3,000–5,000 newborns.
- Inheritance is autosomal dominant, with variable expression. 25% of affected individuals arise as new mutations.
- The cardinal features affect skeletal, cardiovascular, respiratory, and ocular systems. There is a wide clinical variability of expression. Diagnosis is based on typical clinical features and a positive family history.
- In the absence of a positive family history, involvement of the skeletal and at least two other systems with a minimum of one major manifestation (ectopia lentis, aortic dilation/dissection, or dural ectasia) is required. If there is a positive family history, only two organs need be involved for diagnosis.
- Patients presenting in the neonatal period are usually severely affected with arachnodactyly, increased length, and cardiac disease (mitral insufficiency), usually as a result of a de novo mutation.

Clinical features

Skeletal

- Disproportionate length of long bones. Tall, thin with an arm span > their height. Arachnodactyly, ligamentous laxity, narrow high-arched palate with secondary dental overcrowding. Pectus excavatum or carinatum, kyphoscoliosis (10%), and hypermobile joints.

Cardiovascular

- Main cause of morbidity and mortality. Mitral valve prolapse, mitral regurgitation (commonest reason for cardiac surgery), aortic root dilation, and aortic regurgitation.
- Aortic aneurysm and dissection: commonest cause of death.
- ECHO shows about one-third of affected individuals have mitral valve prolapse, aortic root enlargement, or both, despite a normal clinical examination.

Ocular

- Subluxation of the lens (ectopia lentis: 60%), myopia, increased axial globe length, retinal detachment.

Other features

- Dural ectasia (widening of the outer layer of the dural sac and nerve root sleeves) is a widening of the neural canal. Usually occurs in the lumbosacral region and can be associated with back pain. Spinal arachnoid cysts or diverticula.
- Pulmonary blebs and OSA (lax pharyngeal wall).

Perioperative management

- May present for elective orthopaedic, ocular, or cardiovascular surgery.
- Cardiovascular assessment should include ECHO. Patients are treated with prophylactic beta-blockers to slow the rate of aortic root dilation and improve long-term survival. Where these are poorly tolerated, ACE inhibitors are used instead. Labile intraoperative BP may be controlled with glyceryl trinitrate or sodium nitroprusside infusions.
- Intraoperatively, careful positioning, handling, and padding are essential to protect lax joints and avoid dislocations.
- Pulmonary blebs ↑ the incidence of spontaneous pneumothoraces and perioperative lung complications. A preoperative CXR is undertaken. It is advisable to keep peak airway pressures low during IPPV to avoid barotrauma. Patients with significant kyphoscoliosis require lung function tests to determine the extent of their restrictive lung disease.
- Regional anaesthesia may be technically difficult owing to kyphoscoliosis. Ductal ectasia may also potentially alter the dose of LA required to achieve an adequate height of block during spinal anaesthesia.

Mucopolysaccharidoses (MPS)

- Rare group of inherited disorders of metabolism resulting from a deficiency of lysosomal enzymes required for the breakdown of complex carbohydrates known as glycosaminoglycans (GAGs).
- The resultant accumulation of these partially degraded GAGs in connective tissue cells impairs the function of the latter and leads to the clinical manifestations of the diseases. The clinical effects and disease progression depend on the enzyme that is deficient and the sites of deposition.
- Deposition continues throughout life and clinical features worsen with age, except in Sanfilippo syndrome.
- Life expectancy and quality of life are reduced.
- Inheritance is autosomal recessive except for Hunter' syndrome (X-linked disorder).
- Incidence 1:10,000–30,000 live births.
- Classification is based on specific enzyme deficiency.
- Management is mainly supportive; however, recently recombinant DNA technology has enabled IV enzyme replacement therapy to be used to improve symptoms in Hurler, Hurler–Scheie, Hunter, and Morquio A syndromes. BMT has been successfully used to improve life expectancy in Hurler syndrome by slowing progression of cardiorespiratory symptoms.

Clinical features

- Seven major types have been described.
- MPS I (α-L-iduronidase deficiency) has three variants: Hurler syndrome (MPS I H: gargoylism), Scheie syndrome (MPS I S), and Hurler–Scheie syndrome (MPS H/S). Hurler is the severest variant and Scheie the mildest.
- Hurler syndrome (1:100,000 live births) is characterized by dysmorphic features: facial coarseness, short stature, short neck, frontal bossing, hypertelorism, depressed nasal bridge, macroglossia, and gum hypertrophy.
  - Airway: probably the most challenging airway in paediatric anaesthesia.
  - ENT: adenotonsillar hypertrophy, thickened soft tissues in larynx and pharynx with resultant OSA. Deafness.
  - Cardiac involvement is very common and progressive: cardiomyopathy, thickening of the ventricular septum, mitral and aortic valvular insufficiency. Coronary artery disease is progressive.
  - CNS: developmental delay, progressive mental retardation, hydrocephalus, corneal clouding.
  - Hepatosplenomegaly with a protuberant abdomen and a high incidence of inguinal and umbilical hernias.
  - Skeletal: joint stiffness, thoracic and lumbar kyphoscoliosis. Odontoid hypoplasia with atlantoaxial instability.
  - Usually die in the first decade of life secondary to cardiorespiratory failure.

- Scheie syndrome (1:600,000 live births).
  - Characterized by stiff joints, corneal clouding, normal intelligence and stature.
  - Features may be coarse, with excessive body hair, macroglossia, glaucoma, and mitral and/ or aortic incompetence in older patients.
  - Skeletal: carpal tunnel, joint stiffness, back pain, spondylolisthesis.
  - Normal life expectancy.
- Hurler–Scheie syndrome is extremely rare and intermediate in severity. Patients can live into adulthood.
- MPS II: Hunter' syndrome.
  - Rare, X-linked with incidence 1:140,000 male births, mainly Caucasians.
  - Severest form shares many features of Hurler syndrome, but in a milder form. Progressive neurodegeneration results in a vegetative state and death in teenage years.
  - Mild forms are at risk of cervical cord compression secondary to thickening of the dura and ligamentum flavum (MRI to assess compression and stability prior to airway manipulation).
- MPS III: Sanfilippo syndrome (types A, B, C, and D).
  - Commonest variant in UK.
  - Mild dysmorphism, severe mental retardation with difficult aggressive hyperactive behavioural disturbances. Death occurs in second or third decade.
- MPS IV: Morquio syndrome (A and B).
  - Rare. Normal intelligence.
  - Aortic incompetence in adults.
  - Severe bone dysplasia: short-trunk dwarfism, kyphosis (restrictive lung disease), pigeon chest.
  - High risk of cervical cord compression from minimal trauma secondary to a hypoplastic, poorly ossified dens with poor ligamentous support. Often require frequent MRIs and prophylactic occipitocervical fusions. Instability may occur in the lower spine.
  - Life expectancy depends on neurological complications and cardiorespiratory disease secondary to restrictive lung disease.
- MPS VI: Maroteaux–Lamy syndrome.
  - Rare.
  - Normal intelligence.
  - Coarse features. Difficult intubation.
  - Cardiomyopathy, mitral and aortic valve thickening.
  - Kyphoscoliosis, mild joint stiffness and atlantoaxial instability reported.
  - Progressive airway narrowing leading to cor pulmonale and death in early 20s.
- MPS VII: Sly syndrome
  - β-glucuronidase deficiency, extremely rare.
  - Short stature, with possible odontoid hypoplasia and cardiac valvular involvement.

Perioperative management

- Associated with a high morbidity and mortality rate; therefore, surgery is only undertaken in specialist centres familiar with the management of these patients.
- Recent anaesthetic records are useful and imaging of the airway may be available.
- Important risk vs benefit discussions are necessary with the patient (where appropriate), parents, or carers to allow them to be fully informed.
- Coordinate surgical specialties to carry out several procedures under the same GA.
- Always have an experienced ENT surgical team available in theatre.
- Airway obstruction with accompanying difficulty with facemask ventilation, oxygenation and/or laryngoscopy is the most serious potential anaesthetic complication (CICO: can't intubate, can't ventilate). Obstruction can occur anywhere in the upper or lower airways owing to accumulation of GAGs causing macroglossia, adenotonsillar hypertrophy, and thickening of the larynx and pharynx. The trachea and lower airways may also become thickened, distorted, and obstructive, especially under GA.
- Patients with OSA are at high risk of airway emergencies during GA.
- Hurler, Hunter, and Maroteaux–Lamy syndromes commonly present with airways that are difficult to maintain and intubate. This may worsen with age.
- Fibreoptic intubation is frequently necessary but is very challenging because distortion and obstruction of tissue structures make recognition of anatomy potentially difficult.
- Tissues in the airway may be fairly fixed and immobile, making mouth opening and laryngoscopy difficult.
- Awake fibreoptic intubation in this age group is difficult and therefore not commonly performed.
- Airway adjuncts or LMAs may not always improve the airway obstruction.
- ETT sizes may need to be 2 or 3 sizes smaller than the predicted size.
- May have recurrent respiratory tract infections or excessive secretions, or may develop restrictive pulmonary disease secondary to kyphoscoliosis or hepatosplenomegaly. OSA and restrictive lung disease may result in pulmonary hypertension, cor pulmonale, and eventually respiratory failure.
- Cervical cord compression may be present in the cervicocranial region in MPS I, II, IV, and VI. Atlantoaxial instability may also be present in MPS IV and to a lesser extent MPS VI. Neck manipulation during intubation or surgery may result in cord damage and paralysis in these patients. It is essential to have up-to-date information on the current status of any abnormalities.

- CVS: cardiomyopathy, valvular, or coronary artery disease may be difficult to detect in patients owing to poor mobility and communication. Pulmonary hypertension may develop owing to chronic obstructive hypoxic symptoms. Patients may present in heart failure, dysrhythmias, ischaemia, or sudden death. A recent cardiology review is essential.
- Pre- and postoperative care on HDU/ICU.

Muscular dystrophies

- Group of inherited muscle disorders resulting from an abnormality or absence of the muscle-stabilizing protein dystrophin.
- Skeletal, smooth, and cardiac muscles are affected. These muscle fibres undergo a degenerative process and are replaced with fat or connective tissue.
- Presents with progressive muscle weakness. The age of onset and life expectancy are dependent on the type of muscular dystrophy.

Duchenne muscular dystrophy (DMD)

- Sex-linked recessive inheritance.
- Commonest and most severe type. 1:3,500 live male births.
- Presents between 3 and 5 years of age with falls and abnormal waddling (Trendelenburg) gait. Characteristically, children pick themselves up after falls by using their hands to climb up their legs (Gower's sign) because of proximal lower limb and pelvic girdle muscle weakness.
- With disease progression, the calf muscles become pseudohypertrophied. As muscle weakness progresses, flexion contractures develop and 95% of patients are wheelchair-bound by 12 years old.
- Once wheelchair bound, the onset of scoliosis is rapid, forced vital capacity is reduced, distortion of the diaphragm may result in oesophageal reflux and, combined with a poor cough, the risk of aspiration pneumonitis is increased.
- Diagnosis is based on clinical findings, creatinine phosphokinase (CPK) levels (10 times normal) in children not walking by 18 months or showing deterioration of gait, genetic testing (abnormality of chromosome Xp21.2), and muscle biopsy.
- 30% are mentally retarded (non-progressive).
- Dilated cardiomyopathy occurs in >50% by 15 years old and is the leading cause of death. ECG changes are common, with evidence of LVH in younger patients (Q wave in lead III or V6), and commonly in older patients there may be a sinus tachycardia, tall R waves, a short P–R interval, and evidence of RVH.
- Mitral valve prolapse, ventricular wall motion abnormalities, arrhythmias, and sudden death may feature.
- Female carriers are at risk of cardiomyopathy.
- Treatment aims to control symptoms to improve quality of life. Corticosteroids are used to slow the progression of muscle weakness.
- Death is usually due to cardiorespiratory failure in the third decade of life.

Becker's muscular dystrophy

- Sex-linked recessive, less common (1:60,000) and milder than DMD. The abnormality is on the same gene, dystrophin, located at Xp21.
- Onset is later and progression slower than with DMD. Patients may be able to continue walking into their 30s. Up to 50% of patients survive beyond 40 years.
- Mental retardation is less common than in DMD.
- Cardiac muscle may be affected.
- CPK levels, EMG patterns, and muscle biopsy results may be similar to those seen in DMD.

Emery–Dreifuss muscular dystrophy

- Sex-linked recessive inheritance affecting humeral, peroneal, and cardiac muscle. The gene abnormality is at Xp28.
- Symptoms usually develop during childhood or adolescence. Most patients survive into middle age.
- Cardiac involvement may result in heart block and sudden death. Patients usually develop muscle contractures of the Achilles tendon and at their elbows.
- CPK can be normal.

Congenital muscular dystrophy

- Group of conditions that presents as a 'floppy baby' or a myopathic form of arthrogryposis.
- Autosomal recessive affecting both sexes.
- The severe form may be fatal, whereas the more benign forms usually present with orthopaedic complications (contractures, scoliosis, hip dislocation) and may be slow or fail to meet their motor milestones.
- There may be intellectual disability, eye manifestations (cataracts, absent optic nerves, colobomas), brain abnormalities (hydrocephalus, cerebellar cysts, brain stem hypoplasia), and seizures.

Facioscapulohumeral muscular dystrophy

- Autosomal dominant disorder shows marked variations in severity in families.
- It is relatively benign and slowly progressive. Onset is later, with one-third of patients asymptomatic until well into adulthood. It affects abductors of the upper limb, causes facial muscle weakness (with inability to purse lips or close eyes tightly shut), winging of the scapula, sensorineural deafness, and retinopathy.
- Approximately one-half develop leg muscle weakness, with roughly 10% eventually requiring a wheelchair.

Autosomal recessive limb girdle dystrophy

- A wasting weakness with variable rate of progression affecting the big proximal muscle groups of all limbs. Often wheelchair-bound by 30 years of age.
- Both sexes equally affected.
- Calf hypertrophy may occur and CPK is high.

Perioperative management

- The pattern and severity of muscle weakness should be established to help ensure that the benefits of surgery justify the risks of surgery and GA.
- Manage in a centre with a specialist team with access to an ICU.
- A diagnosis is usually present before attending for surgery, allowing the anaesthetist and surgeon to decide on an appropriate perioperative plan and discuss this with the child's parents/carers.
- Occasionally an undiagnosed child presents for incidental surgery or a hypotonic child may require a muscle biopsy. A family history of neuromuscular disease or adverse reaction to GA should provoke suspicion. A neurology opinion should be sought preoperatively, a CK

test may help with diagnosis, and, in the absence of a family history in a hypotonic child with other organ involvement, preoperative lactate levels will help determine if a mitochondrial myopathy is present.

• Assess cardiac function and abnormalities (ECG and ECHO). It can be difficult to assess the physiological reserve of patients who are unable to physically challenge themselves, making traditional stress ECHO unreliable. Cardiac MRI and a dobutamine stress ECHO may give more useful information. ACE inhibitors may be indicated by the cardiologist.

• Respiratory function tests including a baseline ABG may help predict the need for postoperative IPPV. Patients with poor cough, kyphoscoliosis causing restrictive lung disease, and respiratory muscle weakness are more prone to recurrent chest infections. Physiotherapy is used to optimize patients for surgery and is continued postoperatively. Desired targets before elective surgery are FVC >25% predicted and PEFR >30% predicted. Postoperative NIV should be discussed and perhaps trialled preoperatively.

• Have a low threshold for intraoperative invasive monitoring.

• There is no proven link between MH and muscular dystrophy. Occasionally patients with muscular dystrophy may develop dysrhythmias and muscle damage on exposure to volatile anaesthetic agents. The effects are related to release of K^+ from the cells or to release of cellular constituents, e.g. myoglobin. The clinical picture may resemble MH. For this reason, volatile agents are often avoided and a TIVA technique used, although this is not always possible or appropriate. Occasionally a patient may need an inhalational induction before securing IV access for TIVA.

• Anaesthetic-induced rhabdomyolysis (AIR) in muscular dystrophy patients is well described in the literature. This potentially fatal condition may present as an acute hyper-K^+ cardiac arrest, postoperative rhabdomyolysis, a gradual ↑ in HR and temperature, with or without muscle rigidity or signs of hypermetabolism. This may occur intraoperatively or in the recovery period. Suxamethonium is the most potent trigger; its use is contraindicated in patients known or suspected to have muscular dystrophies. A small number of these patients may also develop this with exposure to volatile agents and so, where possible, a 'trigger-free anaesthetic should be given. The role of dantrolene in AIR is unknown—it has no clinical benefit.

• Response to non-depolarizing muscle relaxants is variable, but their use is safe. Reduced doses with neuromuscular monitoring are recommended.

• DMD patients are reported to be at increased risk of bleeding intraoperatively. For major surgery, e.g. scoliosis repair, use a cell saver and an antifibrinolytic agent.

• Regional techniques should be used to ↓ the need for respiratory depressant analgesics postoperatively and improve chest physiotherapy compliance.

• Postoperative ECG monitoring even after minor surgery.

• Have a low threshold for postoperative care in an HDU or PICU.

Myasthenia gravis

- Autoimmune disease caused by IgG autoantibodies blocking the postsynaptic acetylcholine receptors at the nicotinic neuromuscular junction (NMJ); this results in a reduction in the number of functional receptors.
- Cholinergic receptors in smooth and cardiac muscle are unaffected.
- Symptomatic when the number of functional receptors is reduced to approximately 30% of normal.
- Characterized by painless muscular weakness and fatigability of skeletal muscle with exertion. The prevalence is approximately 1:1,000 of the population. Childhood (age <16 years) onset myasthenia gravis accounts for about 10–15% of these patients with a 2M:3F ratio.
- Three main types in childhood:
  - Juvenile myasthenia gravis
  - Transient neonatal myasthenia gravis
  - Congenital myasthenia gravis.

Clinical features

Juvenile myasthenia gravis

- Pubertal and post-pubertal 1M:4.5F, whereas prepubertal 1M:1F.
- Commonest presentation is ptosis, often associated with strabismus, diplopia, lid twitch, and ophthalmoplegia due to involvement of the extraocular muscles. If symptoms are confined to these muscles, then spontaneous remission, especially in prepubertal children, occurs in about 30% of patients.
- Most also develop generalized muscle weakness affecting bulbar, facial, and limb muscles. This results in dysphonia, dysphagia, and proximal limb weakness, which fluctuates in severity, worsens as the day progresses, and improves with rest. Rarely, respiratory muscles are affected; but during a myasthenic crises ventilator support may be required.
- Symptoms may worsen with infection, pyrexia, surgical or emotional stress, and certain drugs (aminoglycosides and anticonvulsants).
- Thymic hyperplasia is implicated in pathogenesis. Thymomas are only found in adults.
- Often there is associated autoimmune diseases, e.g. thyroiditis, systemic lupus erythematosus, and rheumatoid arthritis.
- Diagnosis:
  - Edrophonium test: Atropine is given, then an infusion of edrophonium (fast-onset, short-acting acetylcholinesterase inhibitor). If positive, a rapid improvement of muscle strength occurs for about 5 min.
  - Radioimmunoassay for AChR antibodies. A negative result does not exclude the disease
  - Electrophysiological studies (single-fibre EMG): poorly tolerated
- Treatment:
  - Anticholinesterases. Pyridostigmine bromide (1 mg/kg 4-hourly initially) is used owing to its longer $t_{1/2}$ and better side-effect profile.
  - Immunosuppression with corticosteroids may be used short term for acute exacerbations unresponsive to increased doses

of anticholinesterase. Because of side effects, these may be used in combination with a steroid-sparing immunosuppressant, e.g. azathioprine. Occasionally ciclosporin or cyclophosphamide are used.
- Plasma exchange or IV immunoglobulin may be used preoperatively or in the management of myasthenic crises.
- Thymectomy may lead to an improvement in symptoms and remission in 60–90% of patients.

Neonatal transient myasthenia gravis
- 15% of infants born to myasthenic mothers, secondary to placental transfer of maternal AChR antibodies.
- Symptoms may occur in the first few hours of life but can take several days. The neonate may present with hypotonia, weak cry, feeding difficulties, ptosis, facial weakness, apnoeas, and occasionally respiratory distress requiring IPPV.
- Treatment is supportive.
- Neostigmine is used. Symptoms improve over 4–6 weeks.
- There is no increased incidence of myasthenia gravis in later life.

Congenital myasthenia gravis
- Rare autosomal recessive disorder of the NMJ; a heterogenous disease due to the defect potentially occurring presynaptically, postsynaptically, or at the synapse. There is no autoimmune component.
- Presentation is often at birth, but it may not present until adolescence. Newborns present with severe weakness, hypotonia, recurrent apnoeas, feeding difficulties, and ocular muscle weakness.
- Variable response to anticholinesterases. Patients do not improve with immunosuppressive therapy or thymectomy. The course is often non-progressive, with lifelong mild disease.

Perioperative management
- A multidisciplinary approach involving neurologists, surgeons, intensivists, and anaesthetist is essential.
- Establish the muscle groups affected. In particular, assess respiratory and bulbar involvement. Perform lung function tests.
- Before thymectomy, seek radiological opinion to establish whether there is any tracheal deviation or compression.
- The neurologist and patient should ensure that muscle function is optimized on anticholinesterase therapy. If weakness is severe, preoperative IV immunoglobulin or plasmapheresis therapy may be necessary.
- PICU or HDU admission for IPPV or observation postoperatively must be available and discussed with the patient and their parents/carers.
- Place first on list. Anticholinesterases are omitted the night before surgery.
- If weakness is severe, then therapy is continued up to the time of surgery and glycopyrronium bromide given to ↓ excessive salivation and vagal actions.
- Premedication is best avoided.
- Patients receiving steroids need supplementation intraoperatively.
- The majority require ETT and IPPV during GA.

- Avoid suxamethonium. There is an increased resistance and 3–4 times the normal dose may be required. The incidence of non-depolarizing phase II block is high. Anticholinesterases and plasmapheresis may prolong the action.
- Non-depolarizing muscle relaxants are safe but should be titrated and monitored. As ocular muscles are commonly affected and sensitive to muscle relaxants, facial nerve monitoring is recommended. Atracurium is first choice: dose 10–20% of normal. Descriptions of rocuronium and sugammadex have been widely published in the adult literature, but there is little experience in paediatric cases.
- Maintenance as preferred; avoiding the need for a muscle relaxant is well described.
- Volatile agents are known to ↓ transmission at the NMJ, although there is no clinically significant problem demonstrated. This is not a feature of propofol and so in theory TIVA may be a better choice of technique. Remifentanil is largely metabolized by non-specific tissue esterases.
- Give reversal and extubate once the airway and respiratory muscle function have returned to normal. Head lift for 5 s, vital capacity, and measured inspiratory force are useful measurements where possible. Patients with known bulbar involvement may need airway protection until muscle tone has returned to normal.
- Muscle weakness is exacerbated by hypothermia, hypoK$^+$, aminoglycoside antibiotics, Mg^{2+}, and anticonvulsants.
- Parenteral opioids (infusion or PCA), regional techniques, NSAIDs, and paracetamol are all appropriate analgesic options.
- Restart PO anticholinesterase therapy as soon as possible postoperatively (if need be via an NGT). If the patient has an ileus, use IV neostigmine—titrated slowly to effect up to a maximum equivalent to the patient's normal dose of oral pyridostigmine. 1 mg of IV neostigmine is equivalent to 30 mg of PO pyridostigmine. Seek expert advice!
- Postoperative muscle weakness may result from a myasthenic or cholinergic crisis.
- Myasthenic crises result from a relative ↓ in the amount of ACh at the NMJ. A dose of edrophonium will help differentiate between these and determine the appropriate therapy. Some patients may require postoperative IV immunoglobulins, plasmapheresis, or an IV infusion of neostigmine.
- Cholinergic crises results from excessive administration of acetylcholinesterase inhibitors, resulting in excess ACh at the NMJ. Muscle weakness, sweating, salivation, blurred vision, and diarrhoea occur. Treatment is supportive and further acetylcholinesterase inhibitors are withheld.

Myopathies

- Group of rare muscular diseases where the muscles function abnormally owing to a primary defect within them.
- Classified according to whether they are acquired or inherited. In this section, we will focus solely on the inherited myopathies.
- Classification of the inherited forms is based on identifying specific molecular and enzyme defects often associated with particular histological changes seen in the muscle. There can be marked phenotypic variation in families affecting age of onset and severity.
- Myopathies are multi-organ diseases requiring a careful preoperative assessment of potential cardiovascular or respiratory involvement, which may not always correlate with the degree of muscle weakness.
- Divided into three groups (muscular dystrophies and myotonias are discussed separately):
  - Morphologically defined congenital myopathies:
    —Central core disease
    —Nemaline myopathy.
  - Mitochondrial myopathies:
    —MELAS
    —MERRF syndrome
    —Kearns–Sayre syndrome
    —Leigh syndrome.
  - Metabolic myopathies
    —Muscle glycogenoses.

Morphologically defined congenital myopathies

Central core disease

- Autosomal dominant condition, characterized by the presence of well-defined central cores of myofibrils extending the entire length of type 1 muscle fibres.
- The gene mutation is on chromosome 19 close to the ryanodine receptor gene.
- May present with hypotonia at birth, with proximal muscle weakness and motor delays in infancy. Clinical presentation can vary significantly from fetal akinesia to muscle weakness in adults. There may be associated skeletal deformities, e.g. congenital dislocation of the hips, pes cavus, kyphoscoliosis, joint hypermobility, short neck, and mandibular hypoplasia.
- Symptoms may be mild and muscle biopsy may be required to confirm diagnosis. Creatine kinase levels are normal.
- The condition is non-progressive and intelligence is normal.

Perioperative management

- Muscle weakness is assessed preoperatively.
- Cardiomyopathy is not a feature.
- Closely associated with MH; therefore, treat as susceptible.

Nemaline myopathy

- Characterized by abnormal thread-like or rod-shaped structures called nemaline bodies (mostly α-actinin and actin from breakdown of the Z-discs in the sarcomere) in skeletal muscle fibres.

Bronchiolitis

- An acute infection of the upper and lower respiratory tract. Most commonly symptomatic in children <2yrs. Severe symptoms are due to obstruction of the small airways by respiratory secretions.
- Commonest cause of hospitalization of infants and of acute respiratory failure in UK PICUs.
- Approximately 3–5% of hospitalized infants need PICU. This is greater (30–40%) in high-risk groups.
- In babies with respiratory distress, consider sepsis, airway malacia and CHD (since these can be very similar or concomitant to bronchiolitis).
- If apnoea is the predominant feature, then exclude NAI, pertussis, sepsis, and metabolic conditions.
- Risk factors for severe disease:
  - CHD (particularly lesions associated with pulmonary hypertension).
  - Chronic lung disease (remember to interpret blood gas analysis appropriately if chronic hyperCO_2).
  - Prematurity (<34 weeks corrected gestation at presentation).
  - <6 weeks of age.
  - Immune deficiency.
  - Adenovirus is associated with poorer outcome.
- Clinical features:
  - Moderate: SpO_2 <92% in air, tachypnoea, respiratory distress, tachycardia, poor feeding.
  - Severe: FiO_2 >0.5 to maintain SpO_2 >92%, severe recession, tachypnoea, tachycardia, >2 apnoea/h (not needing bagging).
  - Life-threatening: SpO_2 <88% (despite humidified high-flow nasal cannula O_2 (HHFNC)/CPAP), respiratory acidosis (pH <7.25 despite BiPAP), exhaustion/grunting/marked recession, apnoea (needing bagging) or frequent apnoeas with desaturations and bradycardia.
- Initial management:
  - Manage in resuscitation area e.g. A+E or HDU, with full monitoring (SpO_2/ ECG/ BP/ temperature/ RR).
  - Ensure upper airway patency/nasal suction as required.
  - Stop feeds (2/3 IV fluid maintenance).
  - CXR.
  - Capillary blood gas sample.
  - IV antibiotics if strong evidence of bacterial infection or if severe disease.
  - Trial of HHFNC O_2, e.g. Optiflow/Airvo, aiming for SpO_2 >92%.
  - Consider a trial of nasal CPAP (nCPAP)/BiPAP (aim for PEEP of 5–10 cmH_2O).
  - Insert OGT on free drainage and regularly decompress the stomach.
  - Nebulized treatment is not routinely indicated, but can be trialled (bronchodilators/hypertonic saline).
  - Consider antiviral therapy, e.g. oseltamivir, if severe or life-threatening illness (take local microbiology advice).
  - Consider caffeine 20 mg/kg IV (over 30 min.) for recurrent apnoea (theophylline not routinely recommended).
  - Monitor UO and U+E (risk of hypoNa$^+$).

- Indications for CPAP HHFNC O_2
  - Severe disease unresponsive or deteriorating despite initial treatment.
  - Respiratory acidosis (pH <7.25).
  - Self-limiting apnoeas often improve (not those needing bagging).
  - Significant apnoeas (not self correcting) may respond to nBIPAP with a back up rate but prepare for intubation in parallel
  - If patient is difficult to settle on nCPAP/nBIPAP, consider sedation with 15–30 mg/kg chloral hydrate via OGT (anticipate potential side effects).
- Indication for intubation:
  - Features of life-threatening illness not rapidly improving.
  - Worsening hyperCO$_2$ with respiratory acidosis, despite maximal non-invasive support.
  - Hypoxia, despite maximal non-invasive support.
  - Significant apnoeas (needing frequent bagging) not improving on maximal non-invasive support.
- Drugs for intubation:
  - Consider ketamine 1–2 mg/kg IV bolus, since it is more cardio-stable and also a bronchodilator.
  - Avoid drugs known to precipitate histamine release (if bronchospasm is prominent).
  - Sedation with morphine/fentanyl and midazolam.
  - Paralysis is required to avoid gas trapping and extensive collapse/consolidation.
- Ventilation strategies:
  - Manual IPPV with saline lavage and suction (often frequently repeated) for mucus plugs.
  - Lung protective strategies applied:
    —Limit peak inspiratory pressure to <30 cmH$_2$O.
    —V_T 5–7 mL/kg.
    —PEEP (5–10 cmH$_2$O) dependant on oxygenation
    —Avoid respiratory rates >30/min.
    —Ti 0.7–1.0 s.
    —Aim for SpO$_2$ >92% <97%.
    —Permissive hyperCO$_2$ with pH >7.2.

Convulsive status epilepticus (CSE)

- A generalized convulsion lasting 30 min or longer, or when successive convulsions occur so frequently over a 30 min period, that the patient does not fully recover consciousness between them.
- Simple febrile convulsions are very common in children (1:20). They are usually occur between 6 months to 6 years, last 2-3 mins, usually generalised tonic clonic and have an obvious febrile focus as opposed to complex febrile convulsions.
- Common causes of CSE:
  - Complex febrile convulsion (commonest, ~30%).
  - CNS infection.
  - HypoNa$^+$ or other significant electrolyte abnormality.
  - Hypoglycaemia.
  - Head injury/NAI/CVA/space-occupying lesion/blocked VP shunt.
  - Secondary to hypoxia or hypoperfusion.
  - Toxic substance/poisoning.
  - Inborn error of metabolism (especially if <3 years of age, hepatosplenomegaly, failure to thrive, family history, microcephaly).
  - Idiopathic epilepsy.
- Support A, B, C (➔ Fig. 27.1 for management flow diagram):
  - Maintain airway with adjuncts if necessary.
  - High-flow O$_2$.
  - Gain IV/IO access.
  - Remember to measure glucose: correct hypoglycaemia urgently with 2 mL/kg 10% glucose.
  - 20 mL/kg fluid bolus for signs of shock.
- Stepwise treatment with anticonvulsive drugs (AEDs):
  - Step 1: After 5 min CSE, give benzodiazepines, either 0.1 mg/kg lorazepam IV or 0.5 mg/kg buccal midazolam or diazepam PR if no IV access (remember to consider what prehospital medications have been given).
  - Step 2 – Repeat above dose of benzodiazepine if seizures not terminated 10 min after Step 1.
  - Step 3 – After a further 10 min, re-confirm it is CSE and give phenytoin 20 mg/kg (maximum 1 g) IV over 20 min with continuous cardiac monitoring or phenobarbital 20 mg/kg (maximum 1 g) over 20 min if already taking phenytoin. If no IV/IO access, consider using paraldehyde. Prepare for intubation.
  - Step 4: If CSE is refractory after long-acting AED given, induce GA with thiopental 4–8 mg/kg.
- Important issues to attend to rapidly:
  - Glucose (aim for 4–8 mmol/L).
  - HypoNa$^+$ (consider 2 mL/kg hypertonic saline if Na$^+$ <125 and still convulsing).
  - Cover for meningo/encephalitis with cefotaxime 80 mg/kg, aciclovir (2–10 mg/kg, depending on age: see BNF for Children) and a macrolide (consult local hospital guideline).
  - Treat signs of raised ICP aggressively (clinically or on CT brain).
  - Avoid LP in immediate post-seizure period, since ICP may be raised.
- Indications for intubation:
  - Apnoea.

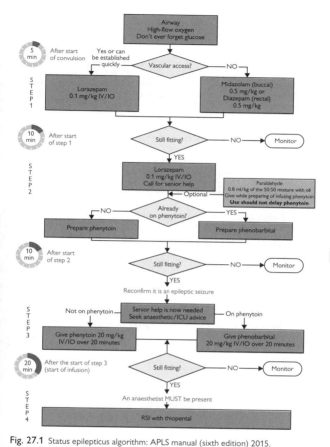

Fig. 27.1 Status epilepticus algorithm: APLS manual (sixth edition) 2015.

Reproduced with permission from Wieteka, S. et al. (2016) *Advanced Paediatric Life Support: A Practical Approach to Emergencies*, 6th Ed. Manchester, UK: Wiley, on behalf of the Advanced Life Support Group. Copyright © 2016 John Wiley and Sons.

- Respiratory depression secondary to anticonvulsant drugs.
- Intractable seizures (Step 4 above).
- To enable neuroimaging (CT or MRI) safely, e.g. when patient is unable to maintain own airway, GCS <13, non-cooperative, hypoxic, and/or hyperCO$_2$.
- Signs of raised ICP.

- Drugs for intubation:
  - Thiopental 4–8 mg/kg is preferred to help control seizure activity.
  - Paralytic agents are only used at induction and during intra/inter-hospital transport, so that seizure activity can be more easily monitored. Ongoing seizure activity should be managed with escalating doses of AED and not more paralysis.
  - Sedation is maintained with morphine and midazolam; however, if early extubation is a possibility, use a shorter-acting agent, e.g. propofol and remifentanil, for transfer, e.g. to and from CT.
- Early extubation of the child with uncomplicated CSE is recommended (reduces the risks associated with transfer and prolonged IPPV, as well as the impact of hospitalization on the family).
- Consider early extubation if:
  - Seizures controlled with long-acting AED.
  - Normal neuro-imaging (CT or MRI) or no changes from previous imaging.
  - Neurological state unchanged from pre-morbid state when sedation is withdrawn.
  - No flexor or extensor posturing.
  - Intact protective airway reflexes.
  - Good respiratory drive and minimal settings on the ventilator.
  - Normal biochemistry and blood glucose.
  - Acid–base balance normalized (raised lactate commonly clears rapidly with seizure termination and small fluid bolus).
  - No concerns about a difficult airway and resources to re-intubate are immediately available.
- Transfer to tertiary centre if unsuitable for early extubation or fails to wake appropriately after 4 h of trying as above (discuss with local transport team/PICU/neurologist) (Fig. 27.1).

Croup (laryngotracheobronchitis)

- Common childhood condition, usually of viral aetiology, occurring between 6 months and 6 years of age.
- It causes mucosal swelling of upper airways. Usually responds to steroids.
- A subgroup can be recurrent and associated with reactive airway disease (with only mild viral symptoms).
- Symptoms: barking cough, fever (mild), hoarse voice, noisy breathing, mild dysphagia.
- Signs: stridor, respiratory distress, tachycardia.
- Differential diagnosis:
  - Infective: epiglottitis, bacterial tracheitis, peri-tonsillar/retropharyngeal abscess, diphtheria.
  - Non-infective: FB, angioneurotic oedema, hypocalcaemic tetany, ingestion of corrosives, mediastinal mass.
- Features of severe croup:
  - Frequent barking cough and prominent inspiratory (often also expiratory) stridor at rest.
  - Marked sternal wall recession.
  - Significant distress and agitation, lethargy, or restlessness.
  - Hypoxaemia.
- Risk factors for intubation in severe croup:
  - History of severe obstruction, or previous severe croup, or known structural upper airway abnormalities, e.g. laryngomalacia.
  - < 6 months of age.
  - Immunocompromised.
  - Poor response to initial treatment.
  - Impending respiratory failure:
    —Decreased level of consciousness.
    —Dusky appearance and hypoxaemia despite O_2.
    —The child who has not improved, but the cough/stridor has become quieter (and recession may have reduced) is about to have complete obstruction.

Anaesthetic management

- Avoid unnecessary interventions that will distress the child, e.g. IV cannulation or CXR (although the appropriate use of LA creams and distraction may allow safe cannulation in some cases).
- SpO_2 monitoring and high-flow O_2.
- Severe cases, nebulized adrenaline (epinephrine) 500 mcg/kg of 1:1000 (max 5mg) ie 0.5 ml/kg (max 5 mls), will improve the child while waiting for theatre. Do not think it has got better—the child still needs to go to theatre. The nebulizer can be repeated, but beware of rebound deterioration.
- Arrange calm transfer to theatre or bring all equipment/personnel to child. Have skilled assistant and appropriate airway equipment available for the transfer.
- Involve consultant ENT surgeon early on.

- Heliox: can provide temporary relief (if available), reduces work of breathing (lower-density gas). Can buy time whilst team/equipment assemble, and some patients may improve enough to avoid intubation.

Intubation
- Have two experienced anaesthetists present.
- Before induction, a focused team brief should occur, including the role of the ENT surgeon and the plan for failure.
- Similar technique as for diagnostic bronchoscopy and removal of inhaled FB.
- Principles of a safe technique are inhalational induction, maintenance of SV, and avoidance of neuromuscular blockade until the airway is secured with an ETT.
- Avoid sedative premedication.
- Induce in position that child prefers (often sitting). Do not force them to lie flat if unwilling.
- THRIVE may be appropriate if it is not distressing.
- Inhalational induction with sevoflurane in 100% O_2.
- Induction is slower than normal. Gentle application of CPAP helps to overcome upper airway obstruction. Total airway obstruction is a risk as muscle tone is progressively lost.
- An IV cannula is inserted (when adequate depth of anaesthesia reached) and atropine (20 mcg/kg) or glycopyrronium bromide (5–10 mcg/kg) given (to dry secretions and protect against bradycardia from airway instrumentation).
- Small and cautious boluses of propofol (e.g. 1 mg/kg) are sometimes used by senior anaesthetists. It allows more rapid deepening of anaesthesia but risks apnoea.
- Once adequately anaesthetized, laryngoscopy and endotracheal intubation are performed under deep inhalational anaesthesia.
- Use smaller ETT (at least 0.5 mm I.D.) than calculated by APLS formula (may need a croup tube—longer than standard in relation to ID) and ensure it is well secured (e.g. Melbourne strapping).
- In epiglottitis, gentle compression of the chest may produce bubbles that give an indication of the position of the laryngeal inlet. An intubation stylet (bougie) with tube railroaded over (used as primary intubation technique) is useful.
- In conditions other than croup, there may be anticipated difficulties with direct visualization of the larynx. In these situations, videolaryngoscopes, rigid bronchoscopes, and flexible fibreoptic scopes are fraught with difficulties and should only be used by those experienced in their use.
- Once intubated, it may be appropriate to change to a nasal ETT (if intubation was not too difficult) to make care in PICU easier. Before transfer to PICU, the child is sedated and paralysed. An NGT, second IV cannula, and an arterial line are usually inserted. Antibiotics are given if appropriate and a CXR to confirm ETT position.
- Occasionally, endotracheal intubation is not possible and a tracheostomy is required with the child maintained on O_2 and volatile breathing spontaneously via a face mask. If a CICO situation develops, this is managed as described in Chapter 9 p. 172.

Diabetic ketoacidosis (DKA)

- For general information on diabetes management, ➲ Chapter 26.

Diagnosis

- Acidosis (pH <7.3 or HCO_3 <18 mmol/L) and ketonaemia (blood β-hydroxybutyrate >3 mmol/L)
- Blood glucose is usually >11 mmol/L, but known IDDM may develop DKA with normal blood glucose levels. If blood ketone measurement is unavailable, use urinary ketones levels.
- Hyperosmolar hyperglycaemic state consists of a very high blood glucose >30 mmol/L and little or no acidosis or ketones. This requires different management than DKA—seek urgent advice.

Severity

- Mild or moderate: pH 7.1–7.3.
- Severe: pH <7.1

Causes of death in DKA

- Cerebral oedema:
  - Unpredictable occurrence.
  - Commoner in younger children and newly diagnosed IDDM.
  - 25% mortality.
  - ↓ risk by slow correction of metabolic abnormalities and maintaining a normal Na^+ level.
  - Reduced GCS is directly related to degree of acidosis, but signs of raised ICP, e.g. headache, irritability, cushings reflex suggest cerebral oedema.
  - Rapidly exclude hypoglycaemia before ascribing neurological symptoms to cerebral oedema.
- $HypoK^+$:
  - Prevent with careful monitoring and management.
  - May need CVL if strong solutions required.
- Aspiration:
  - Assess need to protect airway (may need intubation), consider an NGT.
- Sepsis:
  - May rarely precipitate DKA.
  - Fever is not caused by DKA, but leucocytosis is common.
  - Suspect if pyrexia, hypothermia, hypotension, refractory acidosis or lactic acidosis.

Management

- ABC including 100% O_2.
- Recently, the recommended fluid volumes to be administered have reduced significantly.
- Clinical assessment of degree of dehydration is inaccurate in DKA.
- Use electronic calculator on British Society for Paediatric Endocrinology and Diabetes website (see below).

- If shocked, the circulating volume is restored with 10 mL/kg of 0.9% NaCl. Do not give further fluid boluses without discussion with consultant. Use extreme caution with multiple fluid boluses.
- There is no evidence for other volume expanders/colloids.
- For mild/moderate DKA:
  - No IV fluid bolus.
  - Assume 5% fluid deficit and replace over 48 h.
- For severe DKA:
  - Only give fluid bolus if shocked.
  - Assume 10% fluid deficit and replace over 48 h.
- Maintenance rates are <50% of normal (↓ risk of cerebral oedema):
  - 2 mL/kg/h up to 10 kg.
  - 1 mL/kg/h between 10 and 40 kg.
  - 40 mL/h fixed volume over 40 kg.
  - Remove any bolus fluid volumes from total if >20 mL/kg.
  - Do not routinely give additional fluid for urinary losses.
- Neonates require specialist support and larger volumes.
- 0.9% NaCl with K^+ 40 mmol/L used until glucose <14 mmol/L.
- Insulin:
  - Start only once IV fluids with K^+ administered for 1–2 h.
  - 0.05 or 0.1 units/kg/h.
  - Do not bolus IV insulin.
  - Blood sugar will start to fall with fluid administration
- Bicarbonate: no evidence of benefit.
- Venous thrombosis: significant risk of femoral vein thrombosis in young and very sick who have femoral lines (risk/benefit).

Treatment of cerebral oedema in DKA

- Discuss management with paediatric critical care specialist.
- Treat immediately if child displays any signs or symptoms of possible cerebral oedema.
- Mannitol (0.5 g/kg over 10–15 min), i.e. 2.5–5 mL/kg of 20% solution, or hypertonic NaCl (2.7% or 3%) 2.5–5 mL/kg over 10–15 min.
- Restrict fluids to half of current maintenance rate.
- Secure airway as appropriate (caution against secondary brain injury: ➋ Chapter 21).
- Use hypertonic NaCl (rather than 0.9% NaCl or colloid) if fluid bolus is needed at time of induction (if hypovolaemic).
- If hypotensive despite fluid bolus, start a dopamine infusion.
- Once stable, exclude other diagnoses (thrombosis/haemorrhage/infarction) by CT brain.
- Full guideline: https://www.bsped.org.uk/media/1557/dkaguidelinenov18.pdf
- Fluid and corrected Na^+ calculator: https://www.bsped.org.uk/clinical-resources/guidelines/
- Critical care advice: https://www.evelinalondon.nhs.uk/resources/our-services/hospital/south-thames-retrieval-service/diabetic-ketoacidosis-jan-2018.pdf

Sepsis

- Sepsis and septic shock definitions in adults were revised in 2016 (Sepsis-3). They aim to help the clinician with the detection of sepsis, rapidly identifying septic shock (using a Sequential Organ Failure Assessment score). As yet, these are not validated in paediatrics. The traditional definitions can be confusing and are based more on scientific trials than on clinical 'by the bedside' experience. Both adult and paediatric practice is moving towards simplified rapid clinical recognition of sepsis and protocolled treatments utilizing care bundles.
- The Surviving Sepsis Campaign and the American College of Critical Care Medicine (ACCM) guidelines for hemodynamic support in neonates and children remain the most recognized standards of care for severe sepsis/septic shock. The Paediatric Sepsis Six is the most recently introduced initiative in the UK to improve recognition of sepsis and adherence to guidelines.

Definitions (International Pediatric Sepsis Consensus Conference 2005)

- Systemic inflammatory response syndrome (SIRS): 2 or more of the following:
  - Temperature >38.5°C or <36°C.
  - HR >2 standard deviations above normal, or bradycardia in children <1 year old.
  - RR >2 standard deviations above normal (or $PaCO_2$ <32 mmHg).
  - WCC >12,000 cells/mm^3, <4,000 cells/mm^3, or >10% band forms
- Sepsis: SIRS + suspected/confirmed bacterial, viral, or fungal infection.
- Severe sepsis: sepsis and 1 of the following:
  - CVS dysfunction, or
  - ARDS, or
  - 2 or more other dysfunctions (renal, neurological, hepatic, haematological).
- Septic shock: severe sepsis plus CVS dysfunction (CVS dysfunction being defined as hypotension, tachy/bradycardia, CRT >5 s, lactate >2 × upper limit).

Paediatric Sepsis Six initiative

- Recently, the UK Sepsis Trust has introduced a customized care bundle designed to facilitate prompt recognition of severe sepsis and delivery of an initial six steps of care in a time critical manner (Fig. 27.2).
- It does not replace traditional definitions of sepsis (or senior clinical judgement, which often diverge from the scientific definitions above) but aims to ↑ recognition, speed of treatment, and adherence to guidelines.
- Consider sepsis if there is suspected/proven infection and 2 or more of the following:
  - Temperature >38.5°C or <36°C.
  - Inappropriate tachycardia for age (APLS criteria).
  - Altered mental state, e.g. sleepy, irritable, lethargic, floppy (cf. baseline).
  - Reduced peripheral perfusion or prolonged CRT.
  - Low threshold of suspicion if age <3 months, chronic disease, recent surgery, immunocompromised.

Cardiovascular presentation (compared with adults)

- Loss of vascular tone is not the predominant feature of paediatric sepsis (unlike most adults).
- CVS decompensation with hypotension is a very late (and worrying) sign, since children compensate well initially by constricting capacitance vessels.
- The younger the child, the less the ability to ↑ SV and thus the more HR-dependent is CO.
- Approximately 80% present with 'cold' shock (normal/low CO and high SVR).
- The remainder have 'warm' shock (normal/high CO and low SVR).

General management

- Follow NWTS Sepsis Guideline (Fig. 27.3 Fig 27.3), which is based on American College of Critical Care Medicine—Pediatric Life Support Guidelines for Management of Septic Shock.
- Manage in resuscitation area e.g. A+E or HDU, with full monitoring (SpO₂/ECG/BP/temperature/RR).
- Failure to achieve normal therapeutic endpoints in severe sepsis (HR, BP, mental state, UO >1 mL/kg/h, lactate, oxygenation, etc.) doubles mortality every hour not achieved.
- In infants/neonates, consider that shock may be due to CHD ± superimposed sepsis.
- Specialist paediatric ECHO can exclude CHD and guide fluid/inotrope therapy (if available).
- < 1 hour the following interventions should be initiated:
  - High-flow O₂.
  - IV or IO access and take bloods: glucose, culture, and blood gas (plus lactate/FBC/CRP).
  - IV or IO broad-spectrum antimicrobials (based on local guidance), e.g. cefotaxime and gentamicin.
  - Consider fluid resuscitation to restore circulating volume, e.g. 20 mL/kg crystalloid over 5 min.
  - Involve senior clinicians/specialists early.
  - Consider inotropic support early: if still shocked after 40 mL/kg fluid.

Anaesthetic management

- Initial resuscitation involves a standard ABC approach.
- Gain IV or IO access rapidly (IO indicated after two failed IV attempts or 2 min attempting to get access).
- Early intubation and IPPV should be considered (if >40 mL/kg fluid administered), since they may ↓ myocardial work by up to 40%.
- If intubation and IPPV are required, then prior fluid resuscitation will ↓ the risk of cardiovascular instability. Plan for CVS decompensation and use an acute paediatric intubation checklist. (→ p. 653 and inside back page).
- Ketamine is more cardiovascularly stable than propofol or thiopental.
- Modified RSI (with small Vᴛ breaths whilst awaiting paralysis) is likely to be required (must balance delayed gastric emptying against poor toleration of apnoea with high O₂ demand).
- Fluid resuscitation is directed towards maintaining age-appropriate parameters for HR, BP, and CRT. Repeat boluses of 20 mL/kg crystalloid (or albumin) given over 5–10 min. If signs of overload, e.g. hepatomegaly, pulmonary oedema, start inotropes.

THE UK SEPSIS TRUST **Paediatric Sepsis 6**

Name:

Date of Birth:

Hospital No.:

Affix Hospital Label if available

Recognition of a child at risk:
If a child with suspected or proven Infection AND has at least 2 of the following:

- Core temperature <36°C or >38.5°C
- Inappropriate tachycardia (Refer to local criteria/APLS Guidance)
- Altered mental state (Including: sleepiness/irritability/lethargy/floppiness)
- Reduced peripheral perfusion/prolonged capillary refill

Lower threshold of suspicion for: age <3 months, chronic disease, recent surgery, or immunocompromised

THINK: Could this child have SEVERE SEPSIS, SEPTIC SHOCK or
RED FLAG SEPSIS* - Ask for review by an experienced clinician.

High certainty of Sepsis Respond with Paediatric Sepsis 6:	High certainty NOT Sepsis or Unsure

Complete all elements within 1 hour *Date/Time Sign*

Not Sepsis
Document reasons
Unsure

1. Give high flow oxygen:

2. Obtain IV / IO access & take blood tests:

Review within 1 hour

Not Sepsis
Document reasons
Sepsis
Start Sepsis 6
Unsure

a. Blood cultures
b. Blood glucose - treat low blood glucose
c. Blood gas (+FBC, lactate / CRP as able) *Date/Time Sign*

3. Give IV or IO antibiotics:

Review within 1 hour

Not Sepsis
Document reasons
Sepsis
Start Sepsis 6
Unsure

- Broad spectrum cover as per local policy *Date/Time Sign*

4. Consider fluid resuscitation:

Review within 1 hour

Not Sepsis
Document reasons
Sepsis
Start Sepsis 6
Unsure

- Aim to restore normal circulating volume and physiological parameters
- Titrate 20 mL/kg Isotonic Fluid over 5–10 min and repeat if necessary
- Caution with fluid overload: Examine for crepitations & hepatomegaly *Date/Time Sign*

5. Involve senior clinicians / specialists early:

Review within 1 hour

Not Sepsis
Document reasons
Sepsis
Start Sepsis 6
Unsure

6. Consider inotropic support early:

- If normal physiological parameters are not restored after ≥ 40 mL/kg fluids
- NB adrenaline or dopamine may be given via peripheral IV or IO access

Review within 1 hour

Not Sepsis
Document reasons
Sepsis
Start Sepsis 6

Document reason(s) for variation overleaf

Paediatric: Sepsis 6 version 11.1 August 2015 in collaboration with th UK sepsis Trust Paediatric Group. for further information please contact fora@nta.net

Fig. 27.2 Paediatric Sepsis 6.

Reproduced with permission from Tong, J., et al. *G218(P) The Paediatric Sepsis 6 Initiative*. Copyright © 2014, Published by the BMJ Publishing Group Limited

NWTS
North West & North Wales
Paediatric Transport Service

**Guidelines for Management of
Sepsis in Children**

NHS
North West & North Wales
Paediatric Critical Care Network

Summary Guideline: Paediatric Sepsis - *The First Hour*

0 min

Recognise severe sepsis/septic shock
Begin high flow Oxygen
Establish intravenous (IV) (2–3 minutes) or intra-osseous (IO) access

5 min

Initiate Fluid Resuscitation
20mL/kg 0.9% sodium chloride then 20 mL/kg colloid (reassess & repeat if needed)
Commence appropriate antimicrobial(s) within 1 hour of presentation
Correct hypoglycaemia: 2 mL/kg 10% glucose

Shock not reversed

15 min

*If using dopamine via peripheral line: 3 x wt(kg) Made up to 50 mL with 5% glucose (max - 180 mg/60 mL)

Fluid Refractory Shock (>60mL/kg) - Discuss with NWTS
Anaesthetise for ventilation and invasive monitoring
Hypotension is a risk: NWTS suggest ketamine 1mg/kg +/– fentanyl 1 microgram/kg
+ muscle relaxant either intravenous or introsseous
Begin dopamine via peripheral IV*/IO Dose: up to 10 micrograms/kg/min
Use: www.crashcall.net emergency drug calculator
Discuss with NWTS at earliest opportunity

Goal Directed Therapy
Maintain or restore airway, oxygenation & adequate CO_2 clearance
Restore & maintain normal perfusion:
 • No difference in quality between central & peripheral pulses
 • Warm extremities (caution may have warm shock)
 • HR, BP within normal limits for age
 • Central capillary refill time ≤ 2 seconds
Normal mental status
Urine output returned (>0.5–1 mL/kg/hour)
Serum lactate <2 mmol/L
Central venous saturation ($S_{cv}O_2$) >70% from neck line (ideally)
Normal blood glucose concentration

**Shock not reversed
d/w NWTS**   **CENTRAL ACCESS**

Cold shock with normal blood pressure	Cold shock with low blood pressure	Warm Shock with low blood pressure
Titrate fluid & add adrenaline, Aim $S_{cv}O_2$ > 70%, Hb >100 g/L	Titrate fluid & add adrenaline, Aim $S_{cv}O_2$ > 70%, Hb >100 g/L	Titrate fluid & add noradrenaline, Aim $S_{cv}O_2$ > 70%
If $S_{cv}O_2$ still < 70% NWTS team will consider milrinone with volume loading	If still hypotensive, add noradrenaline If $S_{cv}O_2$ still < 70% NWTS team will consider milrinone	If still hypotensive, add vasopression If $S_{cv}O_2$ still < 70% add low dose adrenaline

60 min

**Shock not reversed
d/w NWTS**

Catecholamine resistant shock
Discuss with NWTS
Consider hydrocortisone (1 mg/kg) if > 2 inotropes/at risk of adrenal insufficiency
Consider calcium gluconate bolus +/– infusion
Continual reassessment to achieve goals
ECMO may be considered

Fig. 27.3 North West and North Wales Paediatric Transport Service (NWTS): Sepsis Guideline (based on ACCM-PALS Guidance 2007). Each UK region will have their own specialist paediatric team to call.

- Consider transfusion if Hb <10 g/dL. Think early about other blood products in case of DIC (major haemorrhage policy may be required).
- Exclude other causes of refractory shock, i.e. pneumothorax, pericardial tamponade, or endocrine emergencies.
- If no response to fluid resuscitation, administer: Inotropes/chronotropes/vasopressors:
  - If 'cold' shock—primarily dopamine or adrenaline (epinephrine).
  - If 'warm' shock—noradrenaline (norepinephrine) followed by vasopressin.
  - Adrenaline or dopamine can initially be given peripherally
  - All can be given via IO until CVL inserted.
  - Specialist advice may add vasodilators, e.g. milrinone
- If suspected adrenal insufficiency or shock refractory to fluid and inotropes, administer IV hydrocortisone.
- Administer antibiotics within 1 h of diagnosing severe sepsis. Blood cultures are preferably taken prior to this, but should not delay actual treatment.
- Administer aciclovir if a high suspicion of herpes infection in older child or empirically in neonate.
- Consider antifungals for immunocompromised child.
- Early and aggressive source control (e.g. interventional radiological drainage of collection) is essential.
- Referral to PICU specialists/transport specialists early for advice/planning.
- Keep family informed with realistic expectations and allow them to be with their child as much as possible.
- Refractory cases may be candidates for ECMO (sepsis is not a contraindication).
- In case of death, ensure bereavement team are involved for family and consider the medical/nursing teams emotional support (and debrief) as well as legal processes.

Further reading

Milési C, Boubal M, Jacquot A, et al. High-flow nasal cannula: recommendations for daily practice in pediatrics. *Ann Intensive Care* 2014;4:29.

NWTS. Algorithm on sepsis. http://www.nwts.nhs.uk/clinicalguidelines

NICE Guideline NG51. Sepsis: recognition, diagnosis and early management. www.nice.org.uk/guidance/ng51

NICE. Sepsis: recognition, diagnosis and early management. www.nice.org.uk/guidance/ng51/resources/algorithm-for-managing-suspected-sepsis-in-children-aged-under-5-years-in-an-acute-hospital-setting-91853485527

Goldstein B, Giroir B, Randolph A. International Pediatric Sepsis Consensus Conference: definitions for sepsis and organ dysfunction in pediatrics. *Pediatr Crit Care Med* 2005;6:2–8.

Dellinger RP, Levy MM, Rhodes A, et al.; Surviving Sepsis Campaign Guidelines Committee including the Paediatric Subgroup. Surviving Sepsis Campaign: international guidelines for management of severe sepsis and septic shock: 2012. *Intensive Care Med* 2013;39:165–228.

Sepsis 6: https://sepsistrust.org/professional-resources/clinical/

Stabilizing and transferring the critically ill child in a general hospital

Pete Murphy and Sarah Stibbards

Stabilization

- Manage in a high-dependency area of ward or equivalent area in ED.
- Assess and resuscitate along ABC principles.
- Obtain senior help early.
- Immediate management includes:
  - ABCDE (airway, breathing, circulation, disability, exposure) + blood sugar measurement.
  - 100% O_2 via a non-rebreathing mask
  - 2 × secure IV or IO access.
  - Fluid bolus of 20 mL/kg crystalloid repeated if required to restore normovolaemia.
  - Correct any underlying hypoglycaemia with 2 mL/kg of 10% glucose.
- Send FBC, U+E, LFT, glucose, blood gases (including lactate), clotting screen, and group and save (plus targeted investigations, e.g. metabolic screens if unexplained coma/seizures) as well as appropriate cultures in cases of suspected sepsis.
- It can be a challenge to assess and treat children owing to their level of understanding, cooperation, and fear/anxiety. A risk/benefit discussion should take place before intubating a child to facilitate adequate therapy, since the procedure carries risks (15% CVS deterioration and 1% failed intubation—NWTS data). Conversely, delaying intubation and failing to rapidly and adequately treat a critically ill child also has risks, e.g. 15% ↑ in mortality per hour in severe sepsis. In general (unless in extremis), there is usually time for a senior anaesthetist and paediatrician to attend.
- Record GCS prior to giving sedation/RSI.
- An example of an acute intubation guide (including decision tree, checklist, sizing chart, and failed intubation algorithm) can be found at www.nwts.nhs.uk/clinicalguidelines. Examples of a checklist and a sizing chart are also given in Fig. 28.1 (available for quick reference on the inside back cover) and Table 6.2, respectively.
- Generally intubate and ventilate if:
  - Patient unable to maintain their airway without assistance.
  - GCS <9.
  - Fluctuating GCS (intervene quickly).
- Patients may require ventilatory support without intubation to:
  - Improve O_2 delivery, using HFHNC O_2, e.g Optiflow/Airvo.
  - Decrease work of breathing using APBiPAP.
  - Aid CO_2 clearance using APBiPAP.
- Place NGT or OGT to prevent a distended stomach splinting the diaphragm.
- Obtain CXR (plus any other X-rays required) and a 12-lead ECG.
- Take detailed history from parents/guardian, including drug history and allergies.
- If fluid boluses are ineffective at maintaining BP, consider inotropes e.g. dopamine (up to 20 mcg/kg/min) or adrenaline (epinephrine) (0.05–2 mcg/kg/min). Both can be given via IO route.
- Check effectiveness of resuscitation, i.e. effects on HR, BP, GCS, metabolic acidosis and UO.
- If sepsis is a potential diagnosis, administer a broad-spectrum IV antibiotic (e.g. a third-generation cephalosporin) within the hour. Consider antivirals and antifungals.

- Discuss patient with PICU and/or receiving specialist in regional centre (in the UK, this is usually facilitated via conference calling with the regional transport service).
- Once patient is stable, establish invasive monitoring.
- Avoid hypothermia (use forced air warmers/overhead radiant heaters).
- Reassess patient following the ABCD rapid clinical assessment.
- Take careful notes of timings, drugs given and any intervention(s) required.
- Keep parents up to date with any changes in condition, reason for transfer, prognosis.
- Use of a checklist helps ensure a safe transfer and avoid omissions (➔ Fig. 28.1 also on inside back cover).

PLANNING / PREPARATION / LOCATION

Alternative airway plan discussed in case of difficulties? Do you need ENT?	☐
C-spine stable? Positioning optimized for age / condition?	☐
Plan for cardiac decompensation?	☐
NG tube / PEG aspirated?	☐
IV / IO—working?	☐
Team roles —Intubator	
Cricoid / airway assistant	
Drugs / runner (minimum 3 people required for RSI)	☐
HELP—who / how / where will it be coming from?	☐
Pre-oxygenation	☐

EQUIPMENT

Face mask / airways (oral and nasal)?	☐
Laryngoscope type/size and checked (preferably 2)?	☐
ETT— above and below expected size available (consider microcuff)?	☐
Breathing circuit (Bag-valve mask available)?	☐
Tube tapes / ties?	☐
Bougie / introducer / Magill's?	☐
Suction (Yankauer and catheter)? NGT / OGT (if not in already)?	☐
Monitoring—**Capnography**, SpO2, stethoscope, BP, ECG?	☐
Alternative airway plan / rescue devices (e.g LMA / cricothyroid etc.)?	☐

DRUGS

Check drug doses and labelling **(www.crashcall.net)**	☐
Induction agent / paralysis (suxamethonium/rocuronium)?	☐
Ongoing sedation/anaesthesia ?	☐
Fluids drawn up? / vasopressor required? / inotrope required?	☐
Crash drugs—adrenaline/ atropine drawn up?	☐

Patients Name:	Date: _/_/_	Team signature:

Fig. 28.1 Acute paediatric intubation checklist.

Inter-hospital transfer

- The principles of inter-hospital transfer are equally valid for intra-hospital transfer, e.g. from ED to CT scan.
- In the UK, definitive specialist paediatric surgical/intensive care mostly occurs in larger tertiary centres; this will entail an inter-hospital transfer.
- In the UK, the Paediatric Intensive Care Society has set a standard of practice for the transport of critically ill children.
- Specialized transport teams improve outcome.
- In the UK, currently >90% of paediatric inter-hospital transport is done by specialist teams.
- There are times when specialist teams are unavailable or when it is more appropriate for the referring general hospital team to perform the transport to minimize delays (e.g. time-critical head injuries). Therefore, general hospitals must have policies, procedures, equipment, and training to perform this (staff- and resource-heavy) task.
- Important considerations for any transfer are:
  - How urgent is the transfer?
  - Is the child in the optimal condition for transfer?
  - Does the benefit of transfer outweigh the risks involved?
  - Who are the most appropriate people to transfer this child?
  - What type and mode of transport is required for this child?
  - Who is covering the base hospital if the local team are performing the transfer?
- Dangers of transfer include:
  - Deranged physiology made worse by movement (acceleration/deceleration leads to cardiovascular instability) and 15% of patients develop avoidable hypoxia and hypotension
  - Vibration leads to failure and inaccuracy of non-invasive monitoring. Consider invasive monitoring if possible
  - Cramped conditions with poor access to the patient, isolation, changes in temperature and pressure
  - Hypothermia, especially in the infant. Use of warming mats, insulating blankets (underneath and then wrapped over the top), and hats help to minimize this.
  - Travel sickness in patients (if awake) and the team.
  - Vehicle crashes. Use of blue lights and road exemptions (e.g. going through red lights) increases the risks of accidents for the ambulance and other road users. It rarely saves significant amounts of total journey time. Discuss with the driver the urgency and risks.
- Referring and receiving units should make notes on their conversations, as well as the names and contact details of the clinicians responsible for current and ongoing care.
- Joint management by the referring hospital and the transport team should commence immediately, since successful initial resuscitation and stabilization is crucial to ultimate outcome. It is the responsibility of the referring hospital to resuscitate and stabilize with the help and guidance of the transport team or receiving hospital.
- Transport team responsibilities:
  - Drugs and infusions (where appropriate made up prior to transfer and labelled).

- Equipment kept in a constant state of readiness and checked at frequent intervals.
  —Monitor to record end-tidal CO_2, SpO_2, ECG, non-invasive BP, temperature (core and peripheral), and RR (activate the alarms and set appropriate limits).
  —Batteries capable of supporting full function for a period of at least twice the maximum anticipated length of the transfer.
- Check parents are up to date prior to transfer and document the discussion. Most transfer teams currently facilitate a parent travelling with the child (if they are medically and emotionally fit to do so); this ↓ parental and child (if awake) anxiety.
- Check parents know where their child is going, including contact numbers for the ward/area, map, and address/postcode.
- Record observations every 10–15 min for ICU patients and every 15–30 min for HDU patients.
- If safeguarding concerns are identified, document and activate local safeguarding team.
- The transport vehicle:
  - Should have adequate space, light, gases, electricity, and communications.
  - Should have appropriate methods to secure the patient to the trolley.
  - Mode of transport: consider urgency, mobilization time, geography, weather, traffic, and costs.
  - Is the same vehicle bringing the transport team back?
  - Consider air transfer (see below) if the distance is >150 miles or there are significant delays due to traffic conditions.

Pre-transfer checks

- Transport of any patient either intra-hospital or inter-hospital requires experienced personnel and attention to detail.
- Airway:
  - Clear? If not, then suction and physio with saline prior to transfer.
  - Check ETT and gastric tube are secure and position adequate on CXR.
  - Re-intubation kit prepared.
- Respiratory:
  - Calculate O_2 requirement and check adequate supply:
    —Spontaneous breathing patient: flow (L/min) × 60 × journey time (min) × 2.
    —Ventilated patient: MV (L/min) × 60 × journey time (min) × 2.
  - Ventilation parameters checked.
  - Bagging circuit and self-inflating bag.
  - ABG prior to departure.
  - Chest drain bottles suitable for transport, e.g. flutter valves/ Pneumostat.
- Cardiovascular:
  - Spare IO needle available.
  - Fluid bolus ± inotropes drawn up and in pumps ready.
  - Lines secured to patient.

- Neurological:
  - GCS if un-intubated.
  - Check pupils.
  - Documented: sedation, analgesia, and paralysis given.
  - Copies of CT scans.
  - Neuroprotection, e.g. hypertonic saline or mannitol prepared for raised ICP.
- Infection:
  - Temperature
  - WCC/CRP, cultures/swabs, specific PCR.
  - Antibiotics given.
- Parents and family: communications, concerns, support, can the family travel with patient? Most transport teams give out written information sheets to parents.
- Communications: direct phone numbers (destination, departure point, emergency contact), mobile phones charged.
- Plan for potential foreseeable emergencies on route (equipment/ divert/advice, vehicle breakdown/accident, etc.).
- Documentation: photocopies of notes, drug/fluid charts, blood results, X-rays, observations, and any recent clinic letters.
- Prior to departure:
  - Check referring unit staff are aware of transfer and who is covering roles/bleeps of the transport team (if not supernumerary)?
  - Phone receiving unit, giving a brief handover and estimated time of arrival.
  - Prepare any emergency equipment and drugs that may be needed.
  - Check transport team have mobile phone, money, and warm clothing.
  - Make sure all kit, including monitors, can be secured in the ambulance.

Air transfers

- Air transfers should only be undertaken by experts after suitable education and training as well as familiarization with the environment and equipment of the specific aircraft to be used.
- At high altitude, the partial pressure of O_2 is reduced, e.g. at 1500 m above sea level, PaO_2 is approx. 10 kPa (75 mmHg) giving SaO_2 of 95% normally.
- Most aircraft are pressurized to a cabin altitude of 1500–2000 m, but the reduced PaO_2 may be critical in a hypoxic patient requiring high $Fi O_2$.
- Decreased barometric pressure leads to expansion of gas-filled spaces and therefore ↑ risk of pneumothoraces, distended bowel.
- Air in the ETT cuff should be replaced by saline (to avoid over-inflation at altitude).
- Pressurizing the cabin to sea level can ↓ these problems but ↑ fuel consumption and costs.
- Helicopters fly at relatively low altitude and therefore avoid some of the problems of airplanes. But there are issues with noise, vibration, space, and number of people who can fly with the patient.

Suggested UK training courses

- APLS: www.alsg.org
- NLS/EPALS: https://www.resus.org.uk/information-on-courses/
- NAPSTaR (Neonatal, Adult and Paediatric Safe Transport and Retrieval course): www.alsg.org
- Transport of the critically ill: https://www.bmsc.co.uk/course/transport-of-the-critically-ill-course/
- Aeromedical training: https://www.ccat-training.org.uk
- Association of Paediatric Anaesthetists list of current courses: https://www.apagbi.org.uk/professionals/courses
- The Paediatric Intensive Care Society has a list of current courses for trainees and nursing staff: http://picsociety.uk/

Resuscitation

Pete Murphy and Sarah Stibbards

Choking

- Suspect choking caused by foreign body if:
  - Sudden onset.
  - No other signs of illness.
  - History to alert the rescuer, e.g. eating or playing with small items immediately prior to event.
- Signs of choking: ➋ Table 29.1.

Table 29.1 Signs of choking

General signs of choking
• Witnessed episode
• Coughing or choking noise
• Sudden onset
• Recent history of playing with or eating small objects

Management

- Remember **SAFE** approach: Shout for help. Approach with caution. Free from danger. Evaluate patient's ABCs.
- Assess if cough is effective: See table below.

Effective cough and conscious

- A spontaneous cough is likely to be more effective and safer than any manoeuvre a rescuer might perform.
- Encourage coughing and continue to check for deterioration.

Ineffective cough and conscious

- Deliver 5 back blows (heal of hand centrally between shoulder blades). In the infant, support in a head-down prone position. In the child, aim for a head-down or forward-leaning position.
- Followed by 5 thrusts (chest for infant, abdominal for child >1 year old). Chest thrusts use the same landmarks as for CPR but are sharper, abdominal thrusts are performed from behind the child, placing a fist between the umbilicus and xiphisternum and grasping it with the other hand before pulling upwards and inwards sharply.
- If choking persists and the victim is still conscious, repeat these steps.

Ineffective coughing	Effective cough
• Unable to vocalize	• Crying or verbal response to questions
• Quiet or silent cough	• Loud cough
• Unable to breathe	• Able to take a breath before coughing
• Cyanosis	• Fully responsive
• Decreasing level of consciousness	

Ineffective cough and unconscious
- If the child is, or becomes unconscious place them on a firm, flat surface.
- Call or send for help.
- Open the mouth and look for any obvious object.
- If one is seen, make an attempt to remove it with a single finger sweep. Do not attempt blind or repeated finger sweeps—these can push the object deeper into the pharynx and cause injury. It may be possible to remove the object with Magill's forceps under direct laryngoscopy.
- Open the airway and attempt 5 rescue breaths.
- Assess the effectiveness of each breath: if a breath does not make the chest rise, reposition the head before making the next attempt.
- Attempt 5 rescue breaths: if there is no response, proceed immediately to chest compression regardless of whether the breaths are successful. Continue using a ratio of 15:2.
- Each time the airway is opened, check for a FB: if visible, attempt removal.
- If the child regains consciousness and is breathing effectively, place in the recovery position and monitor breathing and conscious level whilst awaiting help.

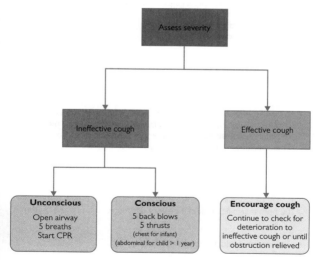

Fig. 29.1 Paediatric choking algorithm 2015.

Reproduced with permission from Maconochie, I. et al. (2015) Resuscitation guidelines: Paediatric basic life support. Copyright © 2015 Resuscitation Council (UK) Available at https://www.resus.org.uk/resuscitation-guidelines/paediatric-basic-life-support/

Dysrhythmias

- Presentation:
  - History of palpitation (verbal child).
  - Poor feeding (non-verbal child).
  - Heart failure or shock.
- Initial assessment:
  - ABCDE: airway, breathing, circulation, disability, and exposure.
  - Ensure airway open: consider airway opening manoeuvres, airway adjuncts, or urgent intubation.
  - High-flow O_2.
  - Monitor ECG:
    —Rate: too fast or too slow?
    —Rhythm: regular or irregular?
    —QRS complexes: narrow or broad?

Bradyarrhythmia

- The rate is usually slow (<60 bpm) and the rhythm usually irregular.
- Causes:
  - Pre-terminal event in hypoxia or shock (commonest).
  - Raised ICP.
  - Conduction pathway damage post cardiac surgery or ablation.
  - Congenital heart block (rare).
  - Poisoning, e.g. digoxin, beta-blockers.
  - Long-QT syndrome.
- Treatment
  - ABC before pharmacological treatment of bradycardia.
  - High-concentration O_2 via bag–valve mask or ETT and IPPV.
  - Volume expansion 20 mL/kg
  - If above is ineffective titrate adrenaline (epinephrine) 10 mcg/kg IV/IO slowly.
  - If above ineffective, infuse adrenaline 0.05–2mcg/kg/min IV/IO
  - If there is evidence of vagal overactivity, give atropine 20 mcg/kg IV/IO (minimum dose 100 mcg; maximum dose 600 mcg). Repeat after 5 min (maximum dose 1 mg child; 2 mg adolescent).
  - Seek expert advice if secondary to poisons (toxbase.org; Tel: 0844 892 0111).

Tachyarrhythmia

- The rate of a significant tachyarrhythmia is age-dependent, but usually >200 bpm is significant. It can be very difficult to assess if the rhythm is irregular.
- Causes:
  - Re-entrant conducting pathway abnormality.
  - CHD and post cardiac surgery.
  - Cardiomyopathies.
  - Poisoning, e.g. tricyclic antidepressants, cocaine, cisapride and macrolide antibiotics are commoner causes (toxbase.org; Tel: 0844 892 0111).
  - Causes of hyperK⁺, e.g. renal disease.
  - Long-QT syndrome (acquired or inherited).

- Clinical indicators of shock:
  - Cool peripheries/prolonged capillary refill time.
  - Significant fall in BP.
  - Reduced conscious level.

Ventricular tachycardia (VT)
- If haemodynamically stable, a careful history is taken to identify the underlying cause and the required treatments. HR is usually between 120 and 250 bpm with wide QRS on ECG.
- Treatment (➲ Fig. 29.2):
  - ABC reassessment and determine haemodynamic stability.
  - If shocked, proceed to synchronized DC shock 1 J/kg; repeat if necessary with 2 J/kg.
  - If not shocked, consult cardiology and consider IV amiodarone 5 mg/kg over 60 min (maximum 300 mg), monitoring ECG and BP.
  - Use synchronous shocks initially, but if these are ineffectual and the child is shocked, subsequent attempts will have to be asynchronous.
  - Torsade de pointe VT is treated with IV magnesium sulfate 25–50 mg/kg (up to 2 g) over 10 min.

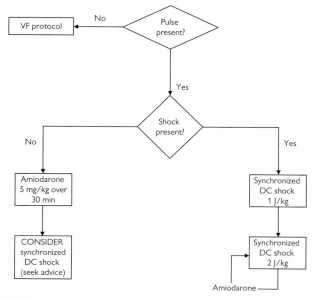

Fig. 29.2 Ventricular tachycardia management algorithm.

Supraventricular tachycardia (SVT)
- Commonest non-arrest arrhythmia.
- Commonest arrhythmia to produce cardiovascular instability in infants.
- HR is >220 bpm in infants, but can often be 250–300 bpm, and >180 bpm in children >3 years.
- The QRS complex is narrow and the rhythm is regular, but P waves may not be visible; however, it may be difficult to differentiate between sinus tachycardia due to shock and SVT.
- Characteristics to distinguish between sinus tachycardia and SVT include:
  - HR is often <200 bpm in infants and children with sinus tachycardia, whereas in SVT, HR is often >220 bpm.
  - If P waves are identifiable, they are usually upright in leads I and aVF in sinus tachycardia and negative in leads II, III, and aVF in SVT.
  - There is often beat-to-beat variability in sinus tachycardia, which is often responsive to stimulation; in SVT, there is no beat-to-beat variability.
  - Termination of SVT is abrupt, but in sinus tachycardia the rate gradually decreases in response to treatment.
- Infants may present with shock, sweatiness, and poor feeding.
- Cardiopulmonary stability is affected by child's age, duration of SVT, prior ventricular function, and ventricular rate.
- Cardiac function deteriorates because of increased myocardial O_2 demand and limited O_2 delivery in the short diastolic phase because of the rapid HR.
- Impaired myocardial function secondary to e.g. cardiomyopathy can cause shock relatively quickly.
- Treatment after reassessing ABC (→ Fig. 29.3):
  - Vagal stimulation with ECG monitoring using the following techniques:
    —For infants, the 'diving reflex' can be used by wrapping the infant in a towel and immersing the face in iced water for up to 5 s.
    —One-sided carotid sinus massage
    —Valsalva manoeuvre for older children, e.g. blowing hard through a 20 mL syringe.
    —The child may know to adopt a certain position.

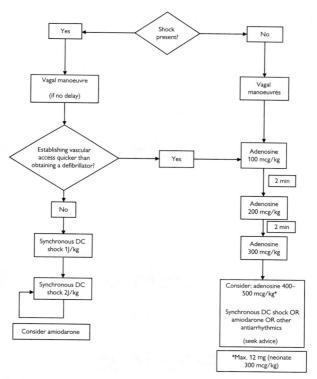

Fig. 29.3 SVT management algorithm.

Basic life support (BLS)

- Resuscitation Council Guidelines (2015) and protocols are used in the UK: follow the algorithm in Fig. 29.4.
- There is limited evidence on paediatric resuscitation. What is known is that cardiopulmonary resuscitation (CPR) should start as soon as possible for optimum outcome.
- The presence or absence of 'signs of life', e.g. response to stimuli, normal breathing (rather than abnormal gasps), or spontaneous movement, must be looked for as part of the child's circulatory assessment.

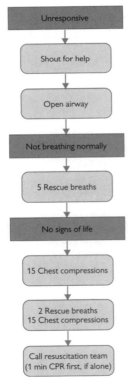

Fig. 29.4 Paediatric basic life support algorithm 2015.

Reproduced with permission from Maconochie, I. et al. (2015) Resuscitation guidelines: Paediatric basic life support. Copyright © 2015 Resuscitation Council (UK) Available at https://www.resus. org.uk/resuscitation-guidelines/paediatric-basic-life-support/

- If a healthcare provider does feel for a pulse in an unresponsive child, they must be certain that one is present for them NOT to start CPR.
- The decision to start CPR should take <10 s: if there is still doubt after that time, start CPR.
- Uninterrupted, high-quality chest compression is vital, including the rate and depth (approximately 4 cm in infants and 5 cm in children) and allowing adequate time for chest recoil to occur (~50% of the whole cycle should be the relaxation phase). The compression rate is 100–120/min. Ideally, chest compressions should be delivered on a firm surface.
- Adopt a **SAFE** approach: Shout for help. Approach with caution. Free from danger. Evaluate patient's ABCs.
- Check responsiveness. Gently stimulate the child and ask loudly, 'Are you all right?'
- Open the airway using head tilt and chin lift (neutral <1 year of age, 'sniffing the morning air' >1 year). Have a low threshold for suspecting injury to the neck. If suspected, try to open the airway using a jaw thrust. If unsuccessful, add head tilt gradually until the airway is open, since establishing an open airway takes priority over the cervical spine.
- Look, Listen, and Feel for chest movements, breathe sounds, and air movement, respectively, for no more than 10 s before deciding—if you have any doubts whether breathing is normal, assume it is abnormal.
- Give 5 initial rescue breaths. For both infants and children, if you have difficulty achieving an effective breath, the airway may be obstructed. Open the child's mouth and remove any visible obstruction. Do not perform a blind finger sweep. Ensure that there is adequate head tilt and chin lift, but also that the neck is not over-extended. If head tilt and chin lift has not opened the airway, try a jaw thrust. Make up to 5 attempts to achieve effective breaths. If still unsuccessful, move on to chest compression.
- If you check the pulse, take no more than 10 s. In a child aged >1 year, feel for the carotid pulse in the neck. In an infant, feel for the brachial pulse. For both infants and children, the femoral pulse in the groin (midway between the anterior superior iliac spine and the symphysis pubis) can be used.
- If there are no signs of life, unless you are CERTAIN that you can feel a definite pulse of >60/min within 10 s, start chest compressions.
- For all children, compress the lower half of the sternum—to avoid compressing the upper abdomen, locate the xiphisternum by finding the angle where the lowest ribs join in the middle. Compress the sternum one finger's breadth above this.
- Chest compression in infants: The lone rescuer should compress the sternum with the tips of two fingers. If there are two or more rescuers, use the encircling technique.
- Chest compression in children aged >1 year: Place the heel of a hand over the lower half of the sternum (as above).
- Allow the chest to return to its resting position before starting the next compression.
- Continue compressions and breaths in a ratio of 15:2.

- Continue resuscitation until:
  - The child shows signs of life (normal breathing, cough, movement or definite pulse of >60/min).
  - Further qualified help arrives.
  - You become exhausted.

Parental presence

- Many want to and should be encouraged to be present during resuscitation attempts.
- Helps them gain a realistic view that all attempts have been made.
- Evidence shows reduced anxiety and depression of parents after a death.
- A dedicated staff member should be with the parents at all times.
- If parental behaviour/presence is impairing the team, they are gently asked to leave.

Safeguarding

- All out-of-hospital cardiac arrests are referred to the local safeguarding team and Police.
- Consider local safeguarding referral in any unexplained cardiac arrest or acute deterioration.

Advanced Paediatric life support

- Most arrests arise from decompensated respiratory or circulatory failure (i.e. they are predominantly secondary cardiorespiratory arrests). Cardiorespiratory arrest generally has a poor outcome in children—hence the identification of the seriously ill or injured child is an absolute priority. The order of assessment and intervention for any seriously ill or injured child follows the ABCDE principles (➲ Fig. 29.5):
  - Airway (and cervical spine stabilization for the injured child).
  - Breathing.
  - Circulation (with haemorrhage control in the injured child).
  - Disability (level of consciousness and neurological status).
  - Exposure to ensure full examination (whilst respecting dignity and conserving temperature).
- Establish BLS.
- Oxygenate, ventilate, and start chest compressions:
  - Ensure patent airway as described in the BLS section.
  - Provide ventilation by bag–mask, using high-concentration O_2 as soon as available. Aim for early intubation with minimal interruption to compressions. Intubation controls the airway and enables chest compression to be given continuously, thus improving coronary perfusion pressure.
  - Cuffed ETTs are optimal (>3 kg) and aid continuous-waveform $ETCO_2$ monitoring. If $ETCO_2$ <2 kPa, ensure compressions are optimal. Current evidence does not support a threshold $ETCO_2$ value as an indicator for stopping resuscitation. A rapid rise in CO_2 level can be an early indication of return of spontaneous circulation (ROSC).
  - Compression rate 100–120/min. If the child has been intubated and compressions are uninterrupted, ensure that ventilation is adequate and use a slow ventilation rate of 10–12/min.
- Attach defibrillator or monitor:
  - Assess and monitor the cardiac rhythm.
  - If using a defibrillator, place one pad on the chest wall just below the right clavicle and one in the mid-axillary line. Children's pads are 8–12 cm in size, and those for infants are 4.5 cm. In infants and small children, it may be best to apply the pads to the front and back of the chest if they cannot be adequately separated in the standard positions.
- Assess rhythm and check for signs of life:
  - Non-shockable (asystole or pulseless electrical activity (PEA).
  - Shockable: ventricular fibrillation (VF) or pulseless ventricular tachycardia (pVT).

Non-shockable (asystole or PEA)

- Commonest rhythm.
- Perform continuous CPR with high-concentration O_2. If ventilating with bag–mask, give 15 chest compressions to 2 ventilations, using a compression rate of 100–120/min. Once patient is intubated and compressions are uninterrupted, use a ventilation rate of 10–12/min. Continue CPR, only pausing briefly every 2 min to check for rhythm change.
- Obtain immediate vascular access either IV or IO and if possible obtain blood glucose, blood gas, FBC, and U+E.

- Give adrenaline (epinephrine) 10 mcg/kg (0.1 mL/kg of 1:10,000 solution, maximum 10 mls); flush with 2–5 mL 0.9% saline.
- Give adrenaline 10 mcg/kg every 3–5 min (i.e. every other cycle), while continuing uninterrupted chest compressions and ventilation.
- Consider and correct reversible causes (4Hs and 4Ts: ↪ Fig. 29.5): Hypovolaemia is implicated relatively frequently (dehydration, septic shock, and haemorrhage), so consider 20 mL/kg isotonic fluid bolus early.

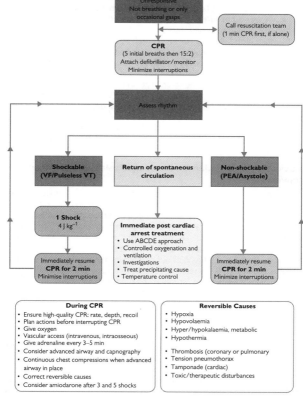

Fig. 29.5 Paediatric advanced life support algorithm 2015.

Reproduced with permission from Maconochie, I. et al. (2015) Resuscitation guidelines: Paediatric basic life support. Copyright © 2015 Resuscitation Council (UK) Available at https://www.resus.org.uk/resuscitation-guidelines/paediatric-basic-life-support/

- If secondary to hyperK$^+$ (usually rare to get arrhythmia with K$^+$ <7.5 mmol/L):
  - 10% calcium gluconate 0.5–1.0 mL/kg (over 5 min, maximum 20 mL), onset few minutes, duration 30–60 min. Side effects hyperCa^{2+} and bradycardia. Can be repeated after 10 min. if required.
  - Salbutamol 4 mcg/kg IV over 5 min, onset 30 min, duration 2–3 h. Side effects tachycardia and hypertension.
  - 10% glucose 500 mg/kg (5mls/kg) rapid bolus, then 500 mg/kg/h if necessary, onset 30 min, duration 1–2 h. Side effect hyperglycaemia: if blood sugar >10 mmol/L add insulin 0.05 IU/kg/h.
  - If significant metabolic acidosis, 8.4% sodium bicarbonate 1–2 mmol/kg IV (over 30 minutes), onset 30 min, duration 1–2 h. Side effects hyperNa$^+$, fluid overload, and alkalosis by separate infusion.
    Maintain blood glucose 10–15 mmol/L by adjusting infusion rate.
    Mixing glucose and insulin for bolus administration is no longer recommended in APLS due to risk of hypoglycemia. Adult ALS maintains treatment with 10iU insulin in 50 mls of 50% glucose (practically this takes time to arrange and is difficult to administer).
  - Calcium polystyrene sulfonate 250 mg/kg PO/PR (maximum 15g), onset 1–4h, duration 4–6 h, Side effect constipation.
  - Dialysis.
- If there is ROSC, the ventilation rate should be 12–20/min. Measure ETCO$_2$ to monitor ventilation and ensure correct ETT placement (see ROSC section).

Shockable (ventricular fibrillation/pulseless ventricular tachycardia)

- Least common scenario, may occur as a secondary event and is likely when there has been a witnessed and sudden collapse. It is seen more often in the ICU and cardiac ward. Continue CPR until a defibrillator is available.
- Charge the defibrillator while chest compressions continue. Once the defibrillator is charged, pause compressions, quickly ensure all rescuers are clear of the patient, and then deliver the shock.
- Give one shock of 4 J/kg. Without reassessing the rhythm or feeling for a pulse, resume CPR immediately, starting with compressions (as the myocardium is likely to be "stunned" by the shock and takes time to hopefully recover and produce ROSC).
- Standard automated external defibrillators (AED's) can be used in children >8yrs. Paediatric pads are ideal but if unavailable placing larger pads anterior and posterior may allow successful defibrillation.
- Consider and correct reversible causes (4Hs and 4Ts: ➜ Fig. 29.5).
- Continue CPR for 2 min, and then pause briefly to check the monitor. If still VF/pVT, give a second shock (4 J/kg). Without reassessing the rhythm or feeling for a pulse, resume CPR immediately, starting with compressions.
- Continue CPR for 2 min, and then pause briefly to check the monitor. If still VF/pVT, give a third shock (4 J/kg). Without reassessing the rhythm or feeling for a pulse, resume CPR immediately, starting with chest compression.
- Give adrenaline 10 mcg/kg and amiodarone 5 mg/kg after the third shock, once chest compressions have resumed.

- Repeat adrenaline every alternate cycle (i.e. every 3–5 min) until ROSC.
- After fifth shock, if still in a shockable rhythm, repeat amiodarone 5 mg/kg once.
- Continue shocks every 2 min, continuing compressions during charging of the defibrillator and minimizing the breaks in chest compression.
- If defibrillation was successful but VF/pVT recurs, resume the CPR sequence and defibrillate. Give an amiodarone bolus (unless two doses have already been administered) and start a continuous infusion.

Newborn life support (NLS)

- Most newborn babies do not require resuscitation.
- Follow guidelines in Fig. 29.6.
- Ideally resuscitation is performed in a warm room with an overhead heater.
- Call for experienced help.
- In the face of anoxia, the infant can maintain an effective circulation throughout the period of primary apnoea, through the gasping phase, and even for a while after the onset of terminal apnoea. Therefore, the most urgent requirement is that the lungs be aerated effectively, allowing oxygenated blood to be conveyed from the aerated lungs to the heart and thus for the brain to be perfused with oxygenated blood. Following this, the respiratory centre will usually function once again and the infant will recover.
- Merely aerating the lungs is sufficient in the vast majority of cases.
- In a few cases, cardiac function will have deteriorated to such an extent that the circulation is inadequate and a brief period of compressions may also be needed.
- In an even smaller number of cases, lung aeration and chest compression will be insufficient, and drugs are required to restore the circulation. The prognosis in this group remains poor.
- Maintain an open airway (head in the neutral position).
- If the infant is not breathing, aerate the lungs with 5 inflation breaths, 3 s long. Confirm response with visible chest movement or an ↑ in HR.
- If no response, check head position and try jaw thrust before repeating 5 inflation breaths and confirming response.
- If still no response, consider oropharyngeal airway followed by repeat jaw thrust and inflation breaths. Consider intubation.
- Continue ventilating apnoeic infants until respiration is established.
- If the heart remains <60 bpm after 5 effective inflation breaths and 30 s of effective ventilation, start compressions and continue a compression : ventilation ratio of 3:1
- If HR not increasing, give adrenaline 10 mcg/kg 1:10,000 via IV/IO or umbilical access.

Updates to NLS guidelines since 2010 edition

- Resuscitation of term infants should commence in air. For preterm infants, an FiO_2 of 21–30% is used initially. If, despite effective ventilation, oxygenation (ideally guided by SpO_2) remains unacceptable, use of a higher concentration of O_2 is considered.
- Attempting to aspirate meconium from the nose and mouth of the unborn infant is not recommended. If presented with a floppy, apnoeic infant born through thick particulate meconium, it is reasonable to inspect the oropharynx rapidly to remove potential obstructions. Tracheal intubation is not routine in the presence of meconium and is only performed for suspected tracheal obstruction.
- Nasal CPAP rather than routine intubation may be used to provide support for spontaneously breathing preterm infants with respiratory distress. Early use of nasal CPAP should be considered in those

spontaneously breathing preterm infants who are at risk of developing respiratory distress syndrome.
- For uncompromised term and preterm infants, a delay in cord clamping of at least 1 min from the complete delivery of the infant is recommended. For infants requiring resuscitation, resuscitative intervention remains the immediate priority.
- Babies <28 weeks gestation should be completely covered up to their necks in a food-grade plastic bag, without drying, immediately after birth.

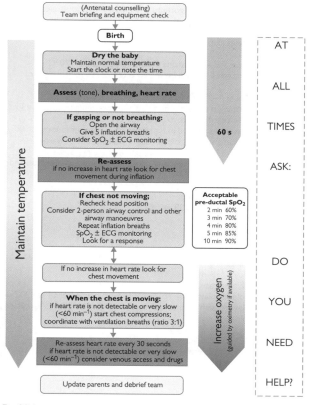

Fig. 29.6 Newborn life support algorithm 2015.

Reproduced with permission from Maconochie, I. et al. (2015) Resuscitation guidelines: Paediatric basic life support. Copyright © 2015 Resuscitation Council (UK) Available at https://www.resus.org.uk/resuscitation-guidelines/paediatric-basic-life-support/

Hypothermia (secondary to drowning)

- Common following drowning, and adversely affects resuscitation unless treated.
- Continue resuscitation until core temperature is at least 32°C, or it cannot be raised despite active measures.
- Obtain a core temperature reading (rectal or oesophageal) urgently.
- Prevent further cooling immediately.
- Arrhythmias are more common, but some, e.g. VF, may be refractory at temperatures <30°C.
- If cardiac arrest, use APLS algorithm and adjust if hypothermic:
  - <30°C: aggressively rewarm, avoid adrenaline (epinephrine)/ amiodarone, maximum 3 defibrillation attempts until >30°C.
  - 30–35°C: defibrillate as usual, double dose interval for resuscitation drugs.
- Avoid adrenaline and amiodarone if core temperature <30°C.
- Rewarming strategies depend on the core temperature and signs of circulation.
- Aim to rewarm at 1–2°C/h to 35°C.
- External rewarming is usually sufficient if the core temperature is >30°C and child is not in cardiac arrest/cardiovascular unstable.
- Active core rewarming added in patients with a core temperature of <30°C/cardiac arrest/cardiovascular instability, but beware of 'rewarming shock'. Most hypothermic patients are hypovolaemic. Hypotension occurs secondary to impaired myocardial dysfunction and a drop in SVR as the core is rewarmed.
- External rewarming:
  - Remove cold, wet clothing.
  - Consider warm IV fluids (38–40°C).
  - Supply warm blankets.
  - Infrared radiant lamp.
  - Heating blanket.
  - Warm-air system.
- Core rewarming:
  - Warm IV fluids (38–40°C).
  - Warm ventilator gases to 42°C to prevent further heat loss.
  - Gastric or bladder lavage with normal (physiological) saline at 42°C.
  - Peritoneal lavage with K^+-free dialysate at 42°C. Use 20 mL/kg cycled every 15 min.
  - CVVH.
  - CPB/ECMO if available.
- The temperature is generally allowed to ↑ by 1°C/h to ↓ haemodynamic instability.
- Data on the use of therapeutic hypothermia in children are insufficient.

Return of spontaneous circulation (ROSC)

- Careful attention should be paid to maintain adequate circulation, ventilation, temperature control, and normoglycaemia following ROSC:
  - Titrate O_2 to achieve normoxaemia, target an SpO_2 of 94–98% unless a specific condition requires a different value, e.g. CHD.
  - The effects of blood CO_2 partial pressure and consequently cerebral perfusion have not been studied after paediatric cardiac arrest; however the usual target pCO_2 in the ventilated child post ROSC is 4.5–5.0 kPa.
  - Shock is common owing to peripheral circulatory failure. Fluids and/ or inotropes are recommended to avoid hypotension, maintaining at least the 5th centile of BP appropriate for age.
  - Avoid hyperglycaemia and hypoglycaemia, although tight glucose control has not shown survival benefits.
- Rescue and post-ROSC use of ECMO may be of benefit for patients with a cardiac cause for the arrest in a setting where it can be rapidly instituted. Benefits for patients with other causes for the arrest remain unclear.
- Therapeutic hypothermia: The Therapeutic Hypothermia After Paediatric Cardiac Arrest (THAPCA) study found no difference in survival or 1-year functional outcome in the two groups (32–34°C vs normal). Active cooling is not recommended in paediatrics, unlike in some adult groups.
- Avoid hyperthermia post ROSC.
- If cold after ROSC, warm slowly (0.25–0.5°C/h) to normothermia. If <32°C, actively rewarm rapidly to 32°C then slowly to normothermia.
- No single prognostic factor is reliable to inform decisions about termination of resuscitation or the outcome if ROSC is achieved. Influencing factors include:
  - Circumstances of the arrest.
  - Initial rhythm.
  - Duration of resuscitation.
  - Presence of hypothermia.
  - Severe metabolic derangement.
- In children with ROSC who fulfil neurological criteria for death, or in whom withdrawal of life-sustaining treatments is planned, consider as potential organ donors. Contact the local Specialist Nurse in Organ Donation (SNOD) for further advice and support.

Emergency drugs: dilutions and doses

Be cautious of maximum doses—in general, a working weight of 50 kg is an adult dose.

- Adenosine: 100–300 mcg/kg rapid IV bolus (maximum 3mg 1st dose, 6mg 2nd dose, 12mg 3rd dose).
- Adrenaline (epinephrine):
  - Cardiac arrest bolus 10 mcg/kg (0.1 mL/kg of 1:10,000 maximum 10 mls).
  - Infusion 0.3 mg/kg in 50 mL of 5% glucose or 0.9% saline: infusion rate of 1 mL/h gives 0.1 mcg/kg/min (range 0.05–2 mcg/kg/min).
  - Nebulized 1–5 mL of 1:1000.
- Aminophylline:
  - Loading dose 5 mg/kg over 20–30 min (maximum 250 mg).
  - Infusion 500 mg in 500 mL of 0.9% saline; 0.5–1 mL/kg/h.
- Amiodarone:
  - Loading dose 5 mg/kg (maximum 300 mg).
  - Infusion 5–15 mcg/kg/min (15 mg/kg in 50 mL of 5% glucose: infusion rate of 1 mL/h gives 5 mcg/kg/min).
- Atracurium: 0.5mg/kg for intubation.
- Atropine: 20 mcg/kg (minimum 100 mcg, maximum 600 mcg).
- Calcium chloride: 0.2 mL/kg of 10% slowly (maximum 10 mls).
- Calcium gluconate: 0.5 mL/kg of 10% slowly (maximum 20 mls).
- Cefotaxime: 50 mg/kg (maximum 2 g)
- Ceftriaxone: 80 mg/kg (>1 months of age) (maximum 2 g).
- Dantrolene: 1 mg/kg repeated every 5–10 min (maximum 10 mg/kg).
- Dexamethasone: 0.1–0.6 mg/kg IV (maximum 8 mg) for airway oedema.
- Glucose: 10% 2 mL/kg for hypoglycaemia.
- Diazepam: 0.5 mg/kg PR; 0.1–0.25 mg/kg IV or IO.
- Dinoprostone (prostaglandin E2):
  - Initial dose of 5–100 nanograms/kg/min.
  - 30 mcg/kg in 50 mL of 5% glucose or 0.9% saline: infusion rate of 1 mL/h gives 10 nanograms/kg/min.
- Dopamine: 3 mg/kg in 50 mL 5% glucose or 0.9% saline: infusion rate of 1 mL/h gives 1 mcg/kg/min.
- Fentanyl:
  - 1–2 mcg/kg IV for intubation.
  - 50 mcg/kg in 50 mL 5% glucose or 0.9% saline; infusion rate of 1–10 mL/h gives 1–10 mcg/kg/h.
- Hydrocortisone: 1mg/kg in refractory sepsis; 4 mg/kg for life-threatening asthma (maximum 100 mg).
- Hypertonic saline: 2–5 mL/kg IV over 10 min for raised ICP.
- Ketamine: 1–2 mg/kg IV induction dose.
- Lidocaine: 1 mg/kg as antiarrhythmic for VT/VF as alternative to amiodarone (maximum100mg).
- Lorazepam: 0.1 mg/kg (maximum 4 mg).
- Magnesium: 40 mg/kg (maximum 2 g) in 50 mL 5% glucose or 0.9% saline over 20 min for severe/life-threatening asthma.
- Mannitol: 250–500 mg/kg (1.25–2.5 mL/kg of 20%) over 30 min.

- Midazolam:
  - 0.5 mg/kg (maximum 20 mg) buccal for status epilepticus.
  - Intubation dose 100–200mcg/kg.
  - Infusion for sedation: 3 mg/kg in 50 mL 5% glucose or 0.9% saline: infusion rate of 1–5 mL/h gives 60–300 mcg/kg/h.
- Milrinone: 0.75 mg/kg in 50 mL of 5% glucose or 0.9% saline: infusion rate of 1–4 mL/h gives 0.25–1 mcg/kg/min.
- Morphine: for sedation, 1 mg/kg in 50 mL of 5% glucose or 0.9% saline: infusion rate of 1–5 mL/h gives 20–100 mcg/kg/h.
- Naloxone: 4 mcg/kg IV (maximum 2mg).
- Neostigmine: 50 mcg/kg (maximum 2.5mg).
- Noradrenaline (norepinephrine): 0.3 mg/kg in 50 mL of 5% glucose or 0.9% saline: infusion rate of 1 mL/h gives 0.1 mcg/kg/min (range 0.05–2 mcg/kg/min).
- Paraldehyde: 0.8 mL/kg PR (of 50:50 mix with oil) (maximum 20 mL).
- Phenylephrine: bolus 2–4 μg/kg, give larger doses according to response
- Phenytoin: loading dose 20 mg/kg IV over 20 min.
- Prednisolone: 1–2 mg/kg (maximum 40 mg).
- Propofol 1%:
  - 2–4 mg/kg for intubation.
  - Infusion 1–5 mg/kg/h (= 0.1–0.5 mL/kg/h of 1% solution).
  - Short-term infusion only—not licensed beware propofol infusion syndrome (PIS).
- Rocuronium: 1.2 mg/kg IV bolus for modified RSI.
- Salbutamol:
  - Nebulized 2.5–5 mg.
  - IV bolus 5 mcg/kg (maximum 250 mcg).
  - Infusion (peripheral) 10 mg in 50 mL 5% glucose or 0.9% saline: infusion rate 0.3 mL/kg/h gives 1 mcg/kg/min (range 1–2 mcg/kg/min). Doses up to 5 mcg/kg/min in PICU setting.
- Sodium bicarbonate: 1 mL/kg of 8.4% for resuscitation (1–2 mmol/kg for severe acidosis).
- Sugammadex: 16 mg/kg for emergency reversal of rocuronium and vecuronium.
- Suxamethonium: 1-2mg/kg for RSI
- Thiopental:
  - 1–5 mg/kg for RSI.
  - Infusion 1–5 mg/kg/h for refractory status.
- Tranexamic acid: 15 mg/kg (maximum 1 g) loading over 10 min, then 2 mg/kg/h infusion.
- Vasopressin: 0.02–0.1 units/kg/h.

Index

Note: Tables, figures, and boxes are indicated by an italic *t*, *f*, and *b* following the page number.